# CARDIOLOGY MCQs
## for Postgraduate and Superspecialty Medical Entrance Examinations

# CARDIOLOGY MCQs
## for Postgraduate and Superspecialty Medical Entrance Examinations

Based on 20th Edition of Harrison's Prinicples of Internal Medicine

**Dr Ajay Mathur**
Senior Professor
Department of Medicine
SMS Medical College and Hospital
Jaipur, Rajasthan, India

*Foreword*
Ramesh Roop Rai

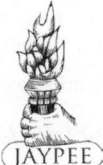

## JAYPEE BROTHERS MEDICAL PUBLISHERS
The Health Sciences Publisher
New Delhi | London | Panama

**Jaypee Brothers Medical Publishers (P) Ltd.**

#### Headquarters
Jaypee Brothers Medical Publishers (P) Ltd
4838/24, Ansari Road, Daryaganj
New Delhi 110 002, India
Phone: +91-11-43574357
Fax: +91-11-43574314
E-mail: jaypee@jaypeebrothers.com

#### Overseas Offices

J.P. Medical Ltd
83, Victoria Street, London
SW1H 0HW (UK)
Phone: +44 20 3170 8910
Fax: +44 (0)20 3008 6180
E-mail: info@jpmedpub.com

Jaypee-Highlights Medical Publishers Inc
City of Knowledge, Bld. 235, 2nd Floor, Clayton
Panama City, Panama
Phone: +1 507-301-0496
Fax: +1 507-301-0499
E-mail: cservice@jphmedical.com

Jaypee Brothers Medical Publishers (P) Ltd
Bhotahity, Kathmandu, Nepal
Phone: +977-9741283608
E-mail: kathmandu@jaypeebrothers.com

Website: www.jaypeebrothers.com
Website: www.jaypeedigital.com

© 2019, Jaypee Brothers Medical Publishers

The views and opinions expressed in this book are solely those of the original contributor(s)/author(s) and do not necessarily represent those of editor(s) of the book.

All rights reserved. No part of this publication may be reproduced, stored or transmitted in any form or by any means, electronic, mechanical, photocopying, recording or otherwise, without the prior permission in writing of the publishers.

All brand names and product names used in this book are trade names, service marks, trademarks or registered trademarks of their respective owners. The publisher is not associated with any product or vendor mentioned in this book.

Medical knowledge and practice change constantly. This book is designed to provide accurate, authoritative information about the subject matter in question. However, readers are advised to check the most current information available on procedures included and check information from the manufacturer of each product to be administered, to verify the recommended dose, formula, method and duration of administration, adverse effects and contraindications. It is the responsibility of the practitioner to take all appropriate safety precautions. Neither the publisher nor the author(s)/editor(s) assume any liability for any injury and/or damage to persons or property arising from or related to use of material in this book.

This book is sold on the understanding that the publisher is not engaged in providing professional medical services. If such advice or services are required, the services of a competent medical professional should be sought.

Every effort has been made where necessary to contact holders of copyright to obtain permission to reproduce copyright material. If any have been inadvertently overlooked, the publisher will be pleased to make the necessary arrangements at the first opportunity. The **CD/DVD-ROM** (if any) provided in the sealed envelope with this book is complimentary and free of cost. **Not meant for sale.**

Inquiries for bulk sales may be solicited at: jaypee@jaypeebrothers.com

### *Cardiology MCQs for Postgraduate and Superspecialty Medical Entrance Examinations*

First Edition: **2019**

ISBN: 978-93-89129-99-1

*Printed at* Sanat Printers

# Foreword

As a professional who has been practicing medicine for over four decades now, I appreciate the value this book brings to the table in times like today. As we move from a largely descriptive era to the bullet-point generation, this academic initiative appears profoundly relevant.

Dr Mathur is bringing to the students and others, Cardiology MCQs in an individual book format. This would be more handy and subject specific. The book has been a reference point for many medical entrance examinations and has left an impact on medical professionals who look for high quality of academic material.

Knowledge is a more processed form of information. Dr Mathur stays true to his pledge by presenting well-digested bytes of knowledge across different fields of medicine. His relying on good old word-of-mouth to make this book a success rather than enthusiastic marketing adds further credibility to his initiative. I recommend this book, without a shadow of doubt, to every medical professional who is looking to continue learning.

**Dr Ramesh Roop Rai**
*Former*, Professor and Head
Department of Gastroenterology
SMS Medical College and Hospital, Jaipur
Past President, Indian Society of Gastroenterology (2008)

# Preface

Medicine, in all its vastness, needs to be understood in a way that makes most sense to how it is applied today. Memorizing each word is elusive and therefore, testing knowledge of a discipline remains an evergreen challenge.

It is a widely accepted fact that taking a quiz soon after studying helps one retain knowledge better and apply the lessons in practice. Multiple Choice Questions (MCQs) are an effective way of remembering the gist of the matter. This is precisely the reason why most examinations today follow this format. This book is committed to honing your skills to retain knowledge, help diagnose medical conditions, and maximize your impact, as a doctor.

A tremendous volume of questions has been generated over the past ten years. As it stands today, the approach needs to be adjusted according to the knowledge available at hand. This time around, my team has decided that each specialism merits its own edition. This will help you to study existing literature with recent advances in medicine and glean deeper insights into the subject matter. Based on the epic 20th edition of Harrison's Principles of Internal Medicine, published by The McGraw-Hill Companies, Inc., this book is dedicated to the field of Cardiology in all its endless scope. This book caters to medical professionals at all levels. Not only can this be used by aspiring doctors to prepare for medical entrance examinations, but also by seasoned physicians to update knowledge long after it has been acquired. The book is sign-posted with references should the reader require elaboration on any given topic.

The book contains 2556 questions and still counting, I continue to keep my promise to continually refine the content of my book and chronicle the advances of medical science.

**Dr Ajay Mathur**

# Contents

1. Dyspnea — 1
2. Hypoxia and Cyanosis — 5
3. Edema — 8
4. Palpitations — 12
5. Basic Biology of the Cardiovascular System — 13
6. Electrocardiography — 18
7. Principles of Electrophysiology — 27
8. The Bradyarrhythmias: Disorders of the Sinoatrial Node — 33
9. The Bradyarrhythmias : Disorders of the Atrioventricular Node — 38
10. Approach to Supraventricular Tachyarrhythmias — 44
11. Physiologic and Nonphysiologic Sinus Tachycardia — 46
12. Focal Atrial Tachycardia — 48
13. Paroxysmal Supraventricular Tachycardias — 50
14. Common Atrial Flutter, Macroreentrant, and Multifocal Atrial Tachycardias — 57
15. Atrial Fibrillation — 59
16. Approach to Ventricular Arrhythmias — 67
17. Premature Ventricular Beats, Non-Sustained Ventricular Tachycardia, and Idioventricular Rhythm — 69
18. Sustained Ventricular Tachycardia — 71
19. Polymorphic Ventricular Tachycardia and Ventricular Fibrillation — 74
20. Electrical Storm and Incessant VT — 79
21. Heart Failure: Pathophysiology and Diagnosis — 84
22. Heart Failure: Management — 90
23. Cardiomyopathy and Myocarditis — 94
24. Aortic Valve Disease — 111
25. Aortic Regurgitation — 116

| 26. | Mitral Stenosis | 119 |
| 27. | Mitral Regurgitation | 125 |
| 28. | Mitral Valve Prolapse | 127 |
| 29. | Tricuspid Valve Disease | 129 |
| 30. | Pulmonic Valve Disease | 131 |
| 31. | Multiple and Mixed Valvular Heart Disease | 132 |
| 32. | Congenital Heart Disease in the Adult | 133 |
| 33. | Pericardial Disease | 146 |
| 34. | Atrial Myxoma and Other Cardiac Tumors | 153 |
| 35. | Non-ST-Segment Elevation Acute Coronary Syndrome (Non-ST-Segment Elevation Myocardial Infarction and Unstable Angina) | 157 |
| 36. | Ischemic Heart Disease | 162 |
| 37. | ST-Segment Elevation Myocardial Infarction | 171 |
| 38. | Hypertensive Vascular Disease | 188 |
| 39. | Renovascular Disease | 204 |
| 40. | Deep Venous Thrombosis and Pulmonary Thromboembolism | 205 |
| 41. | Diseases of the Aorta | 215 |
| 42. | Arterial Diseases of the Extremities | 220 |
| 43. | Chronic Venous Disease and Lymphedema | 224 |
| 44. | Pulmonary Hypertension | 228 |

# CARDIOLOGY

## Dyspnea

1. **Which of the following about dyspnea is false?**
   *Harrison's 20th Ed. Chapter 33 Page 226*
   - A. Self-reported
   - B. Subjective experience of breathing discomfort
   - C. Qualitatively distinct sensations that vary in intensity
   - D. None of the above

   *Dyspnea is a symptom. American Thoracic Society (ATS) defines dyspnea as a "subjective experience of breathing discomfort that consists of qualitatively distinct sensations that vary in intensity. Dyspnea can be perceived only by the person experiencing it and, therefore, must be self-reported.*

2. **Which of the following features of breathing define dyspnea?**
   *S Afr Med J. 2016;106(1):32-36*
   - A. Abnormal
   - B. Uncomfortable
   - C. Awareness
   - D. All of the above

   *Normally, at rest, one is unaware of the act of breathing. With exercise, though aware of breathing, discomfort is expected to be transient. Dyspnea is defined with prefixes before awareness of breathing i.e. abnormally uncomfortable.*

3. **Which of the following is a sign of increased work of breathing?**
   *Harrison's 20th Ed. Chapter 33 Page 226*
   - A. Tachypnea
   - B. Use of accessory muscles of respiration
   - C. Intercostal retraction
   - D. All of the above

4. **Which of the following can cause dyspnea?**
   *Harrison's 20th Ed. Chapter 33 Page 226*
   - A. Pulmonary diseases
   - B. Cardiac diseases
   - C. Neurologic diseases
   - D. All of the above

   *Dyspnea, like hunger or thirst, is a "synthetic sensation" as it often arises from multiple sources of information rather than from stimulation of a single neural receptor.*

5. **Which of the following best relates to dyspnea?**
   *Harrison's 20th Ed. Chapter 33 Page 226*
   - A. Efferent - afferent mismatch
   - B. Efferent - reafferent mismatch
   - C. Afferent - reefferent mismatch
   - D. All of the above

   *Three main components contribute to dyspnea - afferent signals, efferent signals and central information processing. Dyspnea arises when there is a mismatch in integrative signaling between afferent signals from the respiratory system and efferent signals from the CNS. This is termed as "neuro-mechanical" or "efferent-reafferent mismatch".*

6. **Neural signal termed "corollary discharge" is sent to?**
   *Harrison's 20th Ed. Chapter 33 Page 226*
   - A. Sensory cortex
   - B. Motor cortex
   - C. Ventilatory muscles
   - D. All of the above

   *The sensory cortex is simultaneously activated when motor signals are sent to the chest wall, resulting in the conscious sensation of muscular effort and breathlessness. When there is increased work of breathing, increased neural output from the motor cortex is sensed via a neural signal, termed corollary discharge, is sent to the sensory cortex at the same time that motor output is directed to the ventilatory muscles. Corollary discharges are important in shaping the sense of respiratory effort.*

7. **Chemoreceptors in the carotid bodies and medulla are activated by?**
   *Harrison's 20th Ed. Chapter 33 Page 226*
   - A. Hypoxemia
   - B. Acute hypercapnia
   - C. Acidemia
   - D. All of the above

   *Chemoreceptors in the carotid bodies and medulla are activated by hypoxemia, acute hypercapnia, and acidemia.*

8. **The sense of air hunger arises from?**
   *Harrison's 20th Ed. Chapter 33 Page 226*
   - A. Stimulation of chemoreceptors
   - B. J-receptors
   - C. Pulmonary vascular receptors
   - D. All of the above

   *Sensation of air hunger arises from a combination of stimuli that increase drive to breathe such as hypoxemia or hypercapnia (mediated by signals from chemoreceptors in the carotid body and aortic arch), acute hypercapnia or acidemia (mediated by signals from peripheral & central chemoreceptors), airway & interstitial inflammation (mediated by pulmonary afferents), and pulmonary vascular receptors.*

9. **J (juxtacapillary) receptors are found in?**
   *N Engl J Med. 2008;358:1054-9*
   - A. Bronchi
   - B. Terminal brochiole
   - C. Alveolar interstitial space
   - D. All of the above

   *Pulmonary "J Receptors" are sensory cells located within alveolar septa and are "juxtaposed" to the pulmonary capillaries. These cells are activated by physical engorgement of the pulmonary capillaries (left heart dysfunction) or increased pulmonary interstitial volume (pulmonary edema). Dyspnea results from transudation of pulmonary fluid & stretching of pulmonary interstitial juxtacapillary receptors due to combination of increased pulmonary arterial blood flow in concert with elevated pulmonary venous pressures.*

10. **Irritant receptors around the epithelial cells of bronchial walls are activated by?**
    *Am J Respir Crit Care Med. 1999;159:321-340*
    - A. Tactile stimulation in the bronchial mucosa
    - B. High rates of air flow
    - C. Increases in bronchial smooth muscle tone
    - D. All of the above

    *Pulmonary irritant receptors are sensors present within the respiratory epithelium which can sense and respond to a variety of chemical irritants.*

11. **J-receptors are sensitive to?**
    *Harrison's 19th Ed. 47e-1*
    - A. Changes in pulmonary artery pressure
    - B. Acidemia
    - C. Interstitial edema
    - D. Hypercapnia

    *J-receptors or pulmonary C-fiber receptors are sensitive to interstitial edema.*

**12. The sensation of chest tightness results from?**
*Harrison's 20th Ed. Chapter 33 Page 226*

A. Chemoreceptors in medulla
B. Mechanoreceptors in lungs
C. Chemoreceptors in aortic and carotid bodies
D. Afferent fibers in the phrenic nerves

*Mechanoreceptors in the lungs, when stimulated by bronchospasm, lead to a sensation of chest tightness.*

**13. Metaboreceptors are located in?**
*Harrison's 20th Ed. Chapter 33 Page 226, J Physiol. 2007;585(Pt 1):165-174*

A. Medulla
B. Carotid bodies
C. Skeletal muscle
D. All of the above

*Metaboreceptors are located in skeletal muscle. During exercise, accumulation of metabolites within the active skeletal muscle, stimulates group III & IV afferent neurons which evoke a reflex increase in muscle sympathetic nerve activity (MSNA), known as the muscle metaboreflex.*

**14. Which of the following is an ischemic metabolite?**
*J Physiol. 2007;585(Pt 1):165-174*

A. Lactic acid
B. Adenosine
C. Bradykinin
D. All of the above

*Muscle metaboreceptors regulate sympathetic activation during exercise. This reflex is activated by lactic acid, phosphate, K+, H+, adenosine, prostaglandins, and bradykinin released from exercising skeletal muscle. These ischemic metabolites stimulate groups III and IV chemosensitive afferents.*

**15. Which of the following is used to measure dyspnea?**
*Am J Respir Crit Care Med. 1999;159:321-340*

A. Medical Research Council (MRC) Scale
B. Baseline dyspnea index
C. Oxygen Cost Diagram (OCD) scale
D. All of the above

**16. Modified Medical Research Council Dyspnea Scale classifies dyspnea into how many grades?**
*Harrison's 20th Ed. Chapter 33 Page 228 Table 33-1*

A. 3
B. 4
C. 5
D. 6

*Modified Medical Research Council Dyspnea Scale classifies dyspnea into 5 grades i.e. 0 to 4. This scale has been incorporated into GOLD 2017 guidelines as a tool for rating dyspnea in COPD.*

**17. What is the grade of dyspnea if one has to stop to rest after walking 100 meters on level ground?**
*Harrison's 20th Ed. Chapter 33 Page 228 Table 33-1*

A. 1
B. 2
C. 3
D. 4

**18. Chronic dyspnea is defined as symptoms lasting longer than?**
*Harrison's 20th Ed. Chapter 33 Page 226*

A. 1 month
B. 3 months
C. 6 months
D. 12 months

*Chronic dyspnea is defined as symptoms lasting longer than 1 month.*

**19. What proportion of patients have multifactorial reasons underlying dyspnea?**
*Harrison's 20th Ed. Chapter 33 Page 226*

A. 10%
B. 25%
C. 33%
D. 50%

*As many as one-third of patients may have multifactorial reasons underlying dyspnea.*

**20. Breathing discomfort during exercise in anemia is due to stimulation of?**
*Harrison's 20th Ed. Chapter 33 Page 228 Table 33-2*

A. Chemoreceptors
B. Mechanoreceptors
C. Metaboreceptors
D. All of the above

**21. Increased work of breathing (WOB) is the possible mechanism underlying dyspnea in?**
*Harrison's 20th Ed. Chapter 33 Page 228 Table 33-2*

A. COPD
B. Interstitial lung disease
C. Kyphoscoliosis
D. All of the above

**22. Orthopnea is seen in?**
*Harrison's 20th Ed. Chapter 33 Page 227*

A. Congestive heart failure
B. Asthma triggered by esophageal reflux
C. Mechanical impairment of diaphragm in obesity
D. All of the above

**23. "Nocturnal dyspnea" is a feature of which of the following?**
*Harrison's 20th Ed. Chapter 33 Page 227*

A. Chronic heart failure
B. Myocardial ischemia
C. Interstitial lung disease
D. COPD

*CHF or asthma cause nocturnal dyspnea. Circadian variations increase bronchial sensitivity between 2 AM & 4 AM in asthma patients leading to episodes of nocturnal dyspnea.*

**24. Which of the following is most characteristic feature of severe paroxysmal dyspnea of left ventricular failure?**
*N Engl J Med. 2010; 363:1464-1469*

A. Nocturnal episodes
B. Sudden and unexpected
C. Orthopnea
D. All of the above

*Nocturnal episodes of dyspnea are a typical feature of left ventricular failure. Sudden & unexpected dyspneic episodes at rest is more typical of pulmonary embolization, spontaneous pneumothorax, anxiety. Orthopnea is characteristic of congestive heart failure. The differential diagnosis of orthopnea and paroxysmal nocturnal dyspnea includes ischemic heart disease, nonischemic cardiomyopathies, valvular heart disease, constrictive pericarditis, and infiltrative cardiomyopathies.*

25. **Acute intermittent episodes of dyspnea are due to?**
   *Harrison's 20th Ed. Chapter 33 Page 227*
   - A. Myocardial ischemia
   - B. Bronchospasm
   - C. Pulmonary embolism
   - D. All of the above

   Acute intermittent episodes of dyspnea are more likely to reflect episodes of myocardial ischemia, bronchospasm or pulmonary embolism.

26. **Chronic persistent dyspnea is typical of?**
   *Harrison's 20th Ed. Chapter 33 Page 227*
   - A. COPD
   - B. Interstitial lung disease
   - C. Chronic thromboembolic disease
   - D. All of the above

   Chronic persistent dyspnea is typical of COPD, interstitial lung disease and chronic thromboembolic disease.

27. **Platypnea is dyspnea that occurs in which position?**
   *Harrison's 20th Ed. Chapter 33 Page 228*
   - A. Upright
   - B. Sitting
   - C. Supine
   - D. Lateral

   Platypnea is dyspnea that occurs only in upright position with relief in supine position.

28. **Platypnea is a feature of?**
   *Harrison's 20th Ed. Chapter 33 Page 227*
   - A. Hepatopulmonary syndrome
   - B. Emphysema
   - C. Ankylosing spondylitis
   - D. Psychogenic

29. **Platypnea is a feature of?**
   *Harrison's 20th Ed. Chapter 33 Page 227*
   - A. Obesity
   - B. Left atrial myxoma
   - C. Interstitial lung disease
   - D. Chronic thromboembolic disease

   Left atrial myxoma and hepatopulmonary syndrome are the causes of platypnea.

30. **Trepopnea most often occurs in patients with?**
   *N Engl J Med. 1970; 283:266*
   - A. Asthma
   - B. COPD
   - C. Heart disease
   - D. Pleural effusion

   Trepopnea is dyspnea that occurs only in a lateral decubitus position, most often in patients with heart disease due to positional alterations in ventilation-perfusion relationships. Most cardiac patients seem to prefer sleeping on the right side. The reasons given for this preference include "awareness of the heart" and dyspnea. The feature common to most patients seems to be cardiomegaly, and the mechanism of the dyspnea is thought to be positional compression of pulmonary veins. Perhaps trepopnea explains why unilateral pulmonary edema and unilateral pleural effusions, when they occur in these patients, are almost always just on the right.

31. **Which of the following is called "cardiac asthma"?**
   *Harrison's 20th Ed. Chapter 252 Page 1766*
   - A. Paroxysmal nocturnal dyspnea (PND)
   - B. Orthopnea
   - C. Platypnea
   - D. Trepopnea

   PND is also called cardiac asthma. During night, with recumbency, total blood volume is increased due to fluid mobilization from edematous areas leading to pulmonary congestion.

32. **Presence of resting hypoxemia suggests?**
   *Harrison's 20th Ed. Chapter 33 Page 228*
   - A. Ventilation-perfusion mismatch
   - B. Shunt
   - C. Impairment in diffusion capacity
   - D. All of the above

33. **Which of the following indicate increased work of breathing?**
   *Harrison's 20th Ed. Chapter 33 Page 228*
   - A. Supraclavicular retractions
   - B. Use of accessory muscles of ventilation
   - C. Tripod position
   - D. All of the above

   Increased work of breathing is evidenced by supraclavicular retractions, use of accessory muscles of ventilation and tripod position (sitting with hands braced on knees). It is indicative of increased airway resistance or stiffness of the lungs & chest wall.

34. **Paradoxical movement of the abdomen during breathing is suggestive of?**
   *Harrison's 20th Ed. Chapter 33 Page 229*
   - A. Abdominal hernia
   - B. Diaphragmatic weakness
   - C. Pulmonary edema
   - D. Acute asthma

35. **Rounding of the abdomen during exhalation is suggestive of?**
   *Harrison's 20th Ed. Chapter 33 Page 229*
   - A. Abdominal hernia
   - B. Diaphragmatic weakness
   - C. Pulmonary edema
   - D. Acute asthma

   Rounding of the abdomen during exhalation is suggestive of pulmonary edema.

36. **Low lung volumes on a chest radiograph suggests?**
   *Harrison's 20th Ed. Chapter 33 Page 229*
   - A. Interstitial edema or fibrosis
   - B. Diaphragmatic dysfunction
   - C. Impaired chest wall motion
   - D. All of the above

37. **On a chest radiograph, prominent pulmonary vasculature in the upper lung zones indicates?**
   *Harrison's 20th Ed. Chapter 33 Page 229*
   - A. Pulmonary arterial hypertension
   - B. Pulmonary venous hypertension
   - C. Pulmonary embolism
   - D. Any of the above

38. On a chest radiograph, enlarged central pulmonary arteries indicates?

*Harrison's 20th Ed. Chapter 33 Page 229*

A. Pulmonary arterial hypertension
B. Pulmonary venous hypertension
C. Pulmonary embolism
D. Any of the above

39. In cardiopulmonary exercise test (CPET), which of the following suggests respiratory system as the cause of dyspnea?

*Harrison's 20th Ed. Chapter 33 Page 229*

A. Patient achieves predicted maximal ventilation
B. Demonstrates an increase in dead space or hypoxemia
C. Develops bronchospasm
D. All of the above

40. In cardiopulmonary exercise test (CPET), which of the following suggests cardiovascular system as the cause of dyspnea?

*Harrison's 20th Ed. Chapter 33 Page 229*

A. If the heart rate is >85% of the predicted maximum
B. If the anaerobic threshold occurs early
C. If the BP is excessively high or decreases during exercise
D. All of the above

At peak exercise in CPET, if heart rate is >85% of the predicted maximum, if anaerobic threshold occurs early, if BP becomes excessively high or decreases during exercise, if $O_2$ pulse falls, or if there are ischemic changes on ECG, an abnormality of cardiovascular system is likely cause of dyspnea.

41. Cardiopulmonary exercise testing (CPET) provides assessment of the integrative exercise responses involving?

*Postgrad Med J. 2007;83(985):675-682*

A. Pulmonary
B. Cardiovascular
C. Skeletal muscle systems
D. All of the above

Cardiopulmonary exercise testing (CPET) provides assessment of the integrative exercise responses involving the pulmonary, cardiovascular, hematopoietic, neuropsychological, and skeletal muscle systems, which are not adequately reflected through the measurement of individual organ system function.

42. Exercise tolerance is determined by?

*Postgrad Med J. 2007;83(985):675-682*

A. Pulmonary gas exchange
B. Cardiovascular performance
C. Skeletal muscle metabolism
D. All of the above

Peak exercise capacity is defined as "the maximum ability of the cardiovascular system to deliver oxygen to exercising skeletal muscle and of the exercising muscle to extract oxygen from the blood".

43. Oxygen uptake ($VO_2$) is calculated by?

*Postgrad Med J. 2007;83(985):675-682*

A. Bernoulli equation
B. Fick equation
C. Friedewald equation
D. Henderson-Hasselbalch equation

44. One metabolic equivalent (MET) is the resting oxygen uptake in a sitting position and equals?

*Postgrad Med J. 2007;83(985):675-682*

A. 1.5 mL/kg/minute
B. 2.5 mL/kg/minute
C. 3.5 mL/kg/minute
D. 4.5 mL/kg/minute

Oxygen uptake ($VO_2$) equals cardiac output times the arterial minus mixed venous oxygen content or $VO_2 = (SV \times HR) \times (CaO_2 - CvO_2)$, where SV is the stroke volume, HR is the heart rate, $CaO_2$ is the arterial oxygen content, and $CvO_2$ is the mixed venous oxygen content.

45. In dyspnea, supplemental $O_2$ should be administered if?

*Harrison's 20th Ed. Chapter 33 Page 230*

A. Resting $O_2$ saturation is ≤ 88%
B. If patient's saturation drops to ≤ 88% with activity
C. If patient's saturation drops to ≤ 88% with sleep
D. All of the above

46. Which of the following may have a role in managing dyspnea?

*Harrison's 20th Ed. Chapter 33 Page 230*

A. Opioids
B. Anxiolytics
C. Inhaled furosemide
D. All of the above

## Hypoxia and Cyanosis

**47. Pasteur's effect relates to?**
*Harrison's 20th Ed. Chapter 36 Page 234*

- A. Switch from aerobic to anaerobic metabolism
- B. Abnormal hemoglobin derivative
- C. Pulmonary arteriovenous fistulae
- D. Flow rate in vessels

*Pasteur's effect refers to switch from aerobic to anaerobic metabolism.*

**48. Severe hypoxia with inadequate production of ATP leads to?**
*Harrison's 20th Ed. Chapter 36 Page 234*

- A. Uncontrolled Ca++ influx in cells
- B. Activation of Ca++ dependent phospholipases
- C. Activation of Ca++ dependent proteases
- D. All of the above

**49. Which of the following gene is upregulated in adaptation to hypoxia?**
*Harrison's 20th Ed. Chapter 36 Page 234*

- A. Phosphoglycerate kinase
- B. Phosphofructokinase
- C. Glucose transporters Glut-1 and Glut-2
- D. All of the above

*Adaptations to hypoxia are mediated by upregulation of genes encoding glycolytic enzymes like phosphoglycerate kinase & phosphofructokinase & glucose transporters Glut-1 & Glut-2, and by growth factors like vascular endothelial growth factor (VEGF) & erythropoietin (EPO).*

**50. During hypoxia systemic arterioles dilate by opening of?**
*Harrison's 20th Ed. Chapter 36 Page 234*

- A. NaATP channels in vascular smooth-muscle cells
- B. KATP channels in vascular smooth-muscle cells
- C. ClATP channels in vascular smooth-muscle cells
- D. All of the above

*In hypoxia systemic arterioles dilate by opening of KATP channels in vascular smooth-muscle cells.*

**51. During hypoxia, pulmonary vascular smooth-muscle cells contract due to inhibition of?**
*Harrison's 20th Ed. Chapter 36 Page 234*

- A. Na⁺ channels
- B. K⁺ channels
- C. Cl⁻ channels
- D. All of the above

*In pulmonary vascular smooth-muscle cells, inhibition of K⁺ channels causing contraction.*

**52. Acute hypoxia causes a clinical picture resembling?**
*Harrison's 20th Ed. Chapter 36 Page 235*

- A. Partial seizure
- B. Peripheral neuropathy
- C. Acute alcoholism
- D. Migraine

*Clinically, acute hypoxia resembles acute alcoholism (impaired judgment, motor incoordination).*

**53. Headache in high-altitude illness is caused by?**
*Harrison's 20th Ed. Chapter 36 Page 235*

- A. Cerebral vasodilation
- B. Pulmonary arterial constriction
- C. Pulmonary venous constriction
- D. All of the above

*High-altitude illness is characterized by headache secondary to cerebral vasodilation, gastrointestinal symptoms, dizziness, insomnia, fatigue or somnolence. High-altitude cerebral edema (HACE) is manifest by severe headache and papilledema and can cause coma.*

**54. In severe hypoxia, death usually results from?**
*Harrison's 20th Ed. Chapter 36 Page 235*

- A. Respiratory failure
- B. Cardiac arrhythmia
- C. Seizure
- D. Autonomic failure

*In severe hypoxia, centers of brainstem are affected & death results from respiratory failure.*

**55. When hypoxia occurs consequent to respiratory failure, hemoglobin-oxygen dissociation curve is displaced to?**
*Harrison's 20th Ed. Chapter 36 Page 235*

- A. Right
- B. Left
- C. Center
- D. Any of the above

*When hypoxia occurs due to respiratory failure, $PaO_2$ declines, $PaCO_2$ rises & $Hb-O_2$ dissociation curve is displaced to right, with greater quantities of $O_2$ released at any level of tissue $PO_2$.*

**56. Most common cause of respiratory hypoxia is?**
*Harrison's 20th Ed. Chapter 36 Page 235*

- A. Hypoventilation
- B. Ventilation-perfusion mismatch
- C. Intrapulmonary right-to-left shunting
- D. None of the above

*Most common cause of respiratory hypoxia is ventilation-perfusion mismatch.*

**57. High-altitude illness develops when a person ascends rapidly to a height of?**
*Harrison's 20th Ed. Chapter 36 Page 235*

- A. 1000 meters
- B. 2000 meters
- C. 3000 meters
- D. 4000 meters

*High-altitude illness develops when a person ascends rapidly to a height of 3000 meters or ~10,000 feet. At this altitude, the reduction of $O_2$ content of inspired air ($FIO_2$) leads to a decrease in alveolar $PO_2$ to ~60 mm Hg.*

58. In which of the following conditions, PaO$_2$ cannot be restored to normal with inspiration of 100% O$_2$?
   *Harrison's 20th Ed. Chapter 36 Page 235*
   A. Tetralogy of Fallot (TOF)
   B. Transposition of great arteries (TGA)
   C. Eisenmenger's syndrome
   D. All of the above

   *Hypoxia due to congenital cardiac malformations (TOF, TGA & Eisenmenger's syndrome) resembles intrapulmonary right-to-left shunting & PaO$_2$ cannot be restored to normal with 100% O$_2$.*

59. In anemic hypoxia, the PaO$_2$ is?
   *Harrison's 20th Ed. Chapter 36 Page 235*
   A. Normal
   B. Decreased
   C. Increased
   D. Any of the above

   *In anemic hypoxia, PaO$_2$ is normal but due to reduction of Hb concentration, absolute quantity of O$_2$ transported per unit volume of blood is diminished.*

60. Which of the following is false about in anemic hypoxia?
   *Harrison's 20th Ed. Chapter 36 Page 235*
   A. Absolute quantity of O$_2$ transported per unit volume of blood is diminished
   B. Usual quantity of O$_2$ is removed from blood in capillaries
   C. PO$_2$ & saturation in venous blood decline to a greater extent
   D. None of the above

61. In which of the following hypoxia's, venous blood tends to have a high O$_2$?
   *Harrison's 20th Ed. Chapter 36 Page 235*
   A. Excercise induced
   B. Circulatory hypoxia
   C. Cyanide poisoning
   D. Carbon monoxide intoxication

62. Example of "Histotoxic hypoxia" is?
   *Harrison's 20th Ed. Chapter 36 Page 235*
   A. Severe exercise
   B. Cyanide poisoning
   C. Raynaud's phenomenon
   D. High altitude hypoxia

   *Cyanide causes cellular hypoxia because tissues are unable to utilize O$_2$. As a result, venous blood tends to have a high O$_2$ tension. This condition is called histotoxic hypoxia.*

63. Special chemosensitive cells that determine respiratory response to hypoxia are located in?
   *Harrison's 20th Ed. Chapter 36 Page 235*
   A. Carotid bodies
   B. Aortic bodies
   C. Respiratory center in the brainstem
   D. All of the above

64. Which of the following is a feature of chronic mountain sickness?
   *Harrison's 20th Ed. Chapter 36 Page 236*
   A. Reduced ventilation
   B. Cyanosis
   C. Right ventricular enlargement
   D. All of the above

   *In persons with chronic hypoxemia secondary to prolonged residence at a high altitude (>13000 feet or 4200 meters), chronic mountain sickness develops. This is characterized by a blunted respiratory drive, reduced ventilation, erythrocytosis, cyanosis, weakness, right ventricular enlargement secondary to pulmonary hypertension and even stupor.*

65. Cyanosis is usually most marked in?
   *Harrison's 20th Ed. Chapter 36 Page 236*
   A. Nail beds
   B. Ears
   C. Malar eminences
   D. All of the above

   *Cyanosis is usually most marked in the lips, nail beds, ears, and malar eminences.*

66. The degree of cyanosis is modified by?
   *Harrison's 20th Ed. Chapter 36 Page 236*
   A. Color of the cutaneous pigment
   B. Thickness of the skin
   C. State of the cutaneous capillaries
   D. All of the above

67. Cyanosis is apparent when the mean capillary concentration of reduced hemoglobin exceeds?
   *Harrison's 20th Ed. Chapter 36 Page 236*
   A. 2 gram / dL
   B. 3 gram / dL
   C. 4 gram / dL
   D. 5 gram / dL

   *It is the absolute rather than relative quantity of reduced Hb that produces cyanosis. As concentration of total Hb is markedly reduced in severe anemia, absolute quantity of reduced Hb is still small and patients may not become cyanotic even with marked arterial desaturation.*

68. Central and peripheral cyanosis may be present in?
   *Harrison's 20th Ed. Chapter 36 Page 236*
   A. Shock
   B. Congestive failure
   C. Peripheral vascular disease
   D. Cardiogenic shock with pulmonary edema

69. Cyanosis occurs upon ascent to an altitude of?
   *Harrison's 20th Ed. Chapter 36 Page 236*
   A. 2000 meters
   B. 3000 meters
   C. 4000 meters
   D. 5000 meters

   *Cyanosis is manifest in an ascent to 4000 m (13,000 ft). At this height, FIO$_2$ & alveolar PO$_2$ are about 85 & 50 mm Hg, respectively & SaO$_2$ is ~75% leaving more reduced Hb in arterial blood.*

70. Cyanosis can be observed in all except?
   *Harrison's 20th Ed. Chapter 36 Page 237*
   A. Marked polycythemia
   B. Carboxyhemoglobin (COHb)
   C. Methemoglobin
   D. Sulfhemoglobin

   *Patients with marked polycythemia become cyanotic at higher levels of SaO$_2$ than patients with normal hematocrit values. Cyanosis is also observed when nonfunctional hemoglobin (methemoglobin or sulfhemoglobin) is present in blood.*

**71. Most common congenital cardiac lesion associated with cyanosis in adult is?**
*Harrison's 20th Ed. Chapter 234 Page 1667*

A. Tetralogy of Fallot
B. Patent ductus arteriosus
C. Ventricular septal defect
D. Atrial septal defect

*Most common congenital cardiac lesion with cyanosis in the adult is tetralogy of Fallot.*

**72. Differential cyanosis is a feature of?**
*Harrison's 20th Ed. Chapter 234 Page 1667*

A. Tetralogy of Fallot
B. Patent ductus arteriosus
C. Ventricular septal defect
D. Atrial septal defect

*In patent ductus arteriosus, pulmonary hypertension and right-to-left shunt, differential cyanosis results, that is, cyanosis occurs in the lower but not in the upper extremities.*

**73. Which of the following is suspected when blood remains brown after mixing in test tube & exposed to air?**
*Harrison's 20th Ed. Chapter 94 Page 695*

A. Marked polycythemia
B. Carboxyhemoglobin (COHb)
C. Methemoglobin
D. Sulfhemoglobin

*Diagnosis of methemoglobinemia is suspected if blood remains brown after mixing in a test tube & exposure to air. Spectroscopy confirms the diagnosis.*

**74. Acquired methemoglobinemia may occur on exposure to?**
*N Engl J Med. 2000;343:337*

A. Dapsone
B. Nitrates
C. Sulfonamides
D. All of the above

*Acquired methemoglobinemia is a rare consequence of the exposure of normal red cells to oxidizing drugs such as benzocaine, dapsone, nitrates, primaquine and sulfonamides.*

**75. Symptomatic methemoglobinemia should be treated with?**
*N Engl J Med. 1992;327:1461*

A. Methylcobalamin
B. Hexamethylene diisocyanate
C. Methylene blue
D. Toluene diisocyanate

*Symptomatic methemoglobinemia should be treated with intravenous injection of methylene blue (1 to 2 mg per kilogram) or oral methylene blue (60 mg three to four times each day) or ascorbic acid (300 - 600 mg/day).*

**76. Which of the following is false in Eisenmenger syndrome?**
*Harrison's 20th Ed. Chapter 264 Page 1838*

A. Cyanosis
B. Elevated pulmonary vascular resistance
C. Intracardiac communication
D. Pulmonic stenosis

*Elevated pulmonary vascular resistance that produces cyanosis in the presence of intra- & extracardiac communications without pulmonic stenosis is termed Eisenmenger syndrome.*

**77. In peripheral cyanosis of extremities, the arterial blood is?**
*Harrison's 20th Ed. Chapter 36 Page 237*

A. Normally saturated with oxygen
B. Over saturated with oxygen
C. Under saturated with oxygen
D. Any of the above

**78. Clubbing without cyanosis is frequent in?**
*Harrison's 20th Ed. Chapter 36 Page 237*

A. Infective endocarditis
B. Inflammatory bowel disease
C. Jackhammer operators
D. All of the above

*Clubbing without cyanosis is frequent in infective endocarditis, inflammatory bowel disease & in Jackhammer operators.*

## Edema

**79. Edema is defined as a clinically apparent increase in?**
*Harrison's 20th Ed. Chapter 37 Page 237*

A. Intracellular fluid volume
B. Plasma volume
C. Interstitial fluid volume
D. All of the above

*Edema is defined as a clinically apparent increase in interstitial fluid volume.*

**80. Which of the following statements is false?**
*Harrison's 20th Ed. Chapter 37 Page 237*

A. ~ Two-thirds of total body water is intracellular
B. ~ One-third of total body water is extracellular
C. ~ One-fourth of extracellular water is in the plasma and the remainder comprises the interstitial fluid
D. None of the above

**81. Which of the following about movement of water & diffusible solutes from plasma to interstitium is false?**
*Harrison's 20th Ed. Chapter 37 Page 237*

A. Promoted by hydrostatic pressure within the capillaries
B. Promoted by colloid oncotic pressure in the interstitial fluid
C. Most prominent at the arterial origin of the capillary
D. None of the above

**82. Fluid is returned from the interstitial space into the vascular system largely through?**
*Harrison's 20th Ed. Chapter 37 Page 237*

A. Arterial system
B. Venous system
C. Lymphatic system
D. All of the above

*Fluid is returned from the interstitial space into the vascular system largely through the lymphatic system.*

**83. Development of edema occurs due to?**
*Harrison's 20th Ed. Chapter 37 Page 237*

A. Inadequate lymphatic drainage
B. Damage to capillary endothelial barrier
C. Increase in the oncotic pressure in interstitial space
D. All of the above

*Development of edema occurs due to an increase in intracapillary hydrostatic pressure, inadequate lymphatic drainage, reductions in oncotic pressure in plasma, damage to capillary endothelial barrier and increases in the oncotic pressure in interstitial space.*

**84. Which of the following is referred to as "tissue tension"?**
*Harrison's 19th Ed. 250*

A. Hydrostatic pressure within the vascular system
B. Colloid oncotic pressure within the vascular system
C. Hydrostatic pressure within the interstitial fluid
D. All of the above

*Plasma & interstitial fluid are two components of extracellular fluid regulate by Starling forces. Hydrostatic pressure within interstitial fluid is referred to as the tissue tension which promotes the movement of fluid into the vascular compartment.*

**85. Movement of water & diffusible solutes from vascular space into the interstitial space occurs at?**
*Harrison's 20th Ed. Chapter 37 Page 237*

A. Arteriolar end of capillaries
B. Venous end of capillaries
C. Lymphatics
D. All of the above

*Movement of water & diffusible solutes from vascular space into interstitial space occurs at the arteriolar end of capillaries. Fluid is returned from interstitial space into vascular system at the venous end of capillary & by way of lymphatics.*

**86. Which of the following about renal juxtaglomerular cells is false?**
*Harrison's 20th Ed. Chapter 37 Page 237*

A. Secrete renin
B. Specialized myoepithelial cells
C. Surround the afferent renal arteriole
D. None of the above

**87. Which of the following best define renin?**
*Harrison's 20th Ed. Chapter 37 Page 237*

A. Enzyme
B. Pro-hormone
C. Hormone
D. Cofactor

*Renin is an enzyme with a molecular weight of ~40,000 secreted by juxtaglomerular cells.*

**88. Conditions that reduce effective arterial blood volume cause constriction of which of the following?**
*Harrison's 20th Ed. Chapter 37 Page 237*

A. Renal afferent arteriolar constriction
B. Renal efferent arteriolar constriction
C. Renal glomerular capillary constriction
D. All of the above

*Heart failure, nephrotic syndrome & cirrhosis reduce effective arterial blood volume and cause renal efferent arteriolar constriction.*

**89. Which of the following stimulates renin release?**
*Harrison's 20th Ed. Chapter 37 Page 237*

A. Diminished stretch of the juxtaglomerular cells
B. Low sodium chloride load in distal renal tubules
C. Circulating catecholamines
D. All of the above

*Diminished renal blood flow resulting in diminished stretch of juxtaglomerular cells lowers sodium chloride load reaching distal renal tubules signals juxtaglomerular cells to secrete renin. Activation of β-adrenergic receptors in juxtaglomerular cells by sympathetic nervous system & circulating catecholamines stimulates renin release.*

**90. Angiotensinogen is synthesized by?**
*Harrison's 20th Ed. Chapter 37 Page 237*

A. Kidney
B. Liver
C. Pancreas
D. Lung

*Angiotensinogen, an α2 globulin, is synthesized by liver. Renin converts angiotensinogen to a decapeptide angiotensin I, which is broken down to an octapeptide angiotensin II.*

**91. Renal effects of Angiotensin II are mediated by activation of which type of Angiotensin II receptors?**
*Harrison's 20th Ed. Chapter 37 Page 238*

A. Type 1
B. Type 2
C. Type 3
D. Type 4

*Angiotensin II produces renal vasoconstriction & salt and water retention. These renal effects are mediated by activation of Angiotensin II type 1 receptors.*

**92. Which of the following stimulates the production of aldosterone?**
*Harrison's 20th Ed. Chapter 37 Page 238*

A. Angiotensinogen
B. Angiotensin I
C. Angiotensin II
D. All of the above

**93. Aldosterone is produced by?**
*Harrison's 20th Ed. Chapter 37 Page 238*

A. Juxtaglomerular cells of kidney
B. Macula densa cells of kidney
C. Zona glomerulosa of adrenal cortex
D. Zona reticularis of adrenal cortex

*Aldosterone is produced by zona glomerulosa of adrenal cortex & its release is stimulated by Angiotensin II. It is metabolized by liver.*

**94. Site of action of aldosterone is?**
*Harrison's 20th Ed. Chapter 37 Page 238*

A. Proximal convoluted tubule
B. Loop of Henle
C. Distal convoluted tubule
D. Collecting tubule

**95. Blockade of the action of aldosterone can be done by?**
*Harrison's 20th Ed. Chapter 37 Page 238*

A. Spironolactone
B. Eplerenone
C. Amiloride
D. All of the above

**96. In heart failure, aldosterone secretion is elevated due to?**
*Harrison's 20th Ed. Chapter 37 Page 238*

A. Prolongation of biologic half-life
B. Increased secretion
C. Reduced hepatic catabolism
D. All of the above

*In heart failure, levels of aldosterone are raised due to increased secretion, prolonged biologic half-life & reduced hepatic catabolism due to reduced hepatic blood flow, secondary to reduction in cardiac output.*

**97. Activation of Renin-Angiotensin-Aldosterone (RAA) system is most striking in which of the following?**
*Harrison's 20th Ed. Chapter 37 Page 238*

A. Acute, severe heart failure
B. Chronic heart failure
C. Stable heart failure
D. Compensated heart failure

*Activation of RAA system is seen conspicuously in early phase of acute, severe heart failure & is less intense in patients with chronic, stable, compensated heart failure.*

**98. Mineralocorticoid escape phenomenon is best explained by?**
*Harrison's 20th Ed. Chapter 37 Page 238*

A. Deficit in effective arterial blood volume
B. Aldosterone antagonism
C. Pressure natriuresis
D. Blocking of epithelial sodium channels

*Administration of potent mineralocorticoids (deoxycorticosterone acetate or fludrocortisone) leads to salt & water retention. This accumulation is self-limiting, despite continued exposure to steroid, a phenomenon known as mineralocorticoid escape wherein edema does not develop. It is due to an increase in GFR (pressure natriuresis).*

**99. Arginine vasopressin (AVP) is best related to?**
*Harrison's 20th Ed. Chapter 37 Page 238*

A. V1 receptors
B. V2 receptors
C. V3 receptors
D. V4 receptors

*Secretion of arginine vasopressin (AVP) occurs in response to increased intracellular osmolar concentration. By stimulating V2 receptors, AVP increases the reabsorption of free water in the distal tubules and collecting ducts of the kidneys, thereby increasing total-body water.*

**100. Which of the following is an effect of Endothelin-1?**
*Harrison's 20th Ed. Chapter 37 Page 238*

A. Renal vasoconstriction
B. Sodium retention
C. Edema
D. All of the above

*Endothelin-1 is a potent peptide vasoconstrictor released by endothelial cells. Its concentration in the plasma is elevated in patients with severe heart failure and contributes to renal vasoconstriction, sodium retention and edema.*

**101. Atrial natriuretic peptide (ANP) is stored in secretory granules within?**
*Harrison's 20th Ed. Chapter 37 Page 238*

A. Sinoatrial node
B. Atrial myocytes
C. Pulmonary veins
D. All of the above

*Polypeptide ANP is secreted by atrial myocytes secondary to atrial distention and/or sodium load. Its actions are excretion of sodium & water by increasing GFR, inhibiting sodium reabsorption in PCT & inhibiting release of renin & aldosterone. It also antagonizes vasoconstrictor actions of Angiotensin II, AVP & sympathetic stimulation causing arteriolar & venous dilatation.*

**102. Brain natriuretic peptide (BNP) is present in?**
*Harrison's 20th Ed. Chapter 37 Page 238*

A. Cardiac ventricular myocardium
B. Cerebral cortex
C. Cerebellum
D. All of the above

BNP is stored in cardiac ventricular myocardium & is released when ventricular diastolic pressure rises. Its actions are similar to ANP. Circulating levels of ANP & BNP are elevated in CHF.

**103. Released ANP & BNP bind to?**
*Harrison's 20th Ed. Chapter 37 Page 238*

A. Natriuretic receptor-A
B. Natriuretic receptor-B
C. Natriuretic receptor-C
D. Natriuretic receptor-D

Released ANP & BNP bind to the natriuretic receptor-A.

**104. Which of the following is an action of ANP and BNP?**
*Harrison's 20th Ed. Chapter 37 Page 238*

A. Excretion of sodium & water
B. Inhibiting sodium reabsorption
C. Inhibiting release of renin & aldosterone
D. All of the above

Released ANP and BNP lead to excretion of sodium & water by augmenting glomerular filtration rate, inhibiting sodium reabsorption in proximal tubule and inhibiting release of renin & aldosterone.

**105. ANP and BNP antagonize the vasoconstrictor actions of?**
*Harrison's 20th Ed. Chapter 37 Page 238*

A. Angiotensin II
B. Arginine vasopressin
C. Sympathetic stimulation
D. All of the above

Released ANP and BNP also cause dilation of arterioles & venules by antagonizing the vasoconstrictor actions of AII, AVP and sympathetic stimulation. Thus elevated levels of natriuretic peptides have the capacity to oppose sodium retention in hypervolemic and edematous states.

**106. Which of the following is a form of edema?**
*Harrison's 20th Ed. Chapter 37 Page 238*

A. Anasarca
B. Ascites
C. Hydrothorax
D. All of the above

Anasarca refers to gross, generalized edema. Ascites and hydrothorax refer to accumulation of excess fluid in the peritoneal and pleural cavities, respectively and are considered special forms of edema.

**107. Which of the following about edema of renal disease is false?**
*Harrison's 20th Ed. Chapter 37 Page 239*

A. Hypertension
B. Without considerable cardiac enlargement
C. Develop orthopnea
D. Normal cardiac output

**108. NSAIDs and cyclosporine cause edema due to?**
*Harrison's 20th Ed. Chapter 37 Page 239*

A. Renal vasoconstriction
B. Arteriolar dilation
C. Augmented renal sodium reabsorption
D. Capillary damage

**109. Refeeding edema best relates to?**
*Harrison's 20th Ed. Chapter 37 Page 239*

A. Calcium
B. Insulin
C. Paratharmone
D. Oxytocin

Refeeding edema may be linked to increased release of insulin which directly increases tubular sodium reabsorption.

**110. Which of the following is involved in the edema of starvation?**
*Harrison's 20th Ed. Chapter 37 Page 239*

A. Hyponatremia
B. Hypokalemia
C. Hypocalcemia
D. Hypomagnesemia

In addition to hypoalbuminemia, hypokalemia and caloric deficits may be involved in the edema of starvation.

**111. Edema of hypothyroidism best relates to?**
*Harrison's 20th Ed. Chapter 37 Page 240*

A. Glutamic acid
B. Aggrecan
C. Hyaluronic acid
D. Lubricin

Nonpitting edema of hypothyroidism (myxedema) due to deposition of hyaluronic acid.

**112. Causes of facial edema include?**
*Harrison's 20th Ed. Chapter 37 Page 240*

A. Trichinosis
B. Hypoproteinemia
C. Myxedema
D. All of the above

Apart from hypoproteinemia, causes of facial edema include trichinosis (Trichinella spiralis), allergic reactions & myxedema. Trichinosis can also lead to membranous glomerulopathy, proliferative glomerulonephritis & acute pericarditis. Trichinosis is a cause of FUO.

**113. Antihypertensive agents associated with edema formation include all except?**
*Harrison's 20th Ed. Chapter 37 Page 240 Table 37-2*

A. Minoxidil
B. Hydralazine
C. Clonidine
D. Atenolol

**114. Antihypertensive agents associated with edema formation include all except?**
*Harrison's 20th Ed. Chapter 37 Page 240 Table 37-2*

A. Methyldopa
B. Calcium channel antagonists
C. ACE Inhibitors
D. Alpha adrenergic antagonists

**115. Steroid hormones associated with edema formation include all except?**
*Harrison's 20th Ed. Chapter 37 Page 240 Table 37-2*

A. Glucocorticoids
B. Mineralocorticoids
C. Anabolic steroids
D. Estrogens / Progestins

**116. Which of the following is associated with edema formation?**
*Harrison's 20th Ed. Chapter 37 Page 240 Table 37-2*

A. Cyclosporine
B. Growth hormone
C. Interleukin 2
D. All of the above

**117. Which of the following is false about idiopathic edema?**
*N Engl J Med. 1960; 263:1342-1345*

A. Occurs in women
B. Edema unrelated to menstrual cycle
C. Occurs after upright posture
D. None of the above

*Idiopathic cyclic edema occurs almost exclusively in women, is characterized by periodic episodes of edema (unrelated to menstrual cycle), frequently accompanied by abdominal distention orthostatic retention of sodium & water after upright posture.*

**118. Venous pressure in upper extremities is elevated in all except?**
*Harrison's 20th Ed. Chapter 37 Page 240*

A. Advanced heart failure
B. Constrictive pericarditis
C. Tricuspid stenosis
D. Cirrhosis liver

*Venous pressure in upper extremities is elevated in advanced heart failure, constrictive pericarditis or tricuspid stenosis but is normal in cirrhosis. In hepatic cirrhosis, JVP is normal.*

## Palpitations

**119. Palpitations are often noted when the patient is?**
*Harrison's 20th Ed. Chapter 39 Page 249*
- A. Exercising
- B. Quietly resting
- C. Sleeping
- D. Post prandial

*Palpitations are often noted when the patient is quietly resting, when other stimuli are minimal.*

**120. Positional palpitations can be due to?**
*Harrison's 20th Ed. Chapter 39 Page 249*
- A. Atrial myxoma
- B. HOCM
- C. Supravalvular aortic stenosis
- D. All of the above

*Positional palpitations are generally due to a structural process within (atrial myxoma) or adjacent to (mediastinal mass, diaphragmatic hernia, gastric volvulus) the heart.*

**121. Psychiatric illnesses contribute to what proportion of cases of palpitations?**
*Harrison's 20th Ed. Chapter 39 Page 249*
- A. ~ 10%
- B. ~ 20%
- C. ~ 30%
- D. ~ 40%

*Palpitations are caused by cardiac (43%), psychiatric (31%), miscellaneous (10%), and unknown (16%) causes.*

**122. Which of the following is a cause of palpitation?**
*Harrison's 20th Ed. Chapter 39 Page 249*
- A. Mitral valve prolapse
- B. Aortic insufficiency
- C. Pulmonary embolism
- D. All of the above

*Cardiovascular causes of palpitation include premature atrial and ventricular contractions, supraventricular and ventricular arrhythmias, mitral valve prolapse (with or without associated arrhythmias), aortic insufficiency, atrial myxoma, myocarditis, and pulmonary embolism.*

**123. Irregular, sustained palpitations can be caused by?**
*Harrison's 20th Ed. Chapter 39 Page 249*
- A. Atrial fibrillation
- B. Premature atrial contractions
- C. Premature ventricular contractions
- D. Supraventricular tachycardias

*Irregular, sustained palpitations can be caused by atrial fibrillation.*

**124. Palpitation with rapid and irregular rhythm suggest?**
*N Engl J Med. 1998;338(19):1369*
- A. Atrial fibrillation
- B. Atrial flutter
- C. Tachycardia with variable block
- D. Any of the above

**125. Which of the following statements about palpitations is false?**
*Harrison's 20th Ed. Chapter 39 Page 249*
- A. Most arrhythmias are not associated with palpitations
- B. Palpitations are common among athletes
- C. Palpitations due to psychiatric causes have a longer duration of the sensation (>15 minutes)
- D. None of the above

**126. Which of the following enhances the strength of myocardial contraction and cause palpitations?**
*Harrison's 20th Ed. Chapter 39 Page 249*
- A. Tobacco
- B. Cocaine
- C. Amphetamines
- D. All of the above

*Tobacco, caffeine, aminophylline, atropine, thyroxine, cocaine, and amphetamines enhance the strength of myocardial contraction and can cause palpitations.*

**127. Which of the following conditions frequently lead to the sensation of palpitations?**
*Harrison's 20th Ed. Chapter 39 Page 249*
- A. Aortic stenosis
- B. Aortic regurgitation
- C. HOCM
- D. All of the above

*Hyperdynamic cardiovascular states caused by catecholaminergic stimulation as in exercise, stress, or pheochromocytoma can lead to palpitations. Enlarged ventricle of aortic regurgitation & accompanying hyperdynamic precordium frequently lead to the sensation of palpitations.*

**128. Which of the following is the most common structural heart disease leading to palpitations?**
*Am Fam Physician. 2011;84(1):63-69*
- A. Mitral stenosis
- B. Mitral regurgitation
- C. Mitral valve prolapse
- D. Atrial septal defect

*Mitral valve prolapse is the most common structural heart disease leading to palpitations and is likely caused by papillary muscle fibrosis.*

**129. Which of the following arrhythmia has been described with mitral-valve prolapse?**
*N Engl J Med. 1998;338(19):1369*
- A. Supraventricular arrhythmia
- B. Ventricular premature depolarizations
- C. Nonsustained ventricular tachycardia
- D. All of the above

*Virtually every type of supraventricular arrhythmia, as well as ventricular premature depolarizations and nonsustained ventricular tachycardia, has been described with mitral-valve prolapse, and palpitations are nearly ubiquitous in mitral-valve prolapse.*

**130. Which of the following is a cause of palpitations?**
*Harrison's 20th Ed. Chapter 39 Page 249*
- A. Ethanol
- B. Pheochromocytoma
- C. Systemic mastocytosis
- D. All of the above

*Thyrotoxicosis, drugs (aminophylline, atropine, thyroxine, cocaine, amphetamines), ethanol, spontaneous skeletal muscle contractions of chest wall, pheochromocytoma & systemic mastocytosis cause palpitations.*

## Basic Biology of the Cardiovascular System

**131. Cardiac embryogenesis best relates to?**
*Harrison's 20th Ed. Chapter 232 Page 1651*

A. Anterior splanchnic mesoderm
B. Posterior splanchnic mesoderm
C. Medial splanchnic mesoderm
D. Lateral splanchnic mesoderm

*Early cardiac progenitors arise within crescent-shaped fields of lateral splanchnic mesoderm and migrate to midline to form the linear heart tube which is a single layer of endocardium and a single layer of cardiomyocyte precursors.*

**132. "Cardiac jelly" which accumulates within the endocardial cushions best relates to?**
*Harrison's 20th Ed. Chapter 232 Page 1651*

A. Folic acid
B. Hyaluronic acid
C. Citric acid
D. Lactic acid

*Early in development, the single layer of myocardial cells secretes an extracellular matrix rich in hyaluronic acid or "cardiac jelly" which is the precursor of the cardiac valves.*

**133. Proepicardial organ is a derivative of?**
*Harrison's 20th Ed. Chapter 232 Page 1651*

A. Septum transversum
B. Anterior conal septum
C. Septum pellucidum
D. All of the above

*Epicardial cells arise in the transient embryonic structure called proepicardial organ which is a derivative of septum transversum. Septum transversum separates the embryo's thorax from its abdomen, and to the diaphragm and liver. Proepicardial cells contribute smooth-muscle to coronary arteries and are required for proper coronary patterning.*

**134. Neural crest cells are sensitive to which of the following vitamins?**
*Harrison's 20th Ed. Chapter 232 Page 1652*

A. A
B. C
C. D
D. E

*Neural crest cells are sensitive to both vitamin A and folic acid, and congenital heart disease involving abnormal remodeling of aortic arch arteries associates with their maternal deficiencies.*

**135. Neural crest cells form components of?**
*N Engl J Med. 2010;363:1638-47*

A. Peripheral nervous system
B. Craniofacial regions
C. Cardiac outflow tract
D. All of the above

**136. Which of the following cells contribute to cardiac morphogenesis?**
*N Engl J Med. 2010;363:1638-47*

A. Neural-crest cells
B. Cells arising from the second heart field
C. Epicardial progenitors
D. All of the above

**137. Which of the following is a second-heart-field cardiac defect?**
*N Engl J Med. 2010;363:1638-47*

A. Pulmonic stenosis
B. Tetralogy of Fallot
C. Ebstein's anomaly
D. All of the above

**138. Second-heart-field progenitors that express which of the following?**
*N Engl J Med. 2010;363:1638-47*

A. Islet 1
B. Islet 2
C. Islet 3
D. Islet 4

*Second-heart-field progenitors that express islet 1 are multipotent cells that can give rise to smooth-muscle cells at the base of aorta and pulmonary arteries, to endothelial cells, or to myocardium. Cells in second heart field migrate first to pharyngeal regions and express specific marker genes, including the transcription factor islet 1.*

**139. Which of the following statements is false?**
*N Engl J Med. 2010;363:1638-47*

A. Cells that give rise to sinus node express fetal TBX18 gene
B. Cells that give rise to atrioventricular node & Purkinje system express NKX2-5 transcription factor
C. Development of pulmonary-vein myocardium requires PITX2 transcription factor
D. None of the above

**140. Cells from which of the following help in repair of damaged or aging arteries?**
*Harrison's 20th Ed. Chapter 232 Page 1652*

A. Neural crest
B. Mesodermal structures
C. Bone marrow derived endothelial progenitors
D. All of the above

*Bone marrow derived endothelial progenitors may aid repair of damaged or aging arteries.*

**141. Adventitia of arteries consists of?**
*Harrison's 20th Ed. Chapter 232 Page 1652*

A. Fibroblasts
B. Mast cells
C. Nerve terminals
D. All of the above

**142. Pericytes best relate to?**
*Harrison's 20th Ed. Chapter 232 Page 1652*

A. Endothelial cells
B. Smooth-muscle-like cells
C. Fibroblasts
D. All of the above

*The smallest blood vessels i.e. capillaries consist of a monolayer of endothelial cells on a basement membrane, adjacent to a discontinuous layer of smooth-muscle-like cells known as pericytes.*

143. **Vasa vasorum nourishes which of the following?**
   *Harrison's 20th Ed. Chapter 232 Page 1652*

   A. Tunica intima
   B. Tunica media
   C. Tunica adventitia
   D. All of the above

   *Larger arteries the vasa vasorum which nourishes the tunica media.*

144. **Which of the following about blood vessels is false?**
   *Harrison's 20th Ed. Chapter 232 Page 1653 Figure 232-2*

   A. Veins have thin medias and thicker adventitias
   B. Small muscular artery has a prominent tunica media
   C. Larger elastic arteries have cylindrical layers of elastic tissue alternating with concentric rings of smooth muscle cells
   D. None of the above

145. **"Capillary leak" occurs in?**
   *Harrison's 20th Ed. Chapter 232 Page 1653*

   A. Hypertension
   B. Renal disease
   C. Sepsis
   D. All of the above

   *"Capillary leak" occur in atherosclerosis, hypertension, renal disease, pulmonary edema & sepsis.*

146. **Endogenous substance produced by endothelial cells is?**
   *Harrison's 20th Ed. Chapter 231 Page 1653*

   A. Prostacyclin
   B. Nitric oxide (NO)
   C. Hydrogen peroxide ($H_2O_2$)
   D. All of the above

   *Endogenous substances produced by endothelial cells are prostacyclin, endothelium-derived hyperpolarizing factor, nitric oxide (NO), and hydrogen peroxide ($H_2O_2$). These provide tonic vasodilatory stimuli under physiologic conditions in vivo.*

147. **Potent vasoconstrictor substance produced by endothelial cells is?**
   *Harrison's 20th Ed. Chapter 232 Page 1653*

   A. Cathelin
   B. Endoglin
   C. Endothelin
   D. All of the above

   *Potent vasoconstrictor substance produced by endothelial cells is endothelin.*

148. **Which of the following, elaborated by endothelial cells, can inhibit smooth-muscle proliferation?**
   *Harrison's 20th Ed. Chapter 232 Page 1653*

   A. Heparan sulfate proteoglycan
   B. Heparan sulfate glycosaminoglycan
   C. Dermatan sulfate proteoglycan
   D. Dermatan sulfate glycosaminoglycan

   *Heparan sulfate glycosaminoglycans elaborated by endothelial cells inhibits smooth-muscle proliferation.*

149. **Endothelial cells can produce which of the following?**
   *Harrison's 20th Ed. Chapter 232 Page 1653*

   A. Plasminogen activator inhibitor 1 (PAI-1)
   B. Platelet-derived growth factor
   C. Heparan sulfate glycosaminoglycan
   D. All of the above

150. **Which of the following is a neurotransmitter of peptidergic neuronal class?**
   *Harrison's 20th Ed. Chapter 232 Page 1654*

   A. Substance P
   B. Vasoactive intestinal peptide
   C. Calcitonin gene-related peptide
   D. All of the above

151. **Which of the following about cardiomyocyte is false?**
   *Harrison's 20th Ed. Chapter 232 Page 1655*

   A. Normally, 60–140 μm in length & 17–25 μm in diameter
   B. Each cardiomyocyte contains multiple myofibrils
   C. Myofibrils are composed of repeating sarcomeres
   D. None of the above

152. **The structural & functional unit of contraction is?**
   *Harrison's 20th Ed. Chapter 232 Page 1655*

   A. Cardiomyocyte
   B. Myofibril
   C. Sarcomere
   D. All of the above

   *Sarcomere is the structural & functional unit of contraction. It lies between adjacent Z lines. The distance between Z lines ranges between 1.6 and 2.2 μm.*

153. **What is the length of the dark A band?**
   *Harrison's 20th Ed. Chapter 232 Page 1655*

   A. 0.5 μm
   B. 1.0 μm
   C. 1.5 μm
   D. 2.0 μm

154. **With muscle contraction, which of the following occurs?**
   *Harrison's 20th Ed. Chapter 232 Page 1655*

   A. A band remains constant in length
   B. I band shortens
   C. Z lines move toward one another
   D. All of the above

155. **Double helix of two chains of actin molecules are wound on?**
   *Harrison's 20th Ed. Chapter 232 Page 1655*

   A. Tropomyosin
   B. Titin
   C. Actin
   D. Dystrophin

156. **Which of the following connects myosin to the Z line?**
   *Harrison's 20th Ed. Chapter 232 Page 1655*

   A. Tropomyosin
   B. Titin
   C. Actin
   D. Dystrophin

   *Flexible myofibrillar protein, Titin connects myosin to the Z line.*

157. During activation of the cardiac myocyte, Ca++ binds to which of the following?

    *Harrison's 20th Ed. Chapter 232 Page 1655*

    A. Troponin C
    B. Troponin I
    C. Troponin T
    D. All of the above

    During activation of the cardiac myocyte, Ca++ binds troponin C, resulting in conformational changes in the regulatory protein tropomyosin and exposing actin cross-bridge interaction sites.

158. The extracellular concentration of calcium is how many times more than the intracellular concentration?

    *N Engl J Med. 2006;355:608*

    A. 2000 times
    B. 5000 times
    C. 10000 times
    D. 20000 times

159. Stretching capability of which myofibrillar protein contributes to the elasticity of heart?

    *Harrison's 20th Ed. Chapter 232 Page 1655*

    A. Titin
    B. Myosin
    C. Actin
    D. All of the above

160. During activation of the myocyte, $Ca^{2+}$ becomes attached to?

    *Harrison's 20th Ed. Chapter 232 Page 1655*

    A. Troponin C
    B. Troponin I
    C. Troponin T
    D. All of the above

161. Acceleration of cardiac relaxation occurs by phosphorylation by cyclic AMP of which protein?

    *Harrison's 20th Ed. Chapter 232 Page 1655*

    A. Troponin C
    B. Troponin I
    C. Troponin T
    D. All of the above

162. Which of the following gene encods titin?

    *N Engl J Med. 2012; 366:619-628*

    A. TIN
    B. TTN
    C. TNN
    D. TTT

    TTN gene encodes the sarcomere protein titin.

163. Which of the following is the largest human protein?

    *N Engl J Med. 2012; 366:619-628*

    A. Dystrophin
    B. Titin
    C. Myosin
    D. Actin

    Titin is the largest human protein, composed of ~33,000 amino acids. It is the third most abundant striated-muscle protein. Titin molecules are anchored at the Z-line and M-line. TTN truncating mutations are the most common known genetic cause of dilated cardiomyopathy.

164. Drugs that enhance relaxation of myocardium are called?

    *Harrison's 20th Ed. Chapter 232 Page 1658*

    A. Dromotropic
    B. Ionotropic
    C. Lusitropic
    D. Cathotropic

165. Which of the following is termed as the "disease of the sarcomere"?

    *N Engl J Med. 2011;364:1643-1656*

    A. Dilated cardiomyopathy
    B. Hypertrophic cardiomyopathy
    C. Arrhythmogenic Right Ventricular Cardiomyopathy (ARVC)
    D. All of the above

166. Which of the following enzyme is responsible for maintaining correct calcium homeostasis in cardiomyocyte?

    *N Engl J Med. 2011; 364:1643-1656*

    A. Diacylglycerol (DAG)
    B. Phosphatidylinositol 4,5-bisphosphate
    C. Sarcoplasmic reticulum Ca++ATPase (SERCA)
    D. Inositol 1,4,5-trisphosphate (IP3)

167. SERCA is regulated by?

    *N Engl J Med. 2011; 364:1643-1656*

    A. Calsequestrin
    B. Phospholamban
    C. Calstabin 2
    D. All of the above

    In cardiac muscle, SERCA (sarco(endo)plasmic reticulum Ca++-ATPase) is regulated by phospholamban (PLB), a small inhibitory phosphoprotein that decreases the Ca++ affinity of SERCA and attenuates contractile strength. cAMP-dependent phosphorylation of PLB reverses Ca++-ATPase inhibition.

168. Which of the following about protein phospholamban is false?

    *Harrison's 20th Ed. Chapter 232 Page 1657*

    A. Situated on the membrane of sarcoplasmic reticulum
    B. Activated by cAMP
    C. Controls rate of uptake of calcium into sarcoplasmic reticulum
    D. None of the above

    Activated by cAMP, protein phospholamban, situated on membrane of sarcoplasmic reticulum (SR), controls the rate of uptake of calcium into SR. The latter effect explains enhanced relaxation (lusitropic effect).

169. Cyclic adenosine monophosphate (cAMP) acts via?

    *Harrison's 20th Ed. Chapter 232 Page 1657*

    A. Nuclear factor-κB
    B. Protein kinase A
    C. Calcium-dependent calcineurin
    D. Phospholipase C

    Cyclic adenosine monophosphate (cAMP) or the second messenger acts via protein kinase A to stimulate metabolism and phosphorylate the Ca++ channel protein.

170. Ca++ is stored in the sarcoplasmic reticulum by forming a complex with?
*Harrison's 20th Ed. Chapter 232 Page 1657*

   A. Calsequestrin
   B. Phospholamban
   C. Calstabin 2
   D. All of the above

171. Inactive cardiac cell has a transmembrane potential of?
*Harrison's 20th Ed. Chapter 232 Page 1657*

   A. –40 to –60 mV
   B. –60 to –80 mV
   C. –80 to –100 mV
   D. –100 to –120 mV

*Inactive cardiac cell has a transmembrane potential (Vm) of –80 to –100 mV. The interior being negatively charged relative to outside of cell.*

172. Plateau phase of action potential corresponds to?
*Harrison's 20th Ed. Chapter 232 Page 1657*

   A. Phase 1
   B. Phase 2
   C. Phase 3
   D. Phase 4

173. Ca++-induced Ca++ release occurs in?
*Harrison's 20th Ed. Chapter 232 Page 1657*

   A. Sarcolemma
   B. Sarcoplasmic reticulum
   C. Nuclear membrane
   D. All of the above

*Absolute quantity of Ca++ entering sarcolemma & T tubules is modest and insufficient to activate contraction fully. However, this Ca++ current, through Ca++-induced Ca++ release, triggers substantial Ca++ release from the sarcoplasmic reticulum, inducing contraction.*

174. Ryanodine receptor (RyR2) best relate to?
*Harrison's 20th Ed. Chapter 232 Page 1657*

   A. Sarcolemma
   B. Sarcoplasmic reticulum
   C. Nuclear membrane
   D. All of the above

*Ca++ is released from sarcoplasmic reticulum through a Ca++ release channel, a cardiac isoform of ryanodine receptor (RyR2).*

175. Which of the following inhibits ryanodine receptor (RyR2)?
*Harrison's 20th Ed. Chapter 232 Page 1657*

   A. Calsequestrin
   B. Phospholamban
   C. Calstabin 2
   D. All of the above

*Calstabin 2 inhibits RyR2 and thus Ca++ release from sarcoplasmic reticulum.*

176. Ca++ released from sarcoplasmic reticulum interacts with?
*Harrison's 20th Ed. Chapter 232 Page 1657*

   A. Troponin C
   B. Troponin I
   C. Troponin T
   D. All of the above

177. Myocardial contractile force is optimal at a sarcomere length of?
*Harrison's 20th Ed. Chapter 232 Page 1657*

   A. ~ 1.8 μm
   B. ~ 2.0 μm
   C. ~ 2.2 μm
   D. ~ 2.4 μm

*Preload determines sarcomere length at the onset of contraction. Myocardial contractile force is optimal at a sarcomere length of ~2.2 μm where myofilament Ca++ sensitivity is maximal. Starling's law of the heart states that within limits, the ventricular contraction force depends on end-diastolic length of cardiac muscle which relates closely to the ventricular end-diastolic volume.*

178. In Starling's law of heart, the force of ventricular contraction is a function of?
*Harrison's 20th Ed. Chapter 232 Page 1658*

   A. End-diastolic length of cardiac muscle
   B. End-systolic length of cardiac muscle
   C. Mid-diastolic length of cardiac muscle
   D. Mid-systolic length of cardiac muscle

179. Afterload is determined by?
*Harrison's 20th Ed. Chapter 232 Page 1658*

   A. Aortic pressure
   B. LV volume
   C. Thickness of LV wall
   D. All of the above

180. Which of the following parameter is included in Laplace's law?
*Harrison's 20th Ed. Chapter 232 Page 1658*

   A. Intracavitary ventricular pressure
   B. Ventricular radius
   C. Wall thickness
   D. All of the above

181. Laplace's law indicates?
*Harrison's 20th Ed. Chapter 232 Page 1658*

   A. Length of myocardial fiber
   B. Tension of myocardial fiber
   C. Diameter of myocardial fiber
   D. All of the above

182. Aortic pressure depends on?
*Harrison's 20th Ed. Chapter 232 Page 1658*

   A. Peripheral vascular resistance
   B. Biomechanics of the arterial tree
   C. Volume of blood at the onset of ejection
   D. All of the above

183. During exercise, which of the following parameters show relatively little change?
*Harrison's 20th Ed. Chapter 232 Page 1659*

   A. LV end-diastolic pressure
   B. Cardiac output
   C. Aortic flow velocity
   D. Rate of ventricular pressure development

184. Ejection fraction is the?
*Harrison's 20th Ed. Chapter 232 Page 1659*

   A. Ratio of stroke volume to end-systolic volume
   B. Ratio of stroke volume to end-diastolic volume
   C. Ratio of end-systolic volume to stroke volume
   D. Ratio of end-diastolic volume to stroke volume

185. Normal value of ejection fraction is?
*Harrison's 20th Ed. Chapter 232 Page 1659*

   A. 47 ± 8%
   B. 57 ± 8%
   C. 67 ± 8%
   D. 77 ± 8%

186. Normal value of ventricular end-diastolic volume is?
*Harrison's 20th Ed. Chapter 232 Page 1659*

   A. 55 ± 20 mL/m$^2$
   B. 65 ± 20 mL/m$^2$
   C. 75 ± 20 mL/m$^2$
   D. 85 ± 20 mL/m2

187. Normal value of ventricular end-systolic volume is?
*Harrison's 20th Ed. Chapter 232 Page 1659*

   A. 15 ± 7 mL/m2
   B. 25 ± 7 mL/m2
   C. 35 ± 7 mL/m2
   D. 45 ± 7 mL/m2

188. Which of the following is of value in the clinical assessment of myocardial function?
*Harrison's 20th Ed. Chapter 232 Page 1659*

   A. Echocardiography
   B. Radionuclide scintigraphy
   C. Cardiac magnetic resonance imaging (MRI)
   D. All of the above

189. Which of the following strongly influence the measurements of CO, EF and ventricular volumes?
*Harrison's 20th Ed. Chapter 232 Page 1659*

   A. Heart rate
   B. Ventricular loading
   C. Arterial oxygen saturation
   D. All of the above

190. Cardiac function variable that is influenced by ventricular loading conditions is?
*Harrison's 20th Ed. Chapter 232 Page 1659*

   A. Cardiac output
   B. Ejection fraction
   C. Ventricular volumes
   D. All of the above

191. Which of the following does not depend on preload and afterload?
*Harrison's 20th Ed. Chapter 232 Page 1659*

   A. End-systolic left ventricular pressure-volume relationship
   B. End-diastolic left ventricular pressure-volume relationship
   C. Cardiac output
   D. Ejection fraction

192. Which of the following best relates to myocardial relaxation?
*Harrison's 20th Ed. Chapter 232 Page 1660*

   A. Rate of uptake of Na$^+$ by the SR
   B. Rate of uptake of K$^+$ by the SR
   C. Rate of uptake of Ca$^{++}$ by the SR
   D. All of the above

193. The heart requires a continuous supply of energy (ATP) for?
*Harrison's 20th Ed. Chapter 232 Page 1660*

   A. Mechanical contraction
   B. Maintaining ionic homeostasis
   C. Maintaining biochemical homeostasis
   D. All of the above

194. Which of the following is a determinant of the heart's energy needs?
*Harrison's 20th Ed. Chapter 232 Page 1660*

   A. Ventricular wall tension
   B. Frequency of contraction
   C. Myocardial contractility
   D. All of the above

195. Which of the following statements is false?
*Harrison's 20th Ed. Chapter 232 Page 1661*

   A. Energy substrates of heart are glucose & free fatty acids
   B. Oxidation of glucose & FFA produce acetyl coenzyme A in cytoplasm
   C. In fasted, resting state, FFA furnish ~70% of heart's acetyl-CoA
   D. In the fed state, glucose furnish heart's acetyl-CoA

*These two principal sources of acetyl coenzyme A in cardiac muscle i.e. glucose & FFA, vary reciprocally. Glucose is broken down in cytoplasm into pyruvate, which passes into mitochondria, where it is metabolized to acetyl-CoA, and undergoes oxidation. FFAs are converted to acyl-CoA in cytoplasm and acetyl-CoA in mitochondria. Acetyl-CoA enters the citric acid (Krebs) cycle to produce ATP. ATP enters cytoplasm from mitochondrial compartment.*

196. Myocardial energy is stored as?
*Harrison's 20th Ed. Chapter 232 Page 1661*

   A. Calsequestrin
   B. Creatine phosphate
   C. Phospholamban
   D. All of the above

*Myocardial energy is stored as creatine phosphate (CP) or phosphocreatine, which is in equilibrium with ATP, the immediate energy source.*

# Electrocardiography

**197. ECG leads displays?**
*Harrison's 20th Ed. Chapter 235 Page 1675*

A. Instantaneous differences in electrical potential between electrodes
B. Differences in electrical potential between electrode and neutral
C. Differences in electrical potential between electrode & maximum positive charge
D. Differences in electrical potential between electrode & maximum negative charge

*ECG leads display instantaneous differences in potential between electrodes.*

**198. Electric currents that spread through the heart can be produced by?**
*Harrison's 20th Ed. Chapter 235 Page 1675*

A. Cardiac pacemaker cells
B. Specialized conduction tissue
C. Heart muscle
D. All of the above

*Depolarization of the heart is the initiating event for cardiac contraction. The electric currents that spread through the heart are produced by cardiac pacemaker cells, specialized conduction tissue, and heart muscle. The ECG records only the depolarization (stimulation) and repolarization (recovery) potentials generated by the atrial and ventricular myocardium.*

**199. AV junction is constituted by?**
*Harrison's 20th Ed. Chapter 235 Page 1675*

A. Atrioventricular (AV) node
B. AV node and His-bundle
C. AV node, His-bundle and fascicles
D. AV node, His-bundle, fascicles & Purkinje fibres

*AV nodal region & His-bundle area together constitute AV junction.*

**200. Ventricular repolarization is represented by?**
*Harrison's 20th Ed. Chapter 235 Page 1675*

A. ST segment
B. T wave
C. U wave
D. ST-T-U complex

*QRS complex represents ventricular depolarization & ST-T-U complex (ST segment, T wave & U wave) represents ventricular repolarization.*

**201. J point is the junction between?**
*Harrison's 20th Ed. Chapter 235 Page 1675*

A. End of P wave & beginning of QRS complex
B. End of QRS complex & beginning of ST segment
C. End of ST segment & beginning of T wave
D. End of T wave & beginning of U wave

*J point is the junction between the end of QRS complex and the beginning of ST segment.*

**202. Atrial repolarization wave may become apparent in?**
*Harrison's 20th Ed. Chapter 235 Page 1675*

A. Acute pericarditis
B. Cardiomyopathy
C. PSVT
D. Wandering pacemaker

**203. Atrial repolarization wave may become apparent in?**
*Harrison's 20th Ed. Chapter 235 Page 1675*

A. Acute rheumatic fever
B. Cardiomyopathy
C. PSVT
D. Atrial infarction

**204. Atrial repolarization wave may become apparent in?**
*Harrison's 20th Ed. Chapter 235 Page 1675*

A. Acute pericarditis
B. Atrial infarction
C. AV heart block
D. All of the above

*Atrial repolarization is usually too low in amplitude to be detected, but it may become apparent in acute pericarditis, atrial infarction and AV heart block.*

**205. Rapid upstroke of the action potential that corresponds to the onset of QRS is called?**
*Harrison's 20th Ed. Chapter 235 Page 1675*

A. Phase 0
B. Phase 1
C. Phase 2
D. Phase 3

**206. Plateau of the action potential that corresponds to isoelectric ST segment is called?**
*Harrison's 20th Ed. Chapter 235 Page 1675*

A. Phase 0
B. Phase 1
C. Phase 2
D. Phase 3

*The QRS-T waveforms of the surface ECG correspond with the different phases of simultaneously obtained ventricular action potentials. Rapid upstroke (phase 0) of the action potential corresponds to the onset of QRS. Plateau (phase 2) corresponds to the isoelectric ST segment, and active repolarization (phase 3) corresponds to the inscription of the T wave.*

**207. Which of the following prolong phase 2 of the cardiac muscle action potential and increase the QT interval?**
*Harrison's 20th Ed. Chapter 235 Page 1675*

A. Hyperkalemia
B. Amiodarone
C. Digitalis
D. Hypercalcemia

*Factors that decrease slope of phase 0 by impairing influx of Na+ (hyperkalemia & flecainide) tend to increase QRS duration. Conditions that prolong phase 2 (amiodarone, hypocalcemia) increase QT interval. Shortening of ventricular repolarization (phase 2) by digitalis administration or hypercalcemia, abbreviates ST segment.*

### 208. The action potential of the His-Purkinje system and ventricular myocardium has?
*Harrison's 20th Ed. Chapter 235 Page 1675*

A. Two phases
B. Three phases
C. Four phases
D. Five phases

*Action potential of the His-Purkinje system has five phases.*

### 209. Resting membrane potential in ventricular myocardium is?
*Harrison's 20th Ed. Chapter 235 Page 1675*

A. Phase 1
B. Phase 2
C. Phase 3
D. Phase 4

*Rapid depolarizing current (phase 0) is due to influx of Na+ into myocardial cells followed by influx of $Ca^{++}$. Repolarization phases of action potential (phases 1 to 3) are due to outward flux of $K^+$. Resting membrane potential is phase 4.*

### 210. Which of the following intervals is used to calculate heart rate?
*Harrison's 20th Ed. Chapter 235 Page 1676*

A. RR
B. PR
C. QRS
D. QT

*Heart rate can be computed from the interbeat (RR) interval by dividing number of large (0.20 second) time units between consecutive R waves into 300 or the number of small (0.04 second) units into 1500.*

### 211. Which of the following statements is false?
*Harrison's 20th Ed. Chapter 235 Page 1676*

A. Normal PR interval is 120 - 200 ms
B. Normal QRS interval is < 100 - 110 ms
C. Normal QT interval is ≤ 0.44 s
D. None of the above

### 212. Which of the following statements is false?
*Harrison's 20th Ed. Chapter 235 Page 1676*

A. QT interval varies inversely with the heart rate
B. Rate-related ("corrected") QT interval is calculated as QT/√RR
C. Upper normal limits of QTc is 0.45 s in men & 0.46 s in women
D. None of the above

### 213. Rate-related ("corrected") QT interval (QTc) is calculated by?
*N Engl J Med. 1993; 328:287*

A. Alwyn's formula
B. Bazett's formula
C. Frank's formula
D. Donald's formula

*Original formula for QTc was published in 1920 by Bazett based on the study of 39 patients.*

### 214. Rate-related ("corrected") QT interval (QTc) is calculated by?
*Circ J. 2010;74(8):1663-9*

A. Fridericia's formula
B. Holter's formula
C. Grobbee's formula
D. Wilde's formula

*Fridericia's is a cube-root formula while Bazett's is a square-root formula.*

### 215. Which of the following is the more appropriate measure of ventricular cell repolarization?
*N Engl J Med. 1993; 328:287*

A. RT interval
B. JT interval
C. RU interval
D. JU interval

*JT interval, the more appropriate measure of ventricular cell repolarization, which is the point of attack for most influences altering QT intervals.*

### 216. Automaticity is characteristic of?
*Harrison's 20th Ed. Chapter 238 Page 1717*

A. Sinoatrial (SA)
B. Coronary sinus
C. Pulmonary veins
D. All of the above

*Automaticity is characteristic of pacemaking cells in the sinoatrial (SA) and atrioventricular (AV) nodes, His-Purkinje system, coronary sinus and pulmonary veins. It is the property of a cardiac cell that causes it to depolarize spontaneously during phase 4 of the action potential leading to the generation of an impulse.*

### 217. PR interval is related to?
*Harrison's 20th Ed. Chapter 235 Page 1676*

A. Atrial musculature conduction
B. AV node
C. AV junction area
D. All of the above

*PR interval measures the time (normally 120 - 200 ms) between atrial & ventricular depolarization, which includes the physiologic delay imposed by stimulation of cells in the AV junction area.*

### 218. Extremity ECG leads record potentials transmitted onto?
*Harrison's 20th Ed. Chapter 235 Page 1676*

A. Frontal plane
B. Vertical plane
C. Horizontal plane
D. Diagonal plane

### 219. ECG chest leads record potentials transmitted onto?
*Harrison's 20th Ed. Chapter 235 Page 1676*

A. Frontal plane
B. Vertical plane
C. Horizontal plane
D. Diagonal plane

*Six extremity leads record potentials transmitted onto the frontal plane & the six chest leads record potentials transmitted onto the horizontal plane.*

**220.** Which of the following statements about each ECG lead is false?
*Harrison's 20th Ed. Chapter 235 Page 1676 Figure 235-4*

- A. Each ECG lead has a specific spatial orientation
- B. Each ECG lead has a specific polarity
- C. Positive pole of lead I is labeled as 0°
- D. None of the above

*The positive pole of each lead axis and the negative pole are designated by their angular position relative to the positive pole of lead I (0°) in increments of 30°.*

**221.** In the hexaxial diagram representing frontal plane (limb or extremity) leads, 0° corresponds to which lead?
*Harrison's 20th Ed. Chapter 235 Page 1676 Figure 235-4*

- A. Lead I
- B. Lead II
- C. Lead III
- D. Any of the above

*Each lead axis is designated by their angular position relative to the positive pole of lead I (0°).*

**222.** Additional posterior leads are placed on the same horizontal plane as?
*Harrison's 20th Ed. Chapter 235 Page 1676 Figure 235-5*

- A. V3
- B. V4
- C. V5
- D. V6

*Additional posterior leads are sometimes placed on the same horizontal plane as V4.*

**223.** Which chest lead is placed in posterior axillary line?
*Harrison's 20th Ed. Chapter 235 Page 1676 Figure 235-5*

- A. V6
- B. V7
- C. V8
- D. V9

**224.** Number of intercostal spaces used for placing unipolar chest leads in ECG are?
*Harrison's 20th Ed. Chapter 235 Page 1676*

- A. 1
- B. 2
- C. 3
- D. 4

*IV and V intercostal spaces.*

**225.** In ECG, if the mean orientation of the depolarization vector is at right angles to a given lead axis, which of the following will happen?
*Harrison's 20th Ed. Chapter 235 Page 1676*

- A. Positive wave will be recorded
- B. Negative wave will be recorded
- C. Biphasic wave will be recorded
- D. Flat wave will be recorded

*ECG leads are configured so that a positive (upright) deflection is recorded in a lead if a wave of depolarization spreads toward the positive pole of that lead, and a negative deflection if the wave spreads toward the negative pole. If the mean orientation of depolarization vector is at right angles to a given lead axis, a biphasic (equally positive & negative) deflection is recorded.*

**226.** ECG leads I, II, and III are called?
*Harrison's 20th Ed. Chapter 235 Page 1676*

- A. Unipolar leads
- B. Bipolar leads
- C. Tripolar leads
- D. Multipolar leads

**227.** ECG leads aVR, aVL, and aVF are called?
*Harrison's 20th Ed. Chapter 235 Page 1676*

- A. Unipolar leads
- B. Bipolar leads
- C. Tripolar leads
- D. Multipolar leads

*Six extremity leads are 3 bipolar leads (I, II & III) and 3 unipolar leads (aVR, aVL & aVF) leads. Each bipolar lead measures the difference in potential between electrodes at two extremities.*

**228.** Bipolar lead I measures the difference in potential between?
*Harrison's 20th Ed. Chapter 235 Page 1676*

- A. Left arm-right arm voltages
- B. Left leg-right arm voltages
- C. Left leg-left arm voltages
- D. Left leg-right leg voltages

**229.** Bipolar lead II measures the difference in potential between?
*Harrison's 20th Ed. Chapter 235 Page 1676*

- A. Left arm-right arm voltages
- B. Left leg-right arm voltages
- C. Left leg-left arm voltages
- D. Left leg-right leg voltages

**230.** Bipolar lead III measures the difference in potential between?
*Harrison's 20th Ed. Chapter 235 Page 1676*

- A. Left arm-right arm voltages
- B. Left leg-right arm voltages
- C. Left leg-left arm voltages
- D. Left leg-right leg voltages

*Each bipolar lead measures the difference in potential between electrodes at two extremities: lead I = left arm–right arm voltages, lead II = left leg–right arm, and lead III = left leg–left arm.*

**231.** In unipolar leads, the lowercase "a" stands for?
*Harrison's 20th Ed. Chapter 235 Page 1676*

- A. Added
- B. Augmented
- C. Arithmatic
- D. Apparent

**232.** Electrical augmentation of unipolar potentials in unipolar leads is by?
*Harrison's 20th Ed. Chapter 235 Page 1676*

- A. 25%
- B. 50%
- C. 75%
- D. 100%

*The lowercase "a" indicates that these unipolar potentials are electrically augmented by 50%. The right leg electrode functions as a ground. Unipolar leads measure the voltage at one locus relative to an electrode (called central terminal or indifferent electrode) that has approximately zero potential. Thus, aVR = right arm, aVL = left arm, and aVF = left leg.*

### 233. The normal atrial depolarization vector is oriented?
*Harrison's 20th Ed. Chapter 235 Page 1676*

A. Downward and toward left
B. Upward and toward left
C. Downward and toward right
D. Upward and toward right

Normal atrial depolarization vector (P wave) is oriented downward & toward left, indicating spread of depolarization from sinus node to right & then left atrial myocardium. Since this vector points toward the negative pole of lead aVR, normal P wave will be negative in aVR. Opposite will occur if an ectopic pacemaker is in the lower part of either atrium or in the AV junction region.

### 234. QRS vector 1 points towards?
*Harrison's 20th Ed. Chapter 235 Page 1677 Figure 235-6*

A. Leftward and posteriorly
B. Leftward and anteriorly
C. Rightward and posteriorly
D. Rightward and anteriorly

### 235. QRS vector 2 points towards?
*Harrison's 20th Ed. Chapter 235 Page 1677 Figure 235-6*

A. Leftward and posteriorly
B. Leftward and anteriorly
C. Rightward and posteriorly
D. Rightward and anteriorly

QRS complex represents depolarization of ventricles. Its first phase (vector 1) is depolarization of interventricular septum from left to right & anteriorly. Second phase (vector 2) results from the simultaneous depolarization of right & left ventricles that points leftward & posteriorly due to the more massive left ventricle.

### 236. Above what degree of QRS axis is left axis deviation defined?
*Harrison's 20th Ed. Chapter 235 Page 1676*

A. – 10°
B. – 20°
C. – 30°
D. – 40°

### 237. Above what degree of QRS axis is called right axis deviation?
*Harrison's 20th Ed. Chapter 235 Page 1676*

A. + 80°
B. + 90°
C. + 100°
D. + 110°

Normally, the QRS axis ranges from –30° to +100°. QRS axis more negative than – 30° is referred to as left axis deviation, while an axis more positive than + 100° is referred to as right axis deviation.

### 238. Left axis deviation occurs in?
*Harrison's 20th Ed. Chapter 235 Page 1676*

A. As a normal variant
B. Left ventricular hypertrophy
C. Inferior myocardial infarction
D. All of the above

Left axis deviation may occur as a normal variant but is more commonly associated with left ventricular hypertrophy, left anterior fascicular hemiblock, or inferior myocardial infarction.

### 239. Right axis deviation occurs in?
*Harrison's 20th Ed. Chapter 235 Page 1676*

A. Due to reversal of left and right arm electrodes
B. Right ventricular overload
C. Infarction of lateral wall of left ventricle
D. All of the above

### 240. Right axis deviation (RAD) occurs in?
*Harrison's 20th Ed. Chapter 235 Page 1676*

A. Dextrocardia
B. Left pneumothorax
C. Left posterior hemiblock
D. All of the above

RAD may occur as a normal variant (in children & young adults), as a spurious finding due to reversal of left & right arm electrodes, or in right ventricular overload (acute or chronic), infarction of lateral wall of left ventricle, dextrocardia, left pneumothorax or left posterior fascicular block.

### 241. An abnormal increase in U-wave amplitude is due to which of the following drugs?
*Harrison's 20th Ed. Chapter 235 Page 1677*

A. Quinidine
B. Dofetilide
C. Amiodarone
D. All of the above

### 242. An abnormal increase in U-wave amplitude is due which of the following electrolyte disturbance?
*Harrison's 20th Ed. Chapter 235 Page 1677*

A. Hyponatremia
B. Hyperkalemia
C. Hypokalemia
D. All of the above

Abnormal increase in U-wave amplitude is mostly due to hypokalemia or drugs like dofetilide, amiodarone, sotalol, quinidine.

### 243. Very prominent U waves are a marker of increased susceptibility to which of the following?
*Harrison's 20th Ed. Chapter 235 Page 1677*

A. Torsades de pointes (TDP)
B. AIVR
C. Ventricular flutter
D. Any of the above

Very prominent U waves are a marker of increased susceptibility to TDP type of ventricular tachycardia. Inversion of U wave in precordial leads is abnormal & may be a subtle sign of ischemia.

### 244. P wave amplitude of how many millimeter suggests right atrial overload?
*Harrison's 20th Ed. Chapter 235 Page 1677*

A. ≥ 1.0 mm
B. ≥ 1.5 mm
C. ≥ 2.0 mm
D. ≥ 2.5 mm

Right atrial overload (acute or chronic) may lead to an increase in P wave amplitude (≥ 2.5 mm).

### 245. Ventricular "strain" pattern is due to which abnormality in hypertrophied muscle?
*Harrison's 20th Ed. Chapter 235 Page 1677*

A. Depolarization
B. Repolarization
C. Repolarization & depolarization
D. None of the above

Ventricular "strain" pattern is due to repolarization abnormalities in hypertrophied muscle.

### 246. Which of the following is not a common feature in right ventricular hypertrophy due to pressure load?
*Harrison's 20th Ed. Chapter 235 Page 1677*

A. R ≥ S wave in lead V1
B. Right axis deviation
C. Incomplete or complete right bundle branch block pattern
D. ST depression, T-wave inversion in (R) to midprecordial leads

RVH due to a pressure load (PS, PHT) is characterized by tall R wave in lead V1 (R > S wave), with right axis deviation. ST depression and T-wave inversion in right to midprecordial leads are also often present (ventricular strain pattern). Right ventricular hypertrophy with right ventricular volume overload (ostium secundum ASD) is commonly associated with incomplete or complete right bundle branch block pattern with a rightward QRS axis.

### 247. In acute cor pulmonale due to pulmonary embolism, which of the following is the most common arrhythmia?
*Harrison's 20th Ed. Chapter 235 Page 1677*

A. Sinus tachycardia
B. Atrial fibrillation
C. Atrial flutter
D. PSVT

Acute cor pulmonale due to pulmonary embolism may be associated with a normal ECG. Sinus tachycardia is the most common arrhythmia. Atrial fibrillation or flutter may occur.

### 248. S1Q3T3 pattern is seen in?
*Harrison's 20th Ed. Chapter 235 Page 1677*

A. Acute cor pulmonale due to pulmonary embolism
B. Right bundle branch block
C. Severe mitral stenosis
D. Acute dissection of aorta

S1Q3T3 pattern i.e. prominence of S wave in lead I, Q wave in lead III, T-wave inversion in lead III, is seen in acute cor pulmonale due to pulmonary embolism.

### 249. Poor R-wave progression seen in chronic cor pulmonale due to obstructive lung disease is due to?
*Harrison's 20th Ed. Chapter 235 Page 1677*

A. Hyperaeration of lungs
B. Downward displacement of diaphragm and heart
C. Myocardial ischemia
D. All of the above

Poor R-wave progression is noted in chronic cor pulmonale due to obstructive lung disease despite right ventricular hypertrophy. This is due to downward displacement of diaphragm and heart. Low-voltage complexes are commonly present, owing to hyperaeration of the lungs.

### 250. In ECG, SV1 + (RV5 or RV6) ≥ 35 mm indicates?
*Harrison's 20th Ed. Chapter 235 Page 1677*

A. Right ventricular hypertrophy
B. Left ventricular hypertrophy
C. Biventricular hypertrophy
D. None of the above

SV1 + (RV5 or RV6) ≥ 35 mm indicate LVH by voltage criteria.

### 251. In ECG, RaVL ≥ 11 to 13 mm, RaVF ≥ 20 mm or R1 + SIII ≥ 25 mm indicates?
*Harrison's 20th Ed. Chapter 235 Page 1677*

A. Right ventricular hypertrophy
B. Left ventricular hypertrophy
C. Biventricular hypertrophy
D. None of the above

RaVL ≥ 11 to 13 mm, RaVF ≥ 20 mm, R1+SIII ≥ 25 mm, with or without increased precordial voltage, indicates left ventricular hypertrophy.

### 252. Which of the following statements about left ventricular hypertrophy (LVH) is false?
*Harrison's 20th Ed. Chapter 235 Page 1677*

A. Left atrial abnormality increases likelihood of underlying LVH
B. LVH often progresses to incomplete or complete LBBB
C. Sensitivity of conventional voltage criteria for LVH is decreased in thin persons
D. ECG evidence of LVH is a marker of sudden cardiac death

Presence of left atrial abnormality increases the likelihood of underlying LVH. LVH often progresses to incomplete or complete LBBB. Sensitivity of conventional voltage criteria for LVH is decreased in obese persons & in smokers. ECG evidence for LVH is a major noninvasive marker of increased risk of cardiovascular morbidity & mortality, including sudden cardiac death.

### 253. Which of the following about bundle branches is true?
*J Interv Card Electrophysiol. 2014;39(1):45-56*

A. Left is narrow & cable-like, right is a broad sheet of fibers
B. Left is a broad sheet of fibers & right is narrow & cable-like
C. Left & right bundle branches are broad sheets of fibers
D. Left & right bundle branches are narrow & cable-like

Bundle of His gives rise to a broad sheet of fibers that course over the left side of interventricular septum to form left bundle branch & a narrow cable-like structure on the right side that forms the right bundle branch.

### 254. The infrahisian conduction system is insulated by?
*J Interv Card Electrophysiol. 2014;39(1):45-56*

A. Mucopolysaccharide
B. Elastin
C. Collagen
D. All of the above

The infrahisian conduction system originates at bundle of His and ends at individual Purkinje cell–ventricular myocyte junctions. It is insulated by collagen, which is thick & fibrous in proximal portions, and gradually diminishes such that a delicate insulating layer is seen to surround individual Purkinje fibers.

### 255. The conduction velocity in His-Purkinje system is?
*J Interv Card Electrophysiol. 2014;39(1):45-56*

A. 1.3 m/s
B. 2.3 m/s
C. 3.3 m/s
D. 4.3 m/s

The His-Purkinje system is specialized for rapid conduction, with conduction velocities of 2.3 m/s as compared to 0.75 m/s in ventricular muscle.

### 256. Muscle of Lancisi best relates to?
*J Interv Card Electrophysiol. 2014;39(1):45-56*

A. Septal papillary muscle of the mitral valve
B. Septal papillary muscle of the tricuspid valve
C. Septal papillary muscle of the pulmonary valve
D. Septal papillary muscle of the aortic valve

Lancisi's muscle is the main muscle of medial papillary complex, tension apparatus supporting the antero-septal commissure of the tricuspid valve.

**257. With complete bundle branch blocks the QRS interval is?**
*Harrison's 20th Ed. Chapter 235 Page 1678*

A. ≥ 90 ms in duration
B. ≥ 100 ms in duration
C. ≥ 110 ms in duration
D. ≥ 120 ms in duration

With complete bundle branch blocks the QRS interval is ≥ =120 ms in duration. With incomplete blocks, the QRS interval is between 100 and 120 ms.

**258. In RBBB, the terminal QRS vector is oriented?**
*Harrison's 20th Ed. Chapter 235 Page 1678*

A. Anteriorly and to right
B. Anteriorly and to left
C. Posteriorly and to right
D. Posteriorly and to left

In bundle branch blocks, QRS vector is oriented in the direction of myocardial region where depolarization is delayed. In RBBB, the terminal QRS vector is oriented anteriorly and to the right (rSR´ in V1 & qRS in V6).

**259. In LBBB, the major QRS vector is oriented?**
*Harrison's 20th Ed. Chapter 235 Page 1678*

A. Anteriorly and to right
B. Anteriorly and to left
C. Posteriorly and to right
D. Posteriorly and to left

LBBB alters both early & later phases of ventricular depolarization. Major QRS vector is directed to left & posteriorly. Normal early left to right pattern of septal activation is disrupted so septal depolarization proceeds from right to left. LBBB has wide, predominantly negative (QS) complexes in lead V1 & entirely positive (R) complexes in lead V6. A pattern identical to that of LBBB, preceded by a sharp spike, is seen in cases of electronic right ventricular pacing because of the relative delay in left ventricular activation.

**260. Which of the following about bundle branch blocks is false?**
*Harrison's 20th Ed. Chapter 235 Page 1678*

A. Without structural heart disease, LBBB is more common than RBBB
B. Bundle branch blocks may be chronic or intermittent
C. Bundle branch block may be rate-related
D. LBBB pattern is seen in electronic right ventricular pacing

In subjects without structural heart disease, RBBB is seen more commonly than LBBB.

**261. Left bundle branch block is often a marker of?**
*Harrison's 20th Ed. Chapter 235 Page 1679*

A. Coronary heart disease
B. Severe aortic valve disease
C. Cardiomyopathy
D. All of the above

LBBB is a marker of increased risk of cardiovascular morbidity & mortality (coronary heart disease, hypertensive heart disease, aortic valve disease, and cardiomyopathy).

**262. Examples of bifascicular block include?**
*Harrison's 20th Ed. Chapter 235 Page 1679*

A. RBBB and LPHB
B. RBBB with LAHB
C. Complete LBBB
D. All of the above

**263. Alternation of right & left bundle branch block is a sign of?**
*Harrison's 20th Ed. Chapter 235 Page 1679*

A. Bifascicular disease
B. Trifascicular disease
C. Complete heart block
D. AV Dissociation

Alternation of RBBB & LBBB is a sign of trifascicular disease.

**264. Trifascicular block is the combination of?**
*Harrison's 20th Ed. Chapter 235 Page 1679*

A. Right bundle branch block
B. Left anterior or posterior fascicular block
C. First-degree AV block
D. All of the above

**265. Which of the following statements is false?**
*Harrison's 20th Ed. Chapter 235 Page 1679*

A. Discordance of QRS–T-wave vectors seen in BBB
B. Primary repolarization abnormalities are independent of QRS changes
C. Primary and secondary T-wave changes may coexist
D. None of the above

**266. Intraventricular conduction delays can be caused by?**
*Harrison's 20th Ed. Chapter 235 Page 1679*

A. Hyperkalemia
B. Tricyclic antidepressants
C. Phenothiazines
D. All of the above

Intraventricular conduction delays can be caused by toxic factors that slow ventricular conduction (hyperkalemia, class 1 antiarrhythmic agents, tricyclic antidepressants, phenothiazines).

**267. Which of the following is diagnostic of Wolff-Parkinson-White syndrome?**
*Harrison's 20th Ed. Chapter 235 Page 1679*

A. Wide QRS complex
B. Relatively short PR interval
C. Slurring of initial part of QRS (delta wave)
D. All of the above

Prolongation of QRS duration does not necessarily indicate a conduction delay but may be due to A form of ventricular preexcitation via a bypass tract, Wolff-Parkinson-White (WPW) syndrome is diagnosed by a triad consisting of a wide QRS complex associated with a relatively short PR interval and slurring of the initial part of the QRS (delta wave), with the latter effect being due to aberrant activation of ventricular myocardium.

**268. Which of the following about myocardial ischemia is false?**
*Harrison's 20th Ed. Chapter 235 Page 1679*

A. Complex time-dependent effects on electrical properties of myocardial cells
B. Severe, acute ischemia lengthens duration of action potential
C. Cause a voltage gradient between normal & ischemic zones
D. Leads to flow of currents of injury

Severe, acute ischemia lowers the resting membrane potential & shortens duration of action potential.

**269. Wellens T waves are usually associated with?**
*Harrison's 20th Ed. Chapter 235 Page 1680 Figure 235-12, N Engl J Med. 2015; 372:66*

A. Stenosis of left anterior descending coronary artery
B. Stenosis of posterior descending coronary artery
C. Stenosis of left circumflex coronary artery
D. Stenosis of right coronary artery

Severe anterior wall ischemia (with or without infarction) may cause prominent T-wave inversions in the precordial leads. This pattern referred to as Wellens T waves is usually associated with a high-grade stenosis of the left anterior descending coronary artery.

**270. Wellen's syndrome criteria consists of?**
*J Emerg Trauma Shock. 2009;2(3):206-208*

A. Normal ECG or mild ST ↑ or ↓ during chest pain
B. Deeply inverted or biphasic T-waves in V2 & V3 when pain free
C. Cardiac enzymes are normal or mildly elevated
D. All of the above

Wellen's syndrome criteria consists of prior history of chest pain, EKG is normal or with mild ST elevation or depression during chest pain, or with terminal negative deflection of the T wave in V1 and V2, cardiac enzymes are normal or mildly elevated, no pathologic precordial Q-waves, no loss of precordial R-waves, deeply inverted or biphasic T-waves in V2 and V3, possibly V1, V4, V5 and/or V6 when pain free.

**271. Deep T-wave inversions are seen in which of the following ECG leads in severe obstruction in left anterior descending coronary artery?**
*Harrison's 20th Ed. Chapter 235 Page 1679*

A. I
B. aVL
C. V1 - V4
D. All of the above

**272. ST elevation in lead aVR is seen in?**
*Harrison's 20th Ed. Chapter 235 Page 1679*

A. Ischemia of subendocardium
B. Transmural ischemia
C. Wellen's syndrome
D. Takostubo syndrome

**273. Which of the following may exactly simulate the patterns of STEMI or non-STEMI?**
*Harrison's 20th Ed. Chapter 235 Page 1679*

A. Wellen's syndrome
B. Takostubo syndrome
C. Brugada angina
D. Gorlin's syndrome

Takostubo syndrome may exactly simulate the patterns of STEMI or non-STEMI.

**274. Which of the following is false about Prinzmetal's angina?**
*Harrison's 20th Ed. Chapter 235 Page 1680*

A. Reversible transmural ischemia
B. Coronary vasospasm
C. Transient ST-segment ↑ without development of Q waves
D. None of the above

**275. Which of the following statements is false?**
*Harrison's 20th Ed. Chapter 235 Page 1680*

A. Transmural infarcts may occur without Q waves
B. Subendocardial infarcts may be associated with Q waves
C. Complete normalization of ECG after Q-wave infarction may occur in smaller infarcts
D. None of the above

**276. Atrial infarction may be associated with?**
*Harrison's 20th Ed. Chapter 235 Page 1680*

A. PR-segment deviations
B. Changes in P-wave morphology
C. Atrial arrhythmias
D. All of the above

Atrial infarction may be associated with PR-segment deviations due to an atrial current of injury, changes in P-wave morphology, or atrial arrhythmias.

**277. Diagnostic changes of acute or evolving ischemia are masked by?**
*Harrison's 20th Ed. Chapter 235 Page 1680*

A. Left bundle branch block
B. Electronic ventricular pacemaker patterns
C. Wolff-Parkinson-White preexcitation
D. All of the above

Diagnostic changes of acute or evolving ischemia can be masked by presence of LBBB, electronic ventricular pacemaker patterns & WPW preexcitation.

**278. Osborn wave in ECG is found in?**
*Harrison's 20th Ed. Chapter 235 Page 1681 Table 235-1*

A. Heat stroke
B. Hypothermia
C. Cerebrovascular accident
D. Pneumothorax

Systemic hypothermia also prolongs repolarization, usually with a distinctive convex elevation or "hump" at the J point referred to as Osborn wave. It is due to altered ventricular action potential characteristics.

**279. ST-segment elevations simulating ischemia may occur with?**
*Harrison's 20th Ed. Chapter 235 Page 1681 Table 235-1*

A. Hypercalcemia
B. Hyperkalemia
C. Hypothermia
D. All of the above

**280. ST-segment elevations simulating ischemia may occur with?**
*Harrison's 20th Ed. Chapter 235 Page 1681 Table 235-1*

A. Acute pericarditis
B. Myocarditis
C. Brugada syndrome
D. All of the above

**281. Tall, positive T waves are seen in?**
*Harrison's 20th Ed. Chapter 235 Page 1681*

A. Hyperkalemia
B. Cerebrovascular injury
C. Left ventricular volume overload (MR or AR)
D. All of the above

Tall, positive T waves may be seen in hyperacute ischemic changes, normal variants, hyperkalemia, cerebrovascular injury & left ventricular volume overload due to mitral or aortic regurgitation.

**282. The first ECG change in hyperkalemia is?**
*Harrison's 20th Ed. Chapter 235 Page 1681*

A. Diminution in P-wave amplitude
B. Narrowing & peaking (tenting) of T waves
C. Widening of QRS interval
D. AV conduction disturbances

ECG changes in hyperkalemia usually begin with narrowing and peaking (tenting) of the T waves. Further elevation of extracellular K⁺ leads to AV conduction disturbances, diminution in P-wave amplitude, and widening of the QRS interval. Severe hyperkalemia causes a slow sinusoidal type of mechanism ("sine-wave" pattern) followed by asystole.

**283. ECG changes in hypertrophic cardiomyopathy may simulate?**
*Harrison's 20th Ed. Chapter 235 Page 1681*

A. Anterior MI
B. Lateral MI
C. Inferior MI
D. All of the above

**284. QRS & QT prolongation along with sinus tachycardia can be seen in?**
*Harrison's 20th Ed. Chapter 235 Page 1682 Figure 235-15*

A. Tricyclic antidepressant overdose
B. Quinidine excess
C. Subarachnoid hemorrhage
D. Hyperkalemia

Drugs that prolong QT are quinidine, disopyramide, procainamide, tricyclic antidepressants, phenothiazines, amiodarone, sotalol, ibutilide. QRS & QT prolongation along with sinus tachycardia occur in tricyclic antidepressant overdose.

**285. "CVA T-wave" pattern consists of all except?**
*Harrison's 20th Ed. Chapter 235 Page 1681*

A. Marked QT prolongation
B. Marked PR prolongation
C. Deep T-wave inversions
D. Wide T-wave inversions

Marked QT prolongation, with deep & wide T-wave inversions occur with intracranial bleeds, particularly subarachnoid hemorrhage and are called as "CVA T-wave" pattern.

**286. Systemic hypothermia prolongs?**
*Harrison's 20th Ed. Chapter 235 Page 1681*

A. Depolarization
B. Repolarization
C. Depolarization + repolarization
D. None of the above

Systemic hypothermia also prolongs repolarization with a distinctive convex elevation of the J point called Osborn wave.

**287. Which of the following prolongs the QT interval?**
*Harrison's 20th Ed. Chapter 235 Page 1681*

A. Hypothermia
B. Hypokalemia
C. Hypocalcemia
D. All of the above

**288. Abbreviation of ST segment and shortening of QT interval is found in?**
*Harrison's 20th Ed. Chapter 235 Page 1681*

A. Hypocalcemia
B. Hypercalcemia
C. Hyponatremia
D. Hyperkalemia

Hypocalcemia typically prolongs the QT interval (ST portion), while hypercalcemia shortens it.

**289. Which of the following shortens the QT interval?**
*Harrison's 20th Ed. Chapter 235 Page 1681*

A. Digitalis
B. Disopyramide
C. Ibutilide
D. Procainamide

Digitalis glycosides also shorten the QT interval, often with a characteristic "scooping" of the ST–T-wave complex (digitalis effect).

**290. Low QRS voltage is defined as peak-to-trough QRS amplitudes of?**
*Harrison's 20th Ed. Chapter 235 Page 1681*

A. ≤ 5 mm in 3 limb leads
B. ≤ 5 mm in 4 limb leads
C. ≤ 5 mm in 5 limb leads
D. ≤ 5 mm in 6 limb leads

Low QRS voltage is arbitrarily defined as peak-to-trough QRS amplitudes of ≤5 mm in the six limb leads and/or ≤10 mm in the chest leads.

**291. Q waves in ECG can be seen in all of the following except?**
*Harrison's 20th Ed. Chapter 235 Page 1681*

A. Sarcoidosis
B. Scleroderma
C. SLE
D. Chagas' disease

**292. Q waves in ECG can be seen in all of the following except?**
*Harrison's 20th Ed. Chapter 235 Page 1681*

A. Left pneumothorax
B. Dextrocardia
C. Long QT syndrome
D. Wolff-Parkinson-White syndrome

**293. In ECG, transient nonspecific repolarization changes occur following all except?**
*Harrison's 20th Ed. Chapter 235 Page 1681*

A. Meals
B. Postural (orthostatic) change
C. Hyperventilation
D. Sleep

Transient nonspecific ST–T-wave repolarization changes may occur following a meal or with postural (orthostatic) change, hyperventilation, or exercise in healthy individuals.

**294. In ECG, total electrical alternans (P-QRS-T) with sinus tachycardia is a relatively specific sign of?**
*Harrison's 20th Ed. Chapter 235 Page 1683*

- A. Myocardial ischemia
- B. Myocarditis
- C. Pericardial effusion
- D. Pneumothorax

Total electrical alternans (P-QRS-T) with sinus tachycardia (beat-to-beat alternation in one or more components of ECG) is a relatively specific sign of pericardial effusion with cardiac tamponade due to periodic swinging motion of heart in effusion at a frequency exactly half of heart rate.

**295. Repolarization (ST-T or U wave) alternans is a sign of?**
*Harrison's 20th Ed. Chapter 235 Page 1683*

- A. Mechanical instability of heart
- B. Electrical instability of heart
- C. Serious pulmonary disease
- D. Serious hepatic disease

Repolarization (ST-T or U wave) alternans is a sign of electrical instability & may precede ventricular tachyarrhythmias.

**296. Chronic renal failure (CRF) is suspected if ECG shows?**
*Acta Cardiol Sin. 2015;31(1):83-86*

- A. Peaked T waves
- B. Long QT
- C. Left ventricular hypertrophy (LVH)
- D. All of the above

CRF can have the following ECG features as a triad - peaked T waves (hyperkalemia), long QT due to ST segment lengthening (hypocalcemia) & LVH (systemic hypertension).

**297. "Persistent juvenile T-wave pattern" consists of?**
*Heart. 2018;104:A63*

- A. T-wave inversions in leads $V_1$ - $V_3$
- B. T-wave inversions in leads $V_1$ - $V_4$
- C. T-wave inversions in leads $V_1$ - $V_5$
- D. T-wave inversions in leads $V_1$ - $V_6$

The juvenile ECG pattern is defined as T wave inversion in 2 contiguous anterior leads (V1 to V3) in individuals <16 years of age. This is due to electrical predominance of right ventricle in infancy which gradually resolves with normalisation of T waves post-puberty. Anterior TWI is also the hallmark of arrhythmogenic cardiomyopathy.

**298. Yamaguchi's syndrome best relates to?**
*Acta Cardiol Sin. 2015;31(1):83-86*

- A. Scleroderma
- B. Long QT syndrome
- C. Apical HCM
- D. Dextrocardia

LVH with deep T-wave inversions in limb leads, striking T-wave inversions in precordial leads suggest apical HCM (Yamaguchi's syndrome).

## Principles of Electrophysiology

**299. Electrocardiogram (ECG) was developed by?**
*Harrison's 20th Ed. Chapter 238 Page 1716*

A. Hewlet
B. Judkin
C. Einthoven
D. White

ECG was developed by Einthoven at the turn of the twentieth century.

**300. Body surface ECG is the timed sum of the cellular action potentials in the?**
*Harrison's 20th Ed. Chapter 238 Page 1716*

A. Atria
B. Ventricles
C. Atria and ventricles
D. None of the above

Body surface ECG is the timed sum of the cellular action potentials in the atria & ventricles.

**301. Sinoatrial (SA) node is located at the junction of?**
*Harrison's 20th Ed. Chapter 238 Page 1716*

A. Right atrium and superior vena cava
B. Right atrium and inferior vena cava
C. Right atrium and left atrium
D. Right atrium and coronary sinus

SA node is composed of a cluster of small fusiform cells located in sulcus terminalis on epicardial surface of heart at right atrial - superior vena caval junction where they envelop SA nodal artery.

**302. PR interval of ECG represents time needed for activation of?**
*Harrison's 20th Ed. Chapter 238 Page 1716*

A. Both atria
B. Atrioventricular node (AVN)
C. Both atria + Atrioventricular node (AVN)
D. Both atria + AVN + His Purkinje system

Electrical impulse from SA node is transmitted slowly through nodal tissue to atria, and rapidly on to atrioventricular node (AVN), resulting in the P wave of the ECG.

**303. Which of the following statements is false?**
*Harrison's 20th Ed. Chapter 238 Page 1716*

A. Body surface ECG is the timed sum of cellular action potentials in atria & ventricles
B. Repolarization occurs first on endocardium then proceeds to epicardium
C. Activation of atria & AV node is PR interval
D. QT interval is duration of activation & recovery of ventricles

Repolarization occurs first on the epicardial surface, then proceeds to the endocardium.

**304. Electrophysiologically, there are how many phases of action potential in cardiac myocyte?**
*Circ Arrhythmia Electrophysiol. 2009;2:185-194*

A. 3
B. 4
C. 5
D. 6

**305. Which of the following phase represents resting potential?**
*Circ Arrhythmia Electrophysiol. 2009;2:185-194*

A. 0
B. 2
C. 3
D. 4

Phase 4, or the resting potential, is stable at (-)90 mV in normal working myocardial cells.

**306. Which of the following phase represents plateau phase?**
*Circ Arrhythmia Electrophysiol. 2009;2:185-194*

A. 0
B. 2
C. 3
D. 4

Phase 2, a plateau phase, is the longest phase. It is unique among excitable cells and marks the phase of calcium entry into the cell.

**307. Which of the following is a category of cardiac $K^+$ channel?**
*Circ Arrhythmia Electrophysiol. 2009;2:185-194*

A. Voltage gated
B. Inward rectifier channels
C. Background K+ currents
D. All of the above

Cardiac $K^+$ channels fall into 3 broad categories: Voltage gated (Ito, IKur, IKr, and IKs), inward rectifier channels (IK1, IKAch, and IKATP), and the background $K^+$ currents (TASK-1, TWIK-1/2).

**308. Duration of action potential in cardiac myocytes is?**
*Harrison's 20th Ed. Chapter 238 Page 1716*

A. 20 – 40 ms
B. 80 – 1600 ms
C. 200 – 400 ms
D. 500 – 800 ms

Cardiac myocytes have a characteristically long action potential (200–400 ms) compared to neurons or skeletal muscle cells (1–5 ms).

**309. Which of the following participate in the cardiac myocyte action potential?**
*Harrison's 20th Ed. Chapter 238 Page 1716*

A. Ion channels
B. Pumps, transporters
C. Exchangers
D. All of the above

The action potential of cardiac myocyte results from the activity of multiple distinctive time- and voltage-dependent ionic currents. The currents in turn are carried by transmembrane proteins that passively conduct ions down their electrochemical gradients through selective pores (ion channels), actively transport ions against their electrochemical gradient (pumps, transporters), or electrogenically exchange ionic species (exchangers).

**310. Diastole corresponds to which phase of action potentials?**
*Harrison's 20th Ed. Chapter 238 Page 1717 Figure 238-1*

A. Phase 1
B. Phase 2
C. Phase 3
D. Phase 4

Phase 0 is rapid upstroke, phase 1 is early repolarization, phase 2 is plateau, phase 3 is late repolarization, and phase 4 is diastole.

**311. Which of the following gene is responsible for ventricular repolarization?**
*Harrison's 20th Ed. Chapter 238 Page 1717 Figure 238-1*

A. KCNJ2
B. SCN5A
C. CACNA1C
D. SLC8A1

**312. Which of the following is principal current during phase 4?**
*Harrison's 20th Ed. Chapter 238 Page 1717 Figure 238-1*

A. $I_{K1}$
B. $I_{to}$
C. $I_{Kr}$
D. $I_{Ks}$

**313. Which of the following determines the resting membrane potential of the myocyte?**
*Harrison's 20th Ed. Chapter 238 Page 1717 Figure 238-1*

A. $I_{K1}$
B. $I_{to}$
C. $I_{Kr}$
D. $I_{Ks}$

Potassium current (IK1) is the principal current during phase 4 and determines the resting membrane potential of the myocyte.

**314. Which of the following causes phase 3 repolarization?**
*Harrison's 20th Ed. Chapter 238 Page 1717 Figure 238-1*

A. Inactivation of the calcium current
B. Persistent activation of $I_{Kr}$
C. Persistent activation of $I_{Ks}$
D. All of the above

Inactivation of the calcium current with persistent activation of potassium currents (predominantly IKr and IKs) causes phase 3 repolarization.

**315. Sodium-calcium exchanger transports how many Na⁺ for one $Ca^{2+}$?**
*Harrison's 20th Ed. Chapter 238 Page 1716*

A. 1
B. 2
C. 3
D. 4

Electrogenic sodium-calcium exchanger transports three Na⁺ for one $Ca^{2+}$.

**316. Reestablishing of the negative resting membrane potential of the heart cells is done by?**
*Harrison's 20th Ed. Chapter 238 Page 1716*

A. Inactivation of Na channel
B. Inactivation of Ca channel
C. Activation of K channel
D. All of the above

**317. Automaticity is a property of?**
*Harrison's 20th Ed. Chapter 238 Page 1717*

A. Sinoatrial (SA) node
B. His-Purkinje system
C. Coronary sinus
D. All of the above

Property of automaticity (pacemaking i.e. spontaneous diastolic depolarization) is characteristic of sinoatrial (SA) & atrioventricular (AV) nodes, His-Purkinje system, coronary sinus & pulmonary veins.

**318. Abnormal automaticity may produce which of the following?**
*Harrison's 20th Ed. Chapter 238 Page 1717*

A. Atrial tachycardia
B. Accelerated idioventricular rhythms
C. Ventricular tachycardia
D. All of the above

Abnormal automaticity may produce atrial tachycardia, accelerated idioventricular rhythms, and ventricular tachycardia, particularly associated with ischemia and reperfusion.

**319. Triggered automaticity refers to impulse initiation that is dependent on?**
*Harrison's 20th Ed. Chapter 238 Page 1718*

A. Entrance block
B. Overdrive suppression
C. Afterdepolarizations
D. All of the above

Triggered automaticity or activity refers to impulse initiation that is dependent on afterdepolarizations which are membrane voltage oscillations that occur during (early afterdepolarizations, EADs) or after (delayed afterdepolarizations, DADs) an action potential.

**320. Early afterdepolarizations occur during?**
*Harrison's 20th Ed. Chapter 238 Page 1718*

A. Phases 0 and 1 of the action potential
B. Phases 1 and 2 of the action potential
C. Phases 2 and 3 of the action potential
D. Phases 3 and 4 of the action potential

**321. Delayed afterdepolarizations occur after completion of?**
*Harrison's 20th Ed. Chapter 238 Page 1718*

A. Phase 1 of action potential
B. Phase 2 of action potential
C. Phase 3 of action potential
D. Phase 4 of action potential

Afterdepolarizations are spontaneous depolarizations due to membrane voltage oscillations in cardiac myocytes. Early afterdepolarizations (EAD) occur before the end of the action potential (phases 2 and 3), interrupting repolarization. Delayed afterdepolarizations (DAD) occur during phase 4 of the action potential after completion of repolarization.

322. Cellular feature common to induction of DADs is the presence of?
*Harrison's 20th Ed. Chapter 238 Page 1718*
   A. Increased $Ca^{2+}$ load in the cytosol
   B. Increased $Na^+$ load in the cytosol
   C. Increased $K^+$ load in the cytosol
   D. Increased $Mg^{2+}$ load in the cytosol

The cellular feature common to induction of DADs is the presence of an increased $Ca^{2+}$ load in the cytosol and sarcoplasmic reticulum.

323. Which of the following enhance $Ca^{2+}$ loading sufficiently to produce DADs?
*Harrison's 20th Ed. Chapter 238 Page 1718*
   A. Digitalis glycoside toxicity
   B. Catecholamines
   C. Myocardial ischemia
   D. All of the above

Digitalis glycoside toxicity, catecholamines, and ischemia all can enhance $Ca^{2+}$ loading sufficiently to produce DADs.

324. Which of the following about connexins is false?
*Harrison's 20th Ed. Chapter 30, 438, 238 Page 1718*
   A. Gap junction membrane-spanning protein
   B. CMT1X is caused by mutations in connexin 32 gene
   C. Mutations in connexin 26 causes progressive hearing loss
   D. None of the above

Connexins are gap junction membrane-spanning structural proteins that are important in cell-to-cell communication. They pair across adjacent cells.

325. Which of the following is the principal connexin expressed in the heart?
*Circ Arrhythmia Electrophysiol. 2009;2:185-194*
   A. Connexin 40
   B. Connexin 43
   C. Connexin 45
   D. All of the above

Three types of connexins are expressed in heart and are defined on the basis of their molecular weight: connexin 40, connexin 43, and connexin 45. Connexin 43 is the principal connexin expressed in the heart.

326. Chronically ischemic myocardium exhibits a downregulation of?
*Harrison's 20th Ed. Chapter 238 Page 1719*
   A. Connexin 26
   B. Connexin 31
   C. Connexin 32
   D. Connexin 43

Chronically ischemic myocardium exhibits a downregulation of the gap junction channel protein (connexin 43) that carries intercellular ionic current.

327. Epsilon waves in ECG are a feature of?
*Harrison's 20th Ed. Chapter 238 Page 1720*
   A. Wolff-Parkinson-White (WPW) syndrome
   B. Long QT syndrome
   C. Arrhythmogenic right ventricular dysplasia
   D. Brugada syndrome

328. Right precordial ST-segment abnormalities in ECG are a feature of?
*Harrison's 20th Ed. Chapter 238 Page 1720*
   A. Wolff-Parkinson-White (WPW) syndrome
   B. Long QT syndrome
   C. Arrhythmogenic right ventricular dysplasia
   D. Brugada syndrome

329. Delta waves in ECG are a feature of?
*Harrison's 20th Ed. Chapter 238 Page 1720*
   A. Wolff-Parkinson-White (WPW) syndrome
   B. Long QT syndrome
   C. Arrhythmogenic right ventricular dysplasia
   D. Brugada syndrome

330. Ventricular tachyarrhythmias occur more frequently in patients with?
*Harrison's 20th Ed. Chapter 238 Page 1720*
   A. Ventricular systolic dysfunction
   B. Hypertrophic cardiomyopathy
   C. Sarcoidosis
   D. All of the above

Ventricular tachyarrhythmias occur more frequently in patients with ventricular systolic dysfunction and chamber dilation, in hypertrophic cardiomyopathy, and in infiltrative diseases like sarcoidosis.

331. Supraventricular arrhythmias may be associated with?
*Harrison's 20th Ed. Chapter 238 Page 1720*
   A. Transposition of the great arteries
   B. Ebstein's anomaly
   C. Ostium primum atrial septal defect (ASD)
   D. Ventricular septal defects (VSD)

Supraventricular arrhythmias may be associated with Ebstein's anomaly.

332. Which of the following is a response to Head-up tilt (HUT)?
*Harrison's 20th Ed. Chapter 238 Page 1720*
   A. Initial increase in heart rate
   B. Drop in blood pressure
   C. Late reduction in heart rate
   D. All of the above

Exaggerated activation of a central reflex in response to Head-up tilt (HUT) testing produces a stereotypic response of an initial increase in heart rate, then a drop in blood pressure followed by a reduction in heart rate characteristic of neurally mediated hypotension.

333. Head-up tilt (HUT) is a useful tool in the diagnosis of and therapy for?
*Harrison's 20th Ed. Chapter 238 Page 1720*
   A. Recurrent idiopathic vertigo
   B. Chronic fatigue syndrome
   C. Recurrent transient ischemic attacks
   D. All of the above

HUT is used most often in patients with recurrent syncope. HUT is also a useful tool in the diagnosis of and therapy for recurrent idiopathic vertigo, chronic fatigue syndrome, recurrent transient ischemic attacks, and repeated falls of unknown etiology in the elderly.

**334. Head-up tilt (HUT) testing is relatively contraindicated in?**
*Harrison's 20th Ed. Chapter 238 Page 1720*
- A. Aortic stenosis
- B. Severe mitral stenosis
- C. Severe cerebrovascular disease
- D. All of the above

HUT is relatively contraindicated in the presence of severe CAD with proximal coronary stenoses, severe cerebrovascular disease, severe mitral stenosis, and obstruction to left ventricular outflow (aortic stenosis).

**335. Nationality of Miles Vaughan Williams was?**
*Circulation. 2018;138:1879-1896*
- A. American
- B. British
- C. Canadian
- D. Swedish

Miles Vaughan Williams (1918–2016) was a British cardiac pharmacologist and worked at Hertford College, University of Oxford. Miles was born in Bangalore, India.

**336. Which of the following best relates to classification of antiarrhythmic drug therapy?**
*European Heart Journal 1991;12(10):1112-1131*
- A. Queen's Gambit
- B. Sicilian Gambit
- C. Roman Gambit
- D. Danish Gambit

Sicilian Gambit is a new approach to classify antiarrhythmic drugs. It correlated information on molecular targets, cellular mechanisms, functional targets & clinical arrhythmias for individual drugs with similarities and differences in their effects, accommodating their multiple actions.

**337. Which of the following relates best with Vaughan-Williams class I class of antiarrhythmic drugs?**
*Harrison's 20th Ed. Chapter 238 Page 1721*
- A. Local anesthetic effect due to blockade of Na⁺ current
- B. Interference of catecholamine action at β-adrenergic receptor
- C. Delayed repolarization by K⁺ current inhibition or activation of depolarizing current
- D. Interference with calcium conductance

**338. Which of the following relates best with Vaughan-Williams class II class of antiarrhythmic drugs?**
*Harrison's 20th Ed. Chapter 238 Page 1721*
- A. Local anesthetic effect due to blockade of Na⁺ current
- B. Interference of catecholamine action at β-adrenergic receptor
- C. Delayed repolarization by K⁺ current inhibition or activation of depolarizing current
- D. Interference with calcium conductance

**339. Which of the following relates best with Vaughan-Williams class III class of antiarrhythmic drugs?**
*Harrison's 20th Ed. Chapter 238 Page 1721*
- A. Local anesthetic effect due to blockade of Na⁺ current
- B. Interference of catecholamine action at β-adrenergic receptor
- C. Delayed repolarization by K⁺ current inhibition or activation of depolarizing current
- D. Interference with calcium conductance

**340. Which of the following relates best with Vaughan-Williams class IV class of antiarrhythmic drugs?**
*Harrison's 20th Ed. Chapter 238 Page 1721*
- A. Local anesthetic effect due to blockade of Na⁺ current
- B. Interference of catecholamine action at β-adrenergic receptor
- C. Delayed repolarization by K⁺ current inhibition or activation of depolarizing current
- D. Interference with calcium conductance

Class I exert their antiarrhythmic action by local anesthetic effect by blockade of Na+ current, class II interfere with the action of catecholamines at β-adrenergic receptor, class III cause delay of repolarization due to inhibition of K+ current or activation of depolarizing current and class IV interfere with calcium conductance.

**341. Which of the following is a class Ia antiarrhythmic agent?**
*Harrison's 20th Ed. Chapter 238 Page 1721*
- A. Lidocaine
- B. Mexiletine
- C. Procainamide
- D. Propafenone

Class I antiarrhythmics have been further subdivided based on the kinetics and potency of Na+ channel binding. Class Ia agents (quinidine, procainamide) have moderate potency & intermediate kinetics. Class Ib agents (lidocaine, mexiletine) have low potency and rapid kinetics while class Ic drugs (flecainide, propafenone) have high potency and the slowest kinetics. Class I drugs produce moderate (Ia), weak (Ib), or marked (Ic) Na+ channel block and reduce AP phase 0 slope & overshoot while increasing, reducing, or conserving AP duration (APD) and effective refractory period (ERP), respectively.

**342. Which of the following is a Class 0 antiarrhythmic agent?**
*Circulation. 2018;138:1879-1896*
- A. Ajmaline
- B. Ivabradine
- C. Dronedarone
- D. Dofetilide

**343. Which of the following about Ivabradine is false?**
*Circulation. 2018;138:1879-1896*
- A. Inhibits $I_f$ current
- B. Acts through hyperpolarization activated cyclic nucleotide-gated channel (HCN)
- C. Reduces sinus node automaticity
- D. None of the above

**344. Which of the following is a Class 1a antiarrhythmic agent?**
*Circulation. 2018;138:1879-1896*
- A. Quinidine
- B. Ajmaline
- C. Disopyramide
- D. All of the above

**345. Which of the following is a nonselective K⁺ channel blocker?**
*Circulation. 2018;138:1879-1896*
- A. Ambasilide
- B. Amiodarone
- C. Dronedarone
- D. All of the above

346. Which of the following is a Kv11.1 (HERG) channel–mediated rapid K⁺ current (IKr) blocker?
   *Circulation. 2018;138:1879-1896*
   A. Dofetilide
   B. Ibutilide
   C. Sotalol
   D. All of the above

347. Which of the following is a Kv1.5 channel–mediated, ultrarapid K⁺ current (IKur) blocker?
   *Circulation. 2018;138:1879-1896*
   A. Bepridil
   B. Nicorandil
   C. Vernakalant
   D. All of the above

348. Which of the following is an intracellular Ca⁺⁺ channel blocker?
   *Circulation. 2018;138:1879-1896*
   A. Flecainide
   B. Diltiazem
   C. Verapamil
   D. Bepridil

349. First catheter ablation using a DC energy source was performed in the early 1980s by?
   *Harrison's 20th Ed. Chapter 238 Page 1721*
   A. Scheinman
   B. Hille
   C. Josephson
   D. Zipes

   *First catheter ablation using a DC energy source was performed in the early 1980s by Scheinman and colleagues.*

350. Which of the following produces a reversible local conduction block in catheter-based ablation in the heart?
   *Harrison's 20th Ed. Chapter 238 Page 1721*
   A. Lasers
   B. Ultrasound
   C. Cryoablation
   D. Radio frequency

351. Which of the following increases mortality rates in patients after myocardial infarction?
   *Can J Cardiol. 2010;26(6):303-312*
   A. Late potentials
   B. T wave alternans (TWA) at low heart rates
   C. Decrease in heart rate variability (HRV)
   D. All of the above

352. Which of the following methods is related to autonomic nervous system influence on the heart?
   *Europace. 2016;18(6):925-944*
   A. Late potentials
   B. T wave alternans (TWA) at low heart rates
   C. QT interval variability (QTV)
   D. All of the above

   *Heart rate variability (HRV) & QT interval variability (QTV) provide noninvasive methods to assess autonomic nervous system influence on heart. A decrease in HRV is associated with increased sympathetic nervous system tone and increased mortality rates in patients after myocardial infarction.*

353. 1 metabolic equivalent (MET) is?
   *BMJ. 2002;324(7345):1084-1087*
   A. 1.5 mL oxygen / kg per minute
   B. 2.5 mL oxygen / kg per minute
   C. 3.5 mL oxygen / kg per minute
   D. 4.5 mL oxygen / kg per minute

   *1 MET is 3.5 mL oxygen/kg per minute, which is the oxygen consumption of an average individual at rest.*

354. To carry out the activities of daily living an exercise intensity of at least how many METs is required?
   *BMJ. 2002;324(7345):1084-1087*
   A. 2 METs
   B. 3 METs
   C. 4 METs
   D. 5 METs

   *To carry out the activities of daily living an exercise intensity of at least 5 METs is required.*

355. In stage 1 of Bruce protocol, energy expenditure is estimated to be?
   *BMJ. 2002;324(7345):1084-1087*
   A. 2.8 METs
   B. 3.8 METs
   C. 4.8 METs
   D. 5.8 METs

   *In stage 1 of Bruce protocol, the patient walks at 1.7 mph (2.7 km) up a 10% incline. Energy expenditure is estimated to be 4.8 METs (metabolic equivalents) during this stage.*

356. For men, the maximum predicted heart rate in exercise stress testing is calculated as?
   *BMJ. 2002;324(7345):1084-1087*
   A. 200 minus the patient's age
   B. 210 minus the patient's age
   C. 220 minus the patient's age
   D. 230 minus the patient's age

   *By convention, the maximum predicted heart rate in exercise stress testing is calculated as 220 (210 for women) minus the patient's age.*

357. Which of the following is a normal electrocardiographic change during exercise?
   *BMJ. 2002;324(7345):1084-1087*
   A. P wave increases in height
   B. R wave decreases in height
   C. T wave decreases in height
   D. All of the above

358. Which of the following is a normal electrocardiographic change during exercise?
   *BMJ. 2002;324(7345):1084-1087*
   A. J point becomes depressed
   B. ST segment becomes sharply upsloping
   C. Q-T interval shortens
   D. All of the above

   *Normal electrocardiographic changes during exercise include P wave increases in height, R wave decreases in height, J point becomes depressed, ST segment becomes sharply upsloping, Q-T interval shortens and T wave decreases in height.*

359. **Which of the following is an abnormal electrocardiographic change during exercise?**
   *BMJ. 2002;324(7345):1084-1087*

   A. ST segment depression of >1 mm (horizontal or downsloping)
   B. ST elevation of >1 mm
   C. Inversion of the U wave
   D. All of the above

360. **In exercise stress testing, findings suggesting high probability of coronary artery disease include?**
   *BMJ. 2002;324(7345):1084-1087*

   A. Early positive response within six minutes
   B. Persistence of ST depression for > 6 minutes into recovery
   C. ST segment depression in five or more leads
   D. All of the above

*Findings suggesting high probability of coronary artery disease include horizontal ST segment depression of < 2 mm, downsloping ST segment depression, early positive response within six minutes, persistence of ST depression for > 6 minutes into recovery, ST segment depression in ≥5 leads and exertional hypotension.*

361. **Contraindications to exercise stress testing include?**
   *BMJ. 2002;324(7345):1084-1087*

   A. Severe aortic stenosis
   B. Rest angina within 48 hours
   C. Active infective endocarditis
   D. All of the above

362. **Contraindications to exercise stress testing include?**
   *BMJ. 2002;324(7345):1084-1087*

   A. Acute myocardial infarction (within 4–6 days)
   B. Deep vein thrombosis
   C. Systolic BP > 220 mm Hg/diastolic BP >120 mm Hg
   D. All of the above

## The Bradyarrhythmias: Disorders of the Sinoatrial Node

**363. Electrical activation of the heart can originate in?**
*Harrison's 20th Ed. Chapter 239 Page 1722*

A. Atrioventricular (AV) node
B. Specialized conducting system
C. Muscle
D. All of the above

Electrical activation of the heart normally originates in sinoatrial (SA) node, the predominant pacemaker. Other subsidiary pacemakers in atrioventricular (AV) node, specialized conducting system and muscle may initiate electrical activation if SA node is dysfunctional or suppressed.

**364. Which of the following is false about nodal cells?**
*Harrison's 20th Ed. Chapter 239 Page 1722*

A. Less negative resting membrane potential
B. Most rapid phase 4 depolarization
C. Slow action potential upstrokes (phase 0)
D. Action potential mediated by Na⁺ rather than Ca⁺⁺

In nodal cells, action potential mediated by Ca⁺⁺ rather than Na⁺ current.

**365. Nodal cell action potentials exhibit which of the following?**
*Harrison's 20th Ed. Chapter 239 Page 1723 Figure 239-1*

A. More depolarized resting membrane potentials
B. Slower phase 0 upstrokes
C. Slower phase 4 diastolic depolarization
D. All of the above

Nodal cell action potentials exhibit more depolarized resting membrane potentials, slower phase 0 upstrokes, and phase 4 diastolic depolarization.

**366. Which of the following is not a depolarizing current?**
*Harrison's 20th Ed. Chapter 239 Page 1723 Figure 239-2*

A. $I_{Ca-L}$
B. $I_{Ca-T}$
C. $I_f$
D. $I_{KACh}$

**367. Which of the following is a repolarizing current?**
*Harrison's 20th Ed. Chapter 239 Page 1723 Figure 239-2*

A. $I_K$
B. $I_{K1}$
C. $I_{KACh}$
D. All of the above

**368. Which of the following is the location of SA node?**
*Harrison's 20th Ed. Chapter 239 Page 1723*

A. Coronal sulcus
B. Superior sulcus
C. Sulcus terminalis
D. Sulcus fusiform

SA node is composed of a cluster of small fusiform cells in sulcus terminalis on the epicardial surface of heart at the right atrial - superior vena caval junction, where they envelop the SA nodal artery.

**369. Which of the following is not a feature of SA nodal cells?**
*Harrison's 20th Ed. Chapter 239 Page 1723*

A. Fewer myofibrils
B. No intercalated disks
C. Well developed sarcoplasmic reticulum
D. No T-tubules

SA nodal cells have fewer distinct myofibrils than surrounding atrial myocardium, no intercalated disks, poorly developed sarcoplasmic reticulum, and no T-tubules. There is a relative absence of inward rectifier potassium current ($I_{K1}$) and absence of available fast sodium current ($I_{Na}$).

**370. Intrinsic discharge rate is highest of which of the following potential cardiac pacemakers?**
*Harrison's 20th Ed. Chapter 239 Page 1723*

A. Sinus node
B. Specialized fibers of His-Purkinje system
C. Some specialized atrial fibers
D. None of the above

SA node is normally the dominant cardiac pacemaker because its intrinsic discharge rate is the highest of all potential cardiac pacemakers.

**371. In majority, SA nodal artery arises from?**
*Harrison's 20th Ed. Chapter 239 Page 1723*

A. Right coronary artery
B. Left anterior descending artery
C. Left circumflex artery
D. Posterior descending artery

SA nodal artery arises from RCA in 55 - 60% and left circumflex artery in 40 - 45% of persons.

**372. Membrane potential of SA nodal cells is?**
*Harrison's 20th Ed. Chapter 239 Page 1723*

A. –20 to –40 mV
B. –40 to –60 mV
C. –60 to –80 mV
D. –80 to –100 mV

The action potentials of SA nodal cells are characterized by a relatively depolarized membrane potential of –40 to –60 mV, slow phase 0 upstroke, and relatively rapid phase 4 diastolic depolarization compared to the action potentials recorded in cardiac muscle cells.

**373. In SA node, which of the following is modulated by β-adrenergic stimulation?**
*Harrison's 20th Ed. Chapter 239 Page 1723*

A. $I_{Ca-L}$
B. $I_{Ca-T}$
C. $I_f$
D. All of the above

### 374. In SA node, which of the following is modulated by vagal stimulation?
*Harrison's 20th Ed. Chapter 239 Page 1723*

A. $I_{Ca-L}$
B. $I_{Na}$
C. $I_{K1}$
D. $I_{KAch}$

$I_{Ca-L}$, $I_{Ca-T}$, and If are modulated by β-adrenergic stimulation and $I_{KAch}$ by vagal stimulation.

### 375. Cushing's response is best related to?
*Harrison's 20th Ed. Chapter 239 Page 1724*

A. Visual blurring
B. Accelerated hypertension
C. Increased intracranial pressure
D. Dermopathy

Increased intracranial pressure producing SA nodal dysfunction is called Cushing's response.

### 376. Which of the following is a cause of extrinsic SA node dysfunction?
*Harrison's 20th Ed. Chapter 239 Page 1724*

A. Sleep apnea
B. Increased intracranial pressure
C. Hypothyroidism
D. All of the above

Most common causes of extrinsic SA node dysfunction are drugs & autonomic nervous system influences.

### 377. Which of the following is associated with SA nodal disease?
*Harrison's 20th Ed. Chapter 239 Page 1724*

A. Pericarditis
B. Myocarditis
C. Rheumatic heart disease
D. All of the above

### 378. Which of the following is associated with SA nodal disease?
*Harrison's 20th Ed. Chapter 239 Page 1724*

A. Systemic lupus erythematosus (SLE)
B. Rheumatoid arthritis (RA)
C. Mixed connective tissue disorders (MCTDs)
D. All of the above

### 379. Acute myocardial infarction in which location is associated with transient SA nodal dysfunction?
*Harrison's 20th Ed. Chapter 239 Page 1724-5*

A. Anterior
B. Inferior
C. Lateral
D. All of the above

Sinus bradycardia is common in patients with acute inferior or posterior MI and can be exacerbated by vagal activation induced by pain or the use of morphine. Ischemia of the SA nodal artery occurs in acute coronary syndromes due to involvement with right coronary artery, and even with infarction, the effect on SA node function is transient.

### 380. Senile amyloidosis causing intrinsic sinus node dysfunction typically presents in which decade of life?
*Harrison's 20th Ed. Chapter 239 Page 1724*

A. 6th
B. 7th
C. 8th
D. 9th

Senile amyloidosis is an infiltrative disorder and causes Intrinsic sinus node dysfunction in patients typically in the ninth decade of life.

### 381. Tachycardia-bradycardia variant of sick-sinus syndrome is referred to as?
*Harrison's 20th Ed. Chapter 239 Page 1724*

A. SSS1
B. SSS2
C. SSS3
D. SSS4

Autosomal dominant sinus node dysfunction in conjunction with supraventricular tachycardia - tachycardia-bradycardia variant of sick-sinus syndrome is referred to as SSS2.

### 382. Tachycardia-bradycardia variant of sick-sinus syndrome is related to which of the following gene?
*Harrison's 20th Ed. Chapter 239 Page 1724*

A. SCN5A
B. HCN4
C. MYH6
D. APC

Tachycardia-bradycardia variant of sick-sinus syndrome has been linked to mutations in the pacemaker current ($I_f$) subunit gene HCN4 on chromosome 15.

### 383. Autosomal recessive form of SSS1 is related to which of the following gene?
*Harrison's 20th Ed. Chapter 239 Page 1724*

A. SCN5A
B. HCN4
C. MYH6
D. APC

An autosomal recessive form of SSS1 with prominent feature of atrial inexcitability and absence of P waves on the electrocardiogram (ECG) is caused by mutations in the cardiac sodium channel gene, SCN5A, on chromosome 3.

### 384. Which of the following neuromuscular disease produce SA node disease?
*Harrison's 20th Ed. Chapter 239 Page 1724*

A. Myasthenia gravis
B. Botulism
C. Lambert-Eaton syndrome
D. Kearns-Sayre syndrome

Neuromuscular diseases like Kearns-Sayre syndrome (ophthalmoplegia, pigmentary degeneration of retina & cardiomyopathy) & myotonic dystrophy produce conducting system & SA node disease.

### 385. Patients with the tachycardia-bradycardia variant of SSS are at risk for?
*Harrison's 20th Ed. Chapter 239 Page 1724*

A. Ventricular fibrillation
B. Thromboembolism
C. Myocardial infarction
D. All of the above

Patients with tachycardia-bradycardia variant of SSS, similar to patients with atrial fibrillation, are at risk for thromboembolism. In such patients, overall longevity is not compromised in absence of other significant comorbid conditions.

386. **Sinus rate of how much in awake state & in absence of physical conditioning generally is considered abnormal?**
   *Harrison's 20th Ed. Chapter 239 Page 1724*

   A. < 40 beats / minute
   B. < 50 beats / minute
   C. < 60 beats / minute
   D. < 70 beats / minute

   *A sinus rate of <40 beats/minute in awake state in the absence of physical conditioning generally is considered abnormal.*

387. **Which of the following statements is false?**
   *Harrison's 20th Ed. Chapter 239 Page 1724*

   A. Sinus pause result from failure of SA node to discharge
   B. Sinus arrest result from failure of SA node to discharge
   C. Sinus pauses of up to 3 seconds are common in awake athletes
   D. None of the above

388. **Sinus bradycardia is associated with all except?**
   *Harrison's 20th Ed. Chapter 239 Page 1724*

   A. Hypothyroidism
   B. Advanced liver disease
   C. Trypnosomiasis
   D. Brucellosis

389. **Sinus bradycardia is associated with all except?**
   *Harrison's 20th Ed. Chapter 239 Page 1724*

   A. Typhoid fever
   B. Acute hypertension
   C. Hypercapnia
   D. Alkalosis

390. **Sinus arrest means?**
   *Harrison's 20th Ed. Chapter 239 Page 1724*

   A. Failure of sinus impulse formation
   B. Block of conduction of sinus impulses to atrial tissue
   C. Block of conduction of sinus impulses at AV node
   D. Block of conduction of sinus impulses beyond AV node

391. **Sinus exit block means?**
   *Harrison's 20th Ed. Chapter 239 Page 1724*

   A. Failure of sinus impulse formation
   B. Failure of conduction of sinus impulses to surrounding atrial tissue
   C. Failure of conduction of sinus impulses at AV node
   D. Failure of conduction of sinus impulses beyond AV node

   *Sinus pauses & sinus arrest result from failure of SA node to discharge, causing a pause without P waves visible on ECG. Intermittent failure of conduction from SA node produces sinus exit block.*

392. **Electrocardiographic manifestations of SA node dysfunction include?**
   *Harrison's 20th Ed. Chapter 239 Page 1724*

   A. Sinus pauses
   B. Sinus exit block
   C. Alternating supraventricular tachycardia & bradycardia
   D. All of the above

   *Electrocardiographic manifestations of SA node dysfunction include sinus bradycardia, sinus pauses, sinus arrest, sinus exit block, tachycardia (in SSS), and chronotropic incompetence.*

393. **Which of the following is false about tachycardia-bradycardia variant of SSS?**
   *Harrison's 20th Ed. Chapter 239 Page 1724*

   A. Are at risk for thromboembolism
   B. May have concurrent AV conduction disease
   C. Symptoms may be related to slow & fast heart rates
   D. SA node dysfunction is associated with increased mortality

   *SA node dysfunction is not associated with increased mortality rates.*

394. **Intermittent absence of P waves on ECG is due to?**
   *Harrison's 20th Ed. Chapter 239 Page 1724*

   A. Second-degree SA block
   B. Sinus exit block
   C. Sinus arrest
   D. Sick sinus syndrome

395. **A prolongation of conduction time from SA node to surrounding atrial tissue is called?**
   *Harrison's 20th Ed. Chapter 239 Page 1724*

   A. First-degree sinoatrial exit block
   B. Second-degree sinoatrial exit block
   C. Third-degree sinoatrial exit block
   D. None of the above

396. **The intermittent failure of conduction of sinus impulses to the surrounding atrial tissue is called?**
   *Harrison's 20th Ed. Chapter 239 Page 1724*

   A. First-degree sinoatrial exit block
   B. Second-degree sinoatrial exit block
   C. Third-degree sinoatrial exit block
   D. None of the above

397. **Lack of atrial activity or the presence of an ectopic subsidiary atrial pacemaker is called?**
   *Harrison's 20th Ed. Chapter 239 Page 1724*

   A. First-degree sinoatrial exit block
   B. Second-degree sinoatrial exit block
   C. Third-degree sinoatrial exit block
   D. None of the above

   *Type I second-degree SA block results from progressive prolongation of SA node conduction with intermittent failure of the impulses originating in the sinus node to conduct to the surrounding atrial tissue. Second-degree SA block appears on the ECG as an intermittent absence of P waves. In type II second-degree SA block, there is no change in SA node conduction before the pause. Complete or third-degree SA block results in no P waves on the ECG.*

398. **Sick sinus syndrome refers to a combination of all except?**
   *Harrison's 20th Ed. Chapter 239 Page 1724*

   A. Sinus bradycardia
   B. Sinoatrial block
   C. Sinus arrest
   D. Sinus arrhythmia

   *ECG manifestations of SA node dysfunction include sinus bradycardia, sinus pauses, sinus arrest, sinus exit block, tachycardia (in SSS), and chronotropic incompetence (inability to increase heart rate in response to exercise or other stress appropriately).*

399. **In sinus arrest and in sinus exit block, atrial asystole is of what duration?**
   *Harrison's 20th Ed. Chapter 239 Page 1724*

   A. > 1 seconds
   B. > 1.5 seconds
   C. > 2.5 seconds
   D. > 3 seconds

   *Sinus pauses of up to 3 seconds are common in the awake athlete, & pauses of this duration or longer may be observed in asymptomatic elderly subjects.*

400. **In Tachycardia-bradycardia syndrome, which of the following is the most common tachycardia?**
   *Harrison's 20th Ed. Chapter 239 Page 1724*

   A. Atrial tachycardia
   B. Atrial flutter
   C. Atrial fibrillation
   D. Any of the above

   *Tachycardia-bradycardia syndrome manifests as alternating sinus bradycardia & atrial tachyarrhythmias. Although atrial tachycardia, atrial flutter, and atrial fibrillation may be observed, the latter is the most common tachycardia.*

401. **Which of the following is false about Mobitz type I SA nodal exit block?**
   *Harrison's 20th Ed. Chapter 239 Page 1725 Figure 239-4*

   A. Regularly irregular heart rhythm
   B. Decreasing P-P intervals before the pause
   C. Pause less than twice the cycle length of last sinus interval
   D. None of the above

   *In Mobitz type I SA nodal exit block, there is grouped beating producing a regularly irregular heart rhythm. SA node rate is constant with progressive delay in exit from the node and activation of atria. This produces subtly decreasing P-P intervals before the pause, and the pause is less than twice the cycle length of the last sinus interval.*

402. **Chronotropic incompetence is failure to reach what percentage of predicted maximal heart rate at peak exercise?**
   *Harrison's 20th Ed. Chapter 239 Page 1725*

   A. 55%
   B. 65%
   C. 75%
   D. 85%

   *Exercise testing is useful in discriminating chronotropic incompetence from resting bradycardia. Failure to increase the heart rate with exercise is called chronotropic incompetence. Alternatively defined as a failure to reach 85% of predicted maximal heart rate at peak exercise or failure to achieve a heart rate >100 beats/minute with exercise or a maximal heart rate with exercise less than two standard deviations below that of an age-matched control population.*

403. **Normal values of intrinsic heart rate are calculated by the formula?**
   *Harrison's 20th Ed. Chapter 239 Page 1725*

   A. 116.2 – (0.53 x age) beats per minute
   B. 117.2 – (0.53 x age) beats per minute
   C. 118.2 – (0.53 x age) beats per minute
   D. 119.2 – (0.53 x age) beats per minute

   *Determining the intrinsic heart rate (IHR) may distinguish SA node dysfunction from slow heart rates resulting from high vagal tone. Normal IHR after administration of 0.2 mg/kg propranolol & 0.04 mg/kg atropine is 117.2 – (0.53 x age) in beats/minute. Low IHR is indicative of SA disease.*

404. **Which of the following conditions do not require electrophysiologic tests for diagnosis in 'symptomatic' patients with ECG documentation of?**
   *Harrison's 20th Ed. Chapter 239 Page 1725*

   A. Asystole
   B. Sinoatrial block or arrest
   C. Bradycardia-tachycardia syndrome
   D. All of the above

   *Symptomatic patients with ECG documentation of asystole, sinoatrial block or arrest, or the bradycardia-tachycardia syndrome do not require electrophysiologic tests for diagnosis.*

405. **Which of the following is a sensitive and specific indicator of intrinsic SA node disease?**
   *Harrison's 20th Ed. Chapter 239 Page 1725*

   A. Sinus node recovery time (SNRT)
   B. Sinoatrial conduction time (SACT)
   C. Intrinsic heart rate (IHR)
   D. All of the above

   *Sinus node recovery time (SNRT) is defined as the longest pause after cessation of overdrive pacing of right atrium near SA node (normal <1500 msec. or, corrected for sinus cycle length, <550 msec.). Sinoatrial conduction time (SACT) is defined as one-half the difference between intrinsic sinus cycle length and a noncompensatory pause after a premature atrial stimulus (normal <125 msec.). Combination of an abnormal SNRT, an abnormal SACT, and a low IHR is a sensitive and specific indicator of intrinsic SA node disease.*

406. **In susceptible individual, SA node dysfunction may become manifest in the presence of which of the following?**
   *Harrison's 20th Ed. Chapter 239 Page 1725*

   A. Cardiac glycosides
   B. Amiodarone
   C. Calcium channel blockers
   D. All of the above

   *Cardiac glycosides, beta-blockers, calcium channel blockers, amiodarone may unmask evidence of sinus node dysfunction in susceptible individuals.*

407. **Which of the following pharmacologic agents may improve SA node function?**
   *Harrison's 20th Ed. Chapter 239 Page 1725*

   A. Class I Antiarrhythmics
   B. Class III Antiarrhythmics
   C. Calcium channel blockers
   D. Digitalis

   *Beta blockers and calcium channel blockers increase SNRT in patients with SA node dysfunction, and antiarrhythmic drugs with class I and III action may promote SA node exit block. Digitalis shortens SNRT in SA node dysfunction. Isoproterenol or atropine administered IV may increase sinus rate acutely. Theophylline increases heart rate.*

408. **How many letter codes are used for describing pacemaker modes & function?**
   *Harrison's 20th Ed. Chapter 239 Page 1725*

   A. 3
   B. 4
   C. 5
   D. 6

   *Pacemaker modes & function are named using a five-letter code.*

409. **The first letter in the pacing code indicates?**
   *Harrison's 20th Ed. Chapter 239 Page 1725*
   A. Chamber(s) paced
   B. Chamber in which electrical activity is sensed
   C. The response to a sensed electric signal
   D. Programmability and rate modulation

410. **The second letter in the pacing code indicates?**
   *Harrison's 20th Ed. Chapter 239 Page 1725*
   A. Chamber(s) paced
   B. Chamber in which electrical activity is sensed
   C. The response to a sensed electric signal
   D. Programmability and rate modulation

411. **The third letter in the pacing code indicates?**
   *Harrison's 20th Ed. Chapter 239 Page 1725*
   A. Chamber(s) paced
   B. Chamber in which electrical activity is sensed
   C. The response to a sensed electric signal
   D. Programmability and rate modulation

412. **The fourth letter in the pacing code indicates?**
   *Harrison's 20th Ed. Chapter 239 Page 1725*
   A. Chamber(s) paced
   B. Chamber in which electrical activity is sensed
   C. The response to a sensed electric signal
   D. Programmability and rate modulation

*In pacing code, the first letter indicates the chamber(s) that is paced (O, none; A, atrium; V, ventricle; D, dual; S, single), the second letter indicates the chamber(s) in which sensing occurs (O, none; A, atrium; V, ventricle; D, dual; S, single), the third letter indicates the response to a sensed event (O, none; I, inhibition; T, triggered; D, inhibition + triggered), the fourth letter refers to the programmability or rate response (R, rate responsive), and the fifth refers to the existence of antitachycardia functions if present (O, none; P, antitachycardia pacing; S, shock; D, pace + shock).*

413. **Twiddler's syndrome best relates to?**
   *Harrison's 20th Ed. Chapter 239 Page 1726*
   A. Failing battery of pacemaker
   B. Interference by external stimuli on pacemaker
   C. Rotation of pacemaker pulse generator in its pocket
   D. All of the above

*Rotation of the pacemaker pulse generator in its subcutaneous pocket, either intentionally or inadvertently, often referred to as "twiddler's syndrome" producing dislodgment with failure to sense or pace the heart.*

414. **Pacemaker syndrome is associated in those?**
   *Harrison's 20th Ed. Chapter 239 Page 1726*
   A. Who do not maintain AV synchrony
   B. Who do not have adequate cardiac output
   C. Who have chronic illnesses (HTN, DM)
   D. All of the above

*Pacemaker syndrome is a constellation of signs and symptoms associated with any mode of pacing that does not maintain or restore AV synchrony.*

415. **Pacemaker syndrome includes which of the following?**
   *Harrison's 20th Ed. Chapter 239 Page 1726*
   A. Cough
   B. Confusion
   C. Third heart sound
   D. All of the above

*Pacemaker syndrome includes neck pulsation, fatigue, palpitations, cough, confusion, exertional dyspnea, dizziness, syncope, elevation in jugular venous pressure, canon A waves, and stigmata of congestive heart failure, including edema, rales, and a third heart sound.*

416. **Class I indication for pacing in SA node dysfunction include all except?**
   *Harrison's 20th Ed. Chapter 239 Page 1726*
   A. Documented symptomatic bradycardia
   B. Syncope of unexplained origin with major abnormalities of SA node dysfunction
   C. Sinus node dysfunction associated long-term drug therapy for which there is no alternative
   D. Symptomatic chronotropic incompetence

*Class I indications for pacing in SA node dysfunction include documented symptomatic bradycardia, sinus node dysfunction associated long-term drug therapy for which there is no alternative, or symptomatic chronotropic incompetence.*

# The Bradyarrhythmias : Disorders of the Atrioventricular Node

**417. Phase 0 depolarization in cells in AV node is mediated by?**
*Harrison's 20th Ed. Chapter 240 Page 1727*

A. Sodium
B. Potassium
C. Calcium
D. All of the above

Cells in AV node have slower phase 0 depolarization, mediated by calcium influx in nodal tissue rather than mediated by sodium influx as seen in ventricular tissue.

**418. Transient AV conduction block is common in?**
*Harrison's 20th Ed. Chapter 240 Page 1727*

A. Infants
B. Young
C. Middle age
D. Elderly

Transient AV conduction block is common in the young and is most likely the result of high vagal tone found in ~10% of young adults.

**419. AV conduction axis consists of?**
*Harrison's 20th Ed. Chapter 240 Page 1727*

A. Atria
B. Ventricles
C. AV node
D. All of the above

AV conduction axis involves the atria and ventricles as well as the AV node.

**420. Which of the following about AV node is false?**
*Harrison's 20th Ed. Chapter 240 Page 1727*

A. Subendocardial structure
B. Located in the posterior-inferior right atrium
C. Measure ~1 × 3 × 5 mm
D. None of the above

**421. The AV node lies at the?**
*Harrison's 20th Ed. Chapter 240 Page 1727*

A. Base of interatrial septum just above tricuspid annulus and anterior to coronary sinus
B. Base of interatrial septum just below tricuspid annulus and anterior to coronary sinus
C. Base of interatrial septum just above tricuspid annulus and posterior to coronary sinus
D. Base of the interventricular septum just above tricuspid annulus and anterior to coronary sinus

**422. Which of the following statements is false?**
*Harrison's 20th Ed. Chapter 240 Page 1727*

A. Compact AV node continues as the penetrating AV bundle
B. Superior, medial, & posterior transitional atrionodal bundles converge on the compact AV node
C. Located at the apex of triangle of Koch
D. None of the above

**423. Intra-atrial conduction system of the heart consists of?**
*Cardiology Journal 2011;18 (3):337*

A. Anterior interatrial band or Bachmann's bundle
B. Middle internodal tract or Wenckebach's bundle
C. Posterior internodal tract of Thorel
D. All of the above

**424. Boundaries of triangle of Koch include all except?**
*Harrison's 20th Ed. Chapter 240 Page 1727*

A. Coronary sinus ostium
B. Septal tricuspid valve annulus
C. Septal mitral valve annulus
D. Tendon of Todaro

Triangle of Koch is bordered by coronary sinus ostium posteriorly, septal tricuspid valve annulus anteriorly & tendon of Todaro superiorly.

**425. The penetrating AV bundle is in close proximity to?**
*Harrison's 20th Ed. Chapter 240 Page 1727*

A. Aortic valve annuli
B. Mitral valve annuli
C. Tricuspid valve annuli
D. All of the above

**426. First septal perforator of left anterior descending coronary artery supplies?**
*Harrison's 20th Ed. Chapter 240 Page 1727*

A. Penetrating AV bundle
B. Left bundle branch
C. Right bundle branch
D. All of the above

Bundle branches also have a dual blood supply from the septal perforators of left anterior descending coronary artery & branches of posterior descending coronary artery.

**427. In decremental conduction, with increasingly rapid rates of stimulation, the conduction?**
*Harrison's 20th Ed. Chapter 240 Page 1727*

A. Slows
B. Becomes faster
C. No change
D. Any of the above

Atrionodal transitional connections exhibit decremental conduction, defined as slowing of conduction with increasingly rapid rates of stimulation.

**428. Myocytes that constitute the compact node have a resting membrane potential of about?**
*Harrison's 20th Ed. Chapter 240 Page 1727*

A. - 50 mV
B. - 60 mV
C. - 70 mV
D. - 80 mV

Myocytes that constitute the compact node are depolarized with a resting membrane potential of about –60 mV. Action potentials have low amplitudes, slow upstrokes of phase 0 (<10 V/s), and phase 4 diastolic depolarization, high-input resistance and relative insensitivity to external $[K^+]$.

429. **AV nodal cells lack which of the following?**
*Harrison's 20th Ed. Chapter 240 Page 1727*

   A. $I_{Na}$
   B. $I_{Ca-L}$
   C. $I_{Ca-T}$
   D. $I_f$

AV nodal cells lack $I_{K1}$ and INa. $I_{Ca-L}$ is responsible for phase 0. Phase 4 depolarization reflects the composite activity of the depolarizing currents If, $I_{Ca-L}$, $I_{Ca-T}$, and INCX and the repolarizing currents IKr and IKAch.

430. **Which of the following connexin is present in gap junction channels between cells in the AV node?**
*Harrison's 20th Ed. Chapter 240 Page 1727*

   A. Connexin-23
   B. Connexin-32
   C. Connexin-40
   D. Connexin-43

431. **Which of the following about His bundle & bundle branches is false?**
*Harrison's 20th Ed. Chapter 240 Page 1727*

   A. Minimally influenced by autonomic tone
   B. Have most rapid conduction in heart
   C. Insulated from ventricular myocardium
   D. None of the above

432. **Which of the following about His bundle & bundle branches is false?**
*Harrison's 20th Ed. Chapter 240 Page 1727*

   A. Very rapid upstrokes (phase 0)
   B. Prolonged plateaus (phase 2)
   C. Modest automaticity (phase 4 depolarization)
   D. None of the above

433. **Normal AV node in vivo possesses?**
*Harrison's 19th Ed. 1470*

   A. Automaticity always
   B. Automaticity sometimes
   C. No automaticity
   D. None of the above

434. **Which of the following is associated with SA node slowing and AV conduction block?**
*Harrison's 20th Ed. Chapter 240 Page 1728*

   A. Carotid sinus hypersensitivity
   B. Cough
   C. Micturition syncope
   D. All of the above

Heightened vagal tone during sleep or in well-conditioned individuals can lead to all grades of AV block. Carotid sinus hypersensitivity, vasovagal syncope, and cough and micturition syncope may be associated with SA node slowing and AV conduction block.

435. **Conditions that can produce AV conduction block include?**
*Harrison's 20th Ed. Chapter 240 Page 1728 Table 240-1*

   A. Hypothyroidism
   B. Hypermagnesemia
   C. Adrenal insufficiency
   D. All of the above

436. **Drugs that can produce atrioventricular block include?**
*Harrison's 20th Ed. Chapter 240 Page 1728 Table 240-1*

   A. Lithium
   B. Adenosine
   C. Antiarrhythmics (class I and III)
   D. All of the above

437. **Conditions that can produce AV conduction block include?**
*Harrison's 20th Ed. Chapter 240 Page 1728 Table 240-1*

   A. Tuberculosis
   B. Lyme disease
   C. Diphtheria
   D. All of the above

438. **Conditions that can produce AV conduction block include?**
*Harrison's 20th Ed. Chapter 240 Page 1728 Table 240-1*

   A. Chagas disease
   B. Toxoplasmosis
   C. Syphilis
   D. All of the above

439. **Conditions that can produce AV conduction block include?**
*Harrison's 20th Ed. Chapter 240 Page 1728 Table 240-1*

   A. Sarcoidosis
   B. Systemic lupus erythematosus
   C. Rheumatoid arthritis
   D. All of the above

Infectious diseases that lead to conducting system disturbances include Lyme disease, Chagas' disease, and syphilis. Autoimmune and infiltrative diseases like SLE, RA, MCTD, scleroderma, amyloidosis (primary & secondary), sarcoidosis, and hemochromatosis may produce AV conduction block

440. **AV conduction block has been associated with which of the following?**
*Harrison's 20th Ed. Chapter 240 Page 1728 Table 240-1*

   A. Kearns-Sayre syndrome
   B. Myotonic dystrophy
   C. Facioscapulohumeral muscular dystrophy
   D. All of the above

441. **Mutation in which of the following gene causes accelerated forms of progressive familial heart block?**
*Harrison's 20th Ed. Chapter 240 Page 1728*

   A. KCNQ1
   B. KCNH2 (HERG)
   C. SCN5A
   D. ANK2

Accelerated forms of progressive familial heart block have been identified in families with mutations in cardiac sodium channel gene (SCN5A).

**442. Congenital AV block may be seen in which of the following?**
*Harrison's 20th Ed. Chapter 240 Page 1728*

A. Transposition of the great arteries
B. Ostium primum atrial septal defect
C. Ventricular septal defect
D. All of the above

Congenital AV block may be observed in complex congenital cardiac anomalies such as transposition of the great arteries, ostium primum atrial septal defects (ASDs), ventricular septal defects (VSDs), endocardial cushion defects and some single-ventricle defects.

**443. Congenital AV block in a structurally normal heart is seen in children born to mothers with?**
*Harrison's 20th Ed. Chapter 240 Page 1728*

A. SLE
B. Sarcoidosis
C. Rheumatoid arthritis
D. Hemochromatosis

Congenital AV block in a structurally normal heart is seen in children born to mothers with SLE.

**444. In acute MI, AV block transiently develops in what percentage of patients?**
*Harrison's 20th Ed. Chapter 240 Page 1728*

A. 5 - 10%
B. 10 - 25%
C. 20 - 35%
D. 30 - 45%

In acute MI, AV block transiently develops in 10 - 25% of patients.

**445. Level of AV block in inferior MI tends to be in?**
*Harrison's 20th Ed. Chapter 240 Page 1728*

A. AV node
B. Distal AV nodal complex
C. His bundle
D. Bundle branches

Level of AV block in inferior MI tends to be in AV node with more stable, narrow escape rhythms. Acute anterior MI is associated with block in distal AV nodal complex, His bundle or bundle branches & results in wide complex, unstable escape rhythms & a worse prognosis with high mortality rates.

**446. First-degree AV block is determined by?**
*Harrison's 20th Ed. Chapter 240 Page 1728*

A. Atrial activation
B. AV nodal activation
C. His-Purkinje activation
D. All of the above

I° AV block (PR interval > 200 ms) is a slowing of conduction through AV "junction". The site of delay is typically in AV node but may be in atria, AV node bundle of His, or His-Purkinje system.

**447. I° AV block with wide QRS suggests delay in?**
*Harrison's 20th Ed. Chapter 240 Page 1728*

A. Proximal AV node
B. Mid AV node
C. Distal AV node
D. Distal conduction system

I° AV block with wide QRS is suggestive of delay in the distal conduction system, whereas a narrow QRS suggests delay in the AV node proper or, less commonly, in the bundle of His.

**448. Nationality of Woldemar Mobitz was?**
*Circulation. 2004;110:1162-1167*

A. Russian German
B. British American
C. Spanish
D. Anglo Indian

Woldemar Mobitz (1889-1951) was a Russian-German physician.

**449. Mobitz Type I is also named after?**
*Circulation. 2004;110:1162-1167*

A. Karel Frederik Wenckebach
B. John Hay
C. Robert Silverman
D. Jack Upshaw

**450. Mobitz Type II is also named after?**
*Circulation. 2004;110:1162-1167*

A. Karel Frederik Wenckebach
B. John Hay
C. Robert Silverman
D. Jack Upshaw

**451. In presence of a normal duration QRS complex, delay within AV node is the cause of prolonged PR interval if it is?**
*Harrison's 20th Ed. Chapter 240 Page 1728*

A. > 0.21 second
B. > 0.22 second
C. > 0.23 second
D. > 0.24 second

**452. When some atrial impulses fail to conduct to ventricles, the type of AV block is?**
*Harrison's 20th Ed. Chapter 240 Page 1728*

A. First-degree heart block
B. Second-degree heart block
C. Third-degree heart block
D. Sick sinus syndrome

In II° AV block there is an intermittent failure of electrical impulse conduction from atrium to ventricle.

**453. Which of the following statements about Mobitz type I, second degree AV block is false?**
*Harrison's 20th Ed. Chapter 240 Page 1728*

A. Also called AV Wenckebach block
B. Progressive PR prolongation prior to block of an atrial impulse
C. Pause that follows is fully compensatory
D. PR interval of first conducted impulse is shorter than last conducted atrial impulse prior to blocked P wave

In Mobitz type 1 II° AV block, periodic failure of conduction occurs characterized by a progressively lengthening PR interval, shortening of RR interval, & a pause that is < 2 times the immediately preceding RR interval. ECG complex after the pause exhibits a shorter PR interval that immediately preceding the pause.

454. Which of the following statements about Mobitz type I second degree AV block is false?
*Harrison's 20th Ed. Chapter 240 Page 1728*

   A. Usually the difference between the longest & shortest PR intervals exceeds 100 mseconds
   B. Block is almost always localized to AV node
   C. Usually associated with a normal QRS duration
   D. Amiodarone therapy is a frequent cause

455. Which of the following statements about Mobitz type I second degree AV block is false?
*Harrison's 20th Ed. Chapter 240 Page 1728*

   A. Most often occurs transiently with inferior MI
   B. Due to digitalis, β-blockers, and Ca++ channel blockers
   C. Seen in normal individuals with heightened vagal tone
   D. Leads to complete heart block

*In Mobitz type 1 II° AV block, difference between the longest & shortest PR intervals exceeds 100 mseconds. It is almost always localized to AV node & associated with a normal QRS duration. It is seen most often as a transient abnormality with inferior wall infarction or with drug intoxication (digitalis, beta and calcium channel blockers) or in normal individuals with heightened vagal tone. Progression to complete heart block is uncommon, except in acute inferior wall myocardial infarction. Even when it does, this heart block is well tolerated because the escape pacemaker usually arises in the proximal His bundle & provides a stable rhythm & rarely requiring aggressive therapy.*

456. Which of the following statements about Mobitz type II second degree AV block is false?
*Harrison's 20th Ed. Chapter 240 Page 1728*

   A. Conduction fails suddenly and unexpectedly without a preceding change in PR intervals
   B. Due to disease of His-Purkinje system and associated with prolonged QRS duration
   C. When Mobitz type II block occurs with a normal QRS duration, an intra-AV node block should be expected
   D. High incidence of progression to complete heart block with an unstable, slow, lower escape pacemaker

457. Which of the following statements about Mobitz type II second degree AV block is false?
*Harrison's 20th Ed. Chapter 240 Page 1728*

   A. Occur in anteroseptal myocardial infarction
   B. Occur in primary or secondary sclerodegenerative or calcific disorders of fibrous skeleton of heart
   C. Block is usually in AV node
   D. Block is usually in His-Purkinje system

458. Which of the following statements about Mobitz type II second degree AV block is false?
*Harrison's 20th Ed. Chapter 240 Page 1728*

   A. Intermittent failure of conduction of the P wave without changes in the preceding PR intervals
   B. Intermittent failure of conduction of the P wave without changes in the preceding RR intervals
   C. Typically occurs in distal or infra-His conduction system
   D. None of the above

*Type 2 II° AV block is characterized by intermittent failure of conduction of the P wave without changes in the preceding PR or RR intervals. It typically occurs in distal or infra-His conduction system, is often associated with intraventricular conduction delays (bundle branch block), and is more likely to proceed to higher grades of AV block.*

459. It may be difficult to distinguish between type I from type II block when AV block is?
*Harrison's 20th Ed. Chapter 240 Page 1728*

   A. 2 : 1
   B. 3 : 1
   C. 4 : 1
   D. 5 : 1

*When AV block is 2:1, it may be difficult to distinguish type I from type II block. The finding of a His bundle electrogram after every atrial electrogram indicates that block is occurring in the distal conduction system. Must obtain a long rhythm strip or use atropine to induce 3:2 block.*

460. Which of the following about Type II second-degree AV block is false?
*Harrison's 20th Ed. Chapter 240 Page 1728*

   A. Occurs in distal or infra-His conduction system
   B. Associated with intraventricular conduction delays
   C. May proceed to higher grades of AV block
   D. None of the above

*Type II second-degree AV block typically occurs in distal or infra-His conduction system and is often associated with intraventricular conduction delays (bundle branch block). It is more likely to proceed to higher grades of AV block than is type I second-degree AV block.*

461. "Paroxysmal AV block" best relates to?
*Harrison's 20th Ed. Chapter 240 Page 1729*

   A. Self correcting AV block
   B. Series of nonconducted P waves
   C. P waves buried in QRS complex
   D. P waves following QRS complex

*Second-degree AV block (particularly type II) may be associated with a series of nonconducted P waves, referred to as paroxysmal AV block. It implies significant conduction system disease and is an indication for permanent pacing.*

462. AV block that is intermediate between second degree & third degree is referred to as?
*Harrison's 20th Ed. Chapter 240 Page 1729*

   A. High-grade AV block
   B. Pre third degree AV block
   C. Post second degree AV block
   D. Paroxysmal AV block

*AV block that is intermediate between second degree & third degree is referred to as high-grade AV block and like CHB implies advanced AV conduction system disease.*

463. Which of the following about Third-degree AV block is false?
*Harrison's 20th Ed. Chapter 240 Page 1729*

   A. No atrial impulse propagates to ventricles
   B. Congenital complete AV block is localized to AV node
   C. In AV nodal block, QRS duration is prolonged
   D. In His bundle block, QRS duration is prolonged

*Complete failure of conduction from atrium to ventricle is called complete or third-degree AV block. It is most often distal to the AV node. A wide QRS escape rhythm implies block in the distal His or bundle branches, while a narrow QRS rhythm implies block in the AV node or proximal His and an escape rhythm originating in the AV junction.*

464. Which of the following argue that the site of block is in the AV node?
*Harrison's 20th Ed. Chapter 240 Page 1729*

   A. Mobitz I
   B. Junctional escape (narrow QRS), faster rate
   C. HR responds to atropine/exercise, vagal
   D. All of the above

*AH becomes progressively long if blockage is in the AV node.*

465. Which of the following argue that the site of block is in the bundle branch / fascicle?
   *Harrison's 20th Ed. Chapter 240 Page 1729*
   A. Concomitant BBB
   B. Slower escape rhythm with wide QRS
   C. No response to Atropine
   D. All of the above

466. Which of the following about Lev's disease is false?
   *Ann Intern Med. 1983;98(3):414*
   A. Calcification & sclerosis of fibrous cardiac skeleton
   B. Frequently involves pulmonary & tricuspid valves
   C. Involves central fibrous body & summit of ventricular septum
   D. Produces AV block

*Lev's disease occurs in older people with progressive fibrosis of the left side of cardiac skeleton. It also involves the mitral and aortic rings.*

467. Which of the following about Lenegre's disease is false?
   *Ann Intern Med. 1983;98(3):414*
   A. Primary sclerodegenerative disease in conducting system
   B. No involvement of myocardium
   C. Involves fibrous skeleton of heart
   D. Cause of isolated chronic heart block in adults

*Lenegre's disease, caused by SCN5A gene mutation, is a progressive sclerosis of the cardiac conduction system in young patients.*

468. Which of the following improve conduction through AV node & impair infranodal conduction?
   *Harrison's 20th Ed. Chapter 240 Page 1729*
   A. Atropine
   B. Isoproterenol
   C. Exercise
   D. All of the above

*Atropine, isoproterenol & exercise improve conduction through AV node & impair infranodal conduction.*

469. Which of the following is false?
   *Harrison's 20th Ed. Chapter 240 Page 1729*
   A. First-degree AV block is intranodal
   B. Mobitz type 1 second-degree AV block is intranodal
   C. Mobitz type 2 second-degree block is infranodal
   D. None of the above

470. To obtain a recording from the bundle of His, the electrode catheter is positioned?
   *Harrison's 20th Ed. Chapter 240 Page 1729*
   A. Across the pulmonary valve
   B. Superior margin of the tricuspid valve
   C. In coronary sinus
   D. In superior vena cava

*Recording of His bundle electrogram by a catheter positioned at superior margin of tricuspid valve annulus provides information about conduction at all levels of AV conduction axis.*

471. Normal AH interval in the His bundle recording is?
   *Harrison's 20th Ed. Chapter 240 Page 1729*
   A. 10 to 50 ms
   B. 60 to 130 ms
   C. 130 to 180 ms
   D. 180 to 250 ms

472. AH interval in the His bundle recording represents an indirect method of assessing?
   *Harrison's 20th Ed. Chapter 240 Page 1729*
   A. AV nodal conduction time
   B. Atrial conduction time
   C. Sinus node activation time
   D. None of the above

*Time from the most rapid deflection of the atrial electrogram in the His bundle recording to the His electrogram (AH interval) represents conduction through the AV node and is normally <130 ms.*

473. HV interval in the His bundle recording represents conduction time through?
   *Harrison's 20th Ed. Chapter 240 Page 1729*
   A. AV node
   B. His bundle
   C. His-Purkinje system
   D. Endocardium to epicardium

474. Normal HV interval in the His bundle recording is?
   *Harrison's 20th Ed. Chapter 240 Page 1730*
   A. 10 to 20 ms
   B. 15 to 35 ms
   C. 35 to 55 ms
   D. 60 to 75 ms

*The time from the His electrogram to the earliest onset of the QRS on the surface ECG (HV interval) represents the conduction time through the His-Purkinje system and is normally ≤55 ms.*

475. Normal PA interval in the His bundle recording is?
   *Harrison's 19th Ed. 1474*
   A. 30 ms
   B. 40 ms
   C. 50 ms
   D. 60 ms

*PA interval is the time from the earliest onset of P wave on surface ECG to onset of atrial deflection on His bundle catheter. It is an index of intra-atrial conduction time & should be 50 ms.*

476. Pacemaker implantation should be performed in any patient with?
   *Harrison's 20th Ed. Chapter 240 Page 1731*
   A. Symptomatic bradycardia
   B. Irreversible second degree AV block
   C. Irreversible third degree AV block
   D. All of the above

*Pacemaker implantation should be performed in any patient with symptomatic bradycardia and irreversible second- or third-degree AV block, regardless of the cause or level of block in the conducting system.*

477. **Anisotropic conduction means impulse propagation is more rapid?**

*Harrison's 19th Ed. 1474*

A. Parallel to fiber orientation than transverse to it
B. Transverse to fiber orientation than parallel to it
C. In a particular fiber type
D. In a particular fiber length

*Impulse propagation is more rapid parallel to fiber orientation than transverse to it. This property is termed anisotropic conduction.*

478. **"Effective" refractory period is defined as that portion of action potential during which?**

*Harrison's 19th Ed. 1474*

A. No stimulus can evoke another response
B. Stimulus can evoke a local, nonpropagated response
C. Stronger stimulus is required to evoke a response
D. Weaker stimulus can evoke a response

*Effective refractory period is that part of the action potential during which a stimulus can evoke only a local, nonpropagated response.*

479. **To obtain a recording of left atrial activity, the electrode catheter is positioned?**

*Harrison's 19th Ed. 1474*

A. Across the pulmonary valve
B. Across the tricuspid valve
C. In the coronary sinus
D. In the superior vena cava

*Left atrial activity is recorded directly via a catheter placed across a patent foramen ovale or indirectly using a catheter inserted into the coronary sinus.*

480. **Escape pacemaker following AV nodal block is usually in?**

A. His bundle
B. Bundle branches
C. Purkinje fibres
D. Ventricular myocardium

*Escape pacemaker following AV nodal block is usually in the His bundle.*

481. **Which of the following statements about escape pacemaker in His bundle is false?**

A. Has a rate of 40 to 60 beats per minute
B. Is associated with a QRS complex of normal duration
C. Is the escape pacemaker following AV nodal block
D. Is unstable

*Escape pacemaker in His bundle is stable with discharge rate of 40 to 60 beats/minute, associated with a QRS complex of normal duration.*

482. **Which of the following statements about escape pacemaker in distal His-Purkinje system is false?**

A. Has a rate of 25 to 45 beats per minute
B. Wide QRS complex of prolonged duration
C. Is the escape pacemaker following AV nodal block
D. Is unstable

*Escape rhythms arising in the distal His-Purkinje system have lower intrinsic rates (25 to 45 beats/minute), manifest wide QRS complexes with prolonged duration and are unstable.*

# Approach to Supraventricular Tachyarrhythmias

**483. Which of the following produces a wide QRS complex during supraventricular tachycardia?**
*Harrison's 20th Ed. Chapter 241 Page 1733*

- A. Conduction block in the left bundle branch
- B. Conduction block in the right bundle branch
- C. Activation of ventricles from an accessory pathway
- D. All of the above

**484. Which of the following is a pathologic supraventricular tachycardia?**
*Harrison's 20th Ed. Chapter 241 Page 1733*

- A. Reentrant arrhythmias dependent on AV nodal conduction
- B. Large reentry circuits within atrial tissue alone
- C. Focal atrial tachycardias due to automaticity or reentry circuits
- D. All of the above

Mechanisms of pathologic supraventricular tachycardia can be reentrant arrhythmias dependent on AV nodal conduction (AV reentry), large reentry circuits within atrial tissue alone (atrial flutter) or focal atrial tachycardias due to automaticity or small reentry circuits.

**485. Paroxysmal supraventricular tachycardia (PSVT) refers to?**
*Harrison's 20th Ed. Chapter 241 Page 1733*

- A. AV node reentry
- B. AV reentry using an accessory pathway
- C. Atrial tachycardia
- D. All of the above

Paroxysmal supraventricular tachycardia (PSVT) refers to a family of tachycardias including AV node reentry, AV reentry using an accessory pathway and atrial tachycardia.

**486. The most common supraventricular tachycardia is?**
*Harrison's 20th Ed. Chapter 241 Page 1733*

- A. Physiologic sinus tachycardia
- B. Inappropriate sinus tachycardia
- C. Focal atrial tachycardia (AT)
- D. Atrial fibrillation

The most common supraventricular tachycardia is sinus tachycardia in response to physiologic stress, such as exercise, but it can also be a manifestation acute illness.

**487. Which of the following is a tachycardia not originating from the atrium?**
*Harrison's 20th Ed. Chapter 241 Page 1733 Table 241-1*

- A. Atrial flutter
- B. Atrial fibrillation
- C. Preexcited tachycardia
- D. Multifocal atrial tachycardia

**488. Which of the following is the most common sustained cardiac arrhythmia in older adults?**
*Harrison's 20th Ed. Chapter 241 Page 1733 Table 241-1*

- A. Atrial flutter
- B. Atrial fibrillation
- C. Preexcited tachycardia
- D. Multifocal atrial tachycardia

**489. Which of the following is the mostly seen in patients with pulmonary disease?**
*Harrison's 20th Ed. Chapter 241 Page 1733 Table 241-1*

- A. Atrial flutter
- B. Atrial fibrillation
- C. Preexcited tachycardia
- D. Multifocal atrial tachycardia

**490. Which of the following is the most common paroxysmal sustained tachycardia in healthy young adults?**
*Harrison's 20th Ed. Chapter 241 Page 1733 Table 241-1*

- A. AV nodal reentry tachycardia (AVNRT)
- B. Atrial fibrillation
- C. Preexcited tachycardia
- D. Multifocal atrial tachycardia

**491. Which of the following is a wide QRS tachycardia with QRS morphology similar to VT?**
*Harrison's 20th Ed. Chapter 241 Page 1733 Table 241-1*

- A. AV nodal reentry tachycardia (AVNRT)
- B. Atrial fibrillation
- C. Preexcited tachycardia
- D. Multifocal atrial tachycardia

**492. Which of the following is a preexcited tachycardia?**
*Harrison's 20th Ed. Chapter 241 Page 1733 Table 241-1*

- A. AV nodal reentry tachycardia (AVNRT)
- B. Orthodromic AV reentry tachycardia
- C. Antidromic AV reentry tachycardia
- D. All of the above

**493. Multiple discrete P waves are seen in which of the following?**
*Harrison's 20th Ed. Chapter 241 Page 1733 Table 241-1*

- A. Atrial flutter
- B. Orthodromic AV reentry tachycardia
- C. Antidromic AV reentry tachycardia
- D. Multifocal atrial tachycardia

**494. Sawtooth waves are seen in which of the following?**
*Harrison's 20th Ed. Chapter 241 Page 1733 Table 241-1*

- A. Atrial flutter
- B. Orthodromic AV reentry tachycardia
- C. Antidromic AV reentry tachycardia
- D. Multifocal atrial tachycardia

**495. Supraventricular arrhythmia may precipitate cardiac arrest in?**
*Harrison's 20th Ed. Chapter 241 Page 1733*

- A. Wolff-Parkinson-White syndrome
- B. Eisenmenger's syndrome
- C. Marfan's syndrome
- D. Osler Weber-Rendu syndrome

Rarely, supraventricular arrhythmia may precipitate cardiac arrest in patients with Wolff-Parkinson-White syndrome or hypertrophic cardiomyopathy.

**496. In narrow complex tachycardia, regular atrial rate is seen in all except?**
*Harrison's 20th Ed. Chapter 241 Page 1734 Figure 241-1*

A. AV nodal reentry tachycardia (AVNRT)
B. Junctional tachycardia
C. Multifocal atrial tachycardia
D. Atrial flutter

**497. AV node blockade with vagal maneuvers, adenosine, verapamil or beta blockers may terminate tachycardia in?**
*Harrison's 20th Ed. Chapter 241 Page 1734 Figure 241-2*

A. AV nodal reentry tachycardia (AVNRT)
B. Orthodromic AV reentry tachycardia (ORT)
C. Focal atrial tachycardia (AT)
D. All of the above

**498. Short R-P tachycardia best relates to?**
*Harrison's 20th Ed. Chapter 241 Page 1735 Table 241-2*

A. AV nodal reentry tachycardia (AVNRT)
B. Orthodromic AV reentry tachycardia (ORT)
C. Focal atrial tachycardia (AT)
D. All of the above

## Physiologic and Nonphysiologic Sinus Tachycardia

**499. Crista terminalis is located in?**
*Harrison's 20th Ed. Chapter 242 Page 1735*

A. Right atrium
B. Left atrium
C. Right ventricle
D. Left ventricle

*Crista terminalis is a thick ridge of muscle and is a natural anatomic barrier of conduction. It is the vertical crest on interior wall of right atrium that separates nontrabeculated posterior right atrium from rest of the trabeculated right atrium.*

**500. Which of the following is an anatomic ridge in heart?**
*Harrison's 18th Ed. 1887*

A. Crista terminalis
B. Valve annuli
C. Limbus of fossa ovalis
D. All of the above

*Anatomic ridges of heart are crista terminalis, valve annuli or limbus of the fossa ovalis.*

**501. Tachyarrhythmias typically refer to?**
*Harrison's 19th Ed. 1476*

A. Isolated premature complexes (depolarizations)
B. Nonsustained forms of tachycardia originating from myocardial foci or reentrant circuits
C. Sustained forms of tachycardia originating from myocardial foci or reentrant circuits
D. All of the above

**502. Sinus P waves are characterized by all except?**
*Harrison's 20th Ed. Chapter 242 Page 1735*

A. Frontal plane axis directed inferiorly & rightward
B. Positive in leads II, III & aVF
C. Negative in aVR
D. Initially positive biphasic P wave in V1

*Sinus P waves are characterized by a frontal plane axis directed inferiorly & leftward, with positive P waves in leads II, III & aVF, a negative P wave in aVR and an initially positive biphasic P wave in V1.*

**503. In sinus tachycardia, the ventricular rate should be?**
*Harrison's 20th Ed. Chapter 242 Page 1735*

A. > 90 beats/minute
B. > 100 beats/minute
C. > 110 beats/minute
D. > 120 beats/minute

*Normal sinus rhythm has a rate of 60-100 beats/minute. Definition of tachycardia is rhythm that produces a ventricular rate >100 beats/minute.*

**504. In sinus bradycardia, the ventricular rate should be?**
*Harrison's 20th Ed. Chapter 242 Page 1735*

A. < 70 beats/minute
B. < 60 beats/minute
C. < 50 beats/minute
D. < 40 beats/minute

*Sinus bradycardia is defined as rates less than 60 beats/minute. Bradycadia can be normal during sleep and in fit individuals.*

**505. In sinus tachycardia, P waves become taller in which of the following ECG leads?**
*Harrison's 20th Ed. Chapter 242 Page 1735*

A. aVR
B. II, III, aVF
C. $V_1 - V_3$
D. $V_4 - V_6$

*In sinus tachycardia, the rate of spontaneous depolarization of sinus node increases & focus of earliest activation within the node shifts more leftward & closer to superior septal aspect of crista terminalis, producing taller P waves in the inferior limb leads when compared to normal sinus rhythm.*

**506. Which of the following is false for physiologic sinus tachycardia?**
*Harrison's 20th Ed. Chapter 242 Page 1735*

A. Present when heart rate exceeds 100 beats/min
B. Heart rate rarely exceeds 200 beats/min
C. Has a gradual onset and offset
D. Carotid sinus pressure produces slowing with sudden return to previous rate upon cessation

*Sinus tachycardia, carotid sinus pressure produces modest & transient slowing but no abrupt termination.*

**507. Which of the following conditions can cause physiologic sinus tachycardia?**
*Harrison's 20th Ed. Chapter 242 Page 1735 Table 242-1*

A. Pulmonary Insufficiency
B. Hyperthyroidism
C. Pheochromocytoma
D. All of the above

**508. Which of the following drugs can cause physiologic sinus tachycardia?**
*Harrison's 20th Ed. Chapter 242 Page 1735 Table 242-1*

A. Tricyclic antidepressants
B. Theophylline
C. Nifedipine
D. All of the above

**509. Which of the following about inappropriate sinus tachycardia is false?**
*Harrison's 20th Ed. Chapter 242 Page 1735*

A. Heart rate increases spontaneously
B. Heart rate increases out of proportion to stress/exercise
C. Therapy is ineffective or poorly tolerated
D. Anxiolytics are the treatment of choice

*In inappropriate sinus tachycardia, heart rate increases either spontaneously or out of proportion to the degree of physiologic stress/exercise. It must be distinguished from appropriate sinus tachycardia and from focal atrial tachycardia.*

**510.** Which of the following about inappropriate sinus tachycardia is false?

*Harrison's 20th Ed. Chapter 242 Page 1735*

A. Sinus rate increases spontaneously at rest
B. Sinus rate out of proportion to physiologic stress or exertion
C. Affects women in third or fourth decade of life
D. None of the above

In "inappropriate sinus tachycardia" the sinus rate increases spontaneously at rest or out of proportion to physiologic stress or exertion. Affected individuals are often women in third or fourth decade of life. It must be distinguished from appropriate sinus tachycardia and from focal atrial tachycardia. Therapy is often ineffective or poorly tolerated with beta blockers and/or calcium channel blockers, clonidine, serotonin reuptake inhibitors and Ivabradine.

**511.** Which of the following drugs block the current that causes sinus node depolarization?

*Harrison's 20th Ed. Chapter 242 Page 1736*

A. Digoxin
B. Mexiletine
C. Ivabradine
D. Midodrine

Ivabradine blocks the $I_f$ current that causes sinus node depolarization.

**512.** Postural orthostatic tachycardia syndrome (POTS) is diagnosed when on standing heart rate increases by?

*Harrison's 20th Ed. Chapter 242 Page 1736*

A. 10 beats / minute
B. 20 beats / minute
C. 30 beats / minute
D. 40 beats / minute

**513.** Postural orthostatic tachycardia syndrome (POTS) is diagnosed when on standing heart rate increases to?

*Harrison's 20th Ed. Chapter 242 Page 1736*

A. > 100 beats / minute
B. > 110 beats / minute
C. > 120 beats / minute
D. > 130 beats / minute

Postural orthostatic tachycardia syndrome (POTS) is characterized by symptomatic orthostatic intolerance without OH, accompanied by either an increase in heart rate to > 120 beats/minute or an increase of 30 beats/minute within 10 minutes of standing. It may occur after a viral illness and resolve spontaneously over 3 - 12 months (postviral dysautonomia).

**514.** Which of the following drugs is of use in postural orthostatic tachycardia syndrome (POTS)?

*Harrison's 20th Ed. Chapter 242 Page 1736*

A. Fludrocortisone
B. Midodrine
C. Volume expansion with salt supplementation
D. All of the above

Volume expansion with salt supplementation, oral fludrocortisone, compression stockings, alpha-agonist midodrine, can be helpful in POTS. Reconditioning and exercise training also improves symptoms.

## Focal Atrial Tachycardia

**515. Focal Atrial Tachycardia can be due to?**
*Harrison's 20th Ed. Chapter 243 Page 1736*

A. Abnormal automaticity
B. Triggered automaticity
C. Small reentry circuit
D. All of the above

**516. Atrial tissue may extend into?**
*Harrison's 20th Ed. Chapter 243 Page 1736*

A. Pulmonary vein
B. Coronary sinus
C. Vena cava
D. All of the above

Focal atrial tachycardia (AT) can be due to abnormal automaticity, triggered automaticity or a small reentry circuit confined to atrium or atrial tissue extending into a pulmonary vein, the coronary sinus or vena cava.

**517. Focal Atrial Tachycardia can be?**
*Harrison's 20th Ed. Chapter 243 Page 1736*

A. Sustained
B. Nonsustained
C. Paroxysmal or incessant
D. Any of the above

**518. Which of the following is false about focal AT?**
*Harrison's 20th Ed. Chapter 243 Page 1736*

A. May lead to atrial fibrillation and flutter
B. Due to atrial fibrosis
C. Sympathetic stimulation is a promoting factor
D. None of the above

**519. Incessant AT can cause?**
*Harrison's 20th Ed. Chapter 243 Page 1736*

A. Complete heart block
B. CHF
C. Tachycardia-induced cardiomyopathy
D. All of the above

Incessant AT can cause tachycardia-induced cardiomyopathy.

**520. Which of the following is false about focal AT?**
*Harrison's 20th Ed. Chapter 243 Page 1736*

A. AT will not terminate with AV block
B. Accelerated warm-up or cool-down phase
C. P waves are often discrete
D. R-P interval shorter than the P-R interval

In focal AT, P-R interval is shorter than the R-P interval. P-wave morphology differs depending on the location of the focus.

**521. Focal AT tends to originate in?**
*Harrison's 20th Ed. Chapter 243 Page 1736*

A. Crista terminalis
B. Valve annuli
C. Atrial septum
D. Any of the above

Focal AT tends to originate in areas of complex atrial anatomy like crista terminalis, valve annuli, atrial septum and atrial muscle extending along cardiac thoracic veins (superior vena cava, coronary sinus and pulmonary veins). The location can be estimated by P-wave morphology.

**522. In focal AT, P wave will resemble that of sinus tachycardia when the focus originates in?**
*Harrison's 20th Ed. Chapter 243 Page 1736*

A. Superior aspect of crista terminalis
B. Superior pulmonary veins
C. Left atrium
D. Ostium of the coronary sinus

AT from the right atrium has a positive P-wave morphology in lead 1 and biphasic P-wave morphology in lead V1. AT from the atrial septum will frequently have a narrower P-wave duration than sinus rhythm. AT from the left atrium will usually have a monophasic, positive P wave in lead V1. AT that originates from superior atrial locations, such as the superior vena cava or superior pulmonary veins, will be positive in the inferior limb leads II, III and aVF, whereas AT from a more inferior location, such as the ostium of the coronary sinus, will inscribe negative P waves in these same leads. When the focus is in the superior aspect of the crista terminalis, close to the sinus node, however, the P wave will resemble that of sinus tachycardia.

**523. Focal ATs can be distinguished by?**
*Harrison's 20th Ed. Chapter 243 Page 1736*

A. Response to adenosine
B. Response to amiodarone
C. Response to verapamil
D. All of the above

Focal ATs can be distinguished by observations made at AT initiation & in response to adenosine.

**524. Which of the following drugs is used to terminate reentrant SVT involving AV node?**
*Harrison's 20th Ed. Chapter 243 Page 1738 Table 243-1*

A. Amiodarone
B. Adenosine
C. Digoxin
D. All of the above

**525. Which of the following drugs is indicated in Long QT syndrome?**
*Harrison's 20th Ed. Chapter 243 Page 1738 Table 243-1*

A. Amiodarone
B. Verapamil
C. Digoxin
D. Metoprolol

526. Which of the following drugs is indicated in Long QT syndrome?
   *Harrison's 20th Ed. Chapter 243 Page 1738 Table 243-2*
   A. Atenolol
   B. Acebutolol
   C. Metoprolol
   D. All of the above

527. Which of the following drugs is indicated in exercise induced VT?
   *Harrison's 20th Ed. Chapter 243 Page 1738 Table 243-1*
   A. Amiodarone
   B. Verapamil
   C. Digoxin
   D. Metoprolol

528. Which of the following drugs is indicated for prevention of atrial fibrillation?
   *Harrison's 20th Ed. Chapter 243 Page 1738 Table 243-2*
   A. Dofetilide
   B. Dronedarone
   C. Disopyramide
   D. All of the above

529. Long QT and Torsades des pointes is the proarrhythmic toxicity of which of the following antiarrhythmic agent?
   *Harrison's 20th Ed. Chapter 243 Page 1738 Table 243-3*
   A. Ibutilide
   B. Amiodarone
   C. Procainamide
   D. All of the above

530. Ataxia, tremor, gait disturbances is the toxicity of which of the following antiarrhythmic agent?
   *Harrison's 20th Ed. Chapter 243 Page 1738 Table 243-3*
   A. Mexiletine
   B. Propafenone
   C. Procainamide
   D. Disopyramide

531. Acute urinary retention is the toxicity of which of the following antiarrhythmic agent?
   *Harrison's 20th Ed. Chapter 243 Page 1738 Table 243-3*
   A. Mexiletine
   B. Propafenone
   C. Procainamide
   D. Disopyramide

532. Taste disturbance is the toxicity of which of the following antiarrhythmic agent?
   *Harrison's 20th Ed. Chapter 243 Page 1738 Table 243-3*
   A. Mexiletine
   B. Propafenone
   C. Procainamide
   D. Disopyramide

533. Lupus erythematosus–like syndrome is the toxicity of which of the following antiarrhythmic agent?
   *Harrison's 20th Ed. Chapter 243 Page 1738 Table 243-3*
   A. Mexiletine
   B. Propafenone
   C. Procainamide
   D. Disopyramide

# Paroxysmal Supraventricular Tachycardias

**534. Supraventricular tachycardia (SVT) refers?**
*Am Fam Physician. 2015;92(9):793-800*

A. Atrioventricular nodal reentrant tachycardia (AVNRT)
B. Atrioventricular reciprocating tachycardia (AVRT)
C. Atrial tachycardia
D. All of the above

Supraventricular tachycardia (SVT) refers to rapid rhythms that originate and are sustained in atrial or atrioventricular nodal tissue, and then transmit through bundle of His and cause rapid ventricular response. Although atrial flutter, atrial fibrillation, and multifocal atrial tachycardia also arise from this area, in practice, SVT refers to atrioventricular nodal reentrant tachycardia (AVNRT), atrioventricular reciprocating tachycardia (AVRT), and atrial tachycardia.

**535. Which of the following about AV nodal reentry tachycardia (AVNRT) is false?**
*Harrison's 20th Ed. Chapter 244 Page 1739*

A. Most common paroxysmal regular SVT
B. More common in men than in women
C. Typically manifests in II to IV decades of life
D. Occur in the absence of structural heart disease

AV nodal reentrant tachycardia is the most common paroxysmal regular SVT. It is more common in women than in men (>2:1). Typically manifests in second to fourth decades of life and tends to occur in the absence of structural heart disease, it is usually well tolerated.

**536. AVNRT is more common during?**
*Am Fam Physician. 2015;92(9):793-800*

A. Follicular phase of the menstrual cycle
B. Luteal phase of the menstrual cycle
C. Pregnancy
D. All of the above

AVNRT incidence in women is twice that in men. It is correlated with lower estrogen levels & higher progesterone levels, and is therefore more common during luteal phase of the menstrual cycle and less common during pregnancy.

**537. Most forms of AVNRT utilize which of the following AV nodal pathway?**
*Harrison's 20th Ed. Chapter 244 Page 1739*

A. Right inferior extension
B. Left inferior extension
C. Right superior extension
D. Left superior extension

Most forms of AVNRT utilize a slowly conducting (α) AV nodal pathway (right inferior extension) that extends from the compact AV node near His bundle, inferiorly along the tricuspid valve annulus to floor of coronary sinus. The reentry wavefront propagates up this slowly conducting pathway to the compact AV node and then exits from the fast pathway at the top of the AV node. The path back to the slow pathway probably involves the left atrial septum which has connections to the coronary sinus musculature.

**538. Which of the following is false about atrioventricular nodal reentrant tachycardia?**
*N Engl J Med. 2016; 374:e17*

A. Regular tachycardia
B. Narrow QRS complex
C. Narrow P waves deforming the terminal QRS complex
D. None of the above

**539. Which of the following is false about atrioventricular nodal reentrant tachycardia (AVNRT)?**
*Am Fam Physician. 2015;92(9):793-800*

A. Antegrade conduction down in slow AV nodal pathway
B. Retrograde conduction up in the fast AV nodal pathway
C. Pseudo–R wave in lead V1 is the P wave
D. None of the above

**540. Which of the following is false about atrioventricular nodal reentrant tachycardia (AVNRT)?**
*N Engl J Med. 2016; 374:e17*

A. Re-entrant rhythm confined to the AV node
B. Fast (β) pathway has fast conduction & long refractory period
C. Slow (α) pathway has slow conduction & short refractory period
D. None of the above

The fast and slow fibres form the circuit for AVNRT. Each revolution of the circuit generates an impulse that exits the AV node via the His bundle to activate the ventricles. Because atria and ventricles are activated simultaneously the P wave is either buried within the QRS complex or inscribed just after it. The P wave is narrower than in sinus rhythm because left and right atria are activated simultaneously not sequentially.

**541. Which of the following relate to atrioventricular nodal reentrant tachycardia?**
*Harrison's 20th Ed. Chapter 244 Page 1739*

A. Pseudo-S wave
B. Pseudo-r' wave
C. Cannon A waves
D. All of the above

In typical forms, the conduction time from the compact AV node region to atrium is similar to that from compact node to His bundle and ventricles. Therefore, atrial activation occurs at about the same time as ventricular activation. P wave is seen at the end of the QRS complex as a pseudo-r' (r' prime) in lead V1 (an appearance similar to incomplete RBBB) and pseudo-S waves in leads II, III, and aVF, typical of slow-fast AVNRT.

**542. "Frog sign" is best related to?**
*N Engl J Med. 2016; 374:e17*

A. Arterial pulse
B. Jugular veins
C. Abdominal pulsations
D. Nail beds

**543. "Frog sign" is best related to?**
*N Engl J Med. 2016; 374:e17*

A. Atrial fibrillation
B. Atrioventricular nodal reentrant tachycardia
C. Ventricular tachycardia
D. All of the above

In atrioventricular nodal reentrant tachycardia, the characteristic flapping or bulging appearance of the neck vein pulsations are felt due to simultaneous atrial & ventricular contraction, and a "frog sign" is identified on physical examination during arrhythmia.

### 544. Which of the following is a symptom of AVNRT?
*Harrison's 20th Ed. Chapter 244 Page 1739*

A. Polydipsia
B. Polyuria
C. Anorexia
D. Polyphagia

*Elevated venous pressures in AVNRT may lead to release of natriuretic peptides that cause post-tachycardia diuresis.*

### 545. Which of the following is a type of AVNRT?
*https://www.ncbi.nlm.nih.gov/books/NBK499936*

A. Slow-Fast AVNRT
B. Fast-Slow AVNRT
C. Slow-Slow AVNRT
D. All of the above

*A Slow-Fast AVNRT accounts for 90% of AVNRTs with anterograde conduction by the slow AV nodal pathway and retrograde conduction by the fast AV nodal pathway.*

### 546. Pseudo-S wave in II, III, AVF and Pseudo-R' in V1 are a feature of?
*https://www.ncbi.nlm.nih.gov/books/NBK499936*

A. Slow-Fast AVNRT
B. Fast-Slow AVNRT
C. Slow-Slow AVNRT
D. All of the above

### 547. P waves between QRS and T waves (QRS-P-T complexes) is a feature of?
*https://www.ncbi.nlm.nih.gov/books/NBK499936*

A. Slow-Fast AVNRT
B. Fast-Slow AVNRT
C. Slow-Slow AVNRT
D. All of the above

### 548. Late P waves after a QRS, appearing as atrial tachycardia is a feature of?
*https://www.ncbi.nlm.nih.gov/books/NBK499936*

A. Slow-Fast AVNRT
B. Fast-Slow AVNRT
C. Slow-Slow AVNRT
D. All of the above

*The anatomy of re-entrant circuit defines the type of AVNRT. A Slow-Fast AVNRT accounts for 90% of AVNRTs with anterograde conduction by slow AV nodal pathway & retrograde conduction by fast AV nodal pathway. Fast-slow AVNRT represents ~5 - 10% of AVNRTs with anterograde conduction by fast AV nodal pathway and retrograde conduction by slow AV nodal pathway. Slow-slow AVNRTs account 1 - 5% of AVNRTs with anterograde conduction by slow AV nodal pathways and retrograde conduction by slow atrial fibers.*

### 549. Which of the following can cause a regular, narrow QRS complex tachycardia?
*https://www.ncbi.nlm.nih.gov/books/NBK499936*

A. Intra-atrial reentrant tachycardia
B. Sinoatrial nodal reentrant tachycardia
C. Junctional ectopic tachycardia
D. All of the above

*A regular, narrow QRS complex tachycardia can be caused by Atrioventricular nodal reentrant tachycardia, Atrioventricular reentrant tachycardia, Intraatrial reentrant tachycardia, Sinoatrial nodal reentrant tachycardia, Junctional ectopic tachycardia, Atrial tachycardia, Atrial flutter, Sinus tachycardia and Inappropriate sinus tachycardia*

### 550. Atrial-His / His-atrial ratio (AH/HA) in typical (slow-fast) AVNRT is?
*Circulation. 2016;134:1655-1663*

A. > 0.25
B. > 0.50
C. > 0.75
D. > 1.00

### 551. HA interval in typical (slow-fast) AVNRT is?
*Circulation. 2016;134:1655-1663*

A. ≤ 70 ms
B. ≤ 90 ms
C. ≤ 110 ms
D. ≤ 130 ms

*Typical (slow-fast) AVNRT was defined by an atrial-His/His-atrial ratio (AH/HA) >1, and HA interval ≤70 ms. Atypical AVNRT was defined by delayed retrograde atrial activation with HA>70 ms. If the AH was <200 ms and the AH<HA, the atypical form was characterized as fast-slow. If AH >200 ms and AH>HA, the atypical form is considered slow-slow. Tachycardias with a prolonged AH interval >200 ms but AH<HA, or with AH<200 ms and AH>HA, or with variable intervals during the same or different episodes, are classified as indeterminate.*

### 552. Which of the following about AVNRT is false?
*Harrison's 20th Ed. Chapter 244 Page 1739*

A. Fast pathway has a longer refractory period
B. Slow pathway lower in the AV node region
C. During sinus rhythm, conduction is through both pathways
D. None of the above

*Fast pathway is in superior part of AV node and has a longer refractory period, whereas pathway lower in AV node region conducts more slowly and has a shorter refractory period. During sinus rhythm, conduction is through both pathways.*

### 553. Which of the following occurs in a typical AV nodal reentrant tachycardia?
*Harrison's 20th Ed. Chapter 244 Page 1739*

A. Repetitive activation up slow and down fast pathway
B. Repetitive activation down slow and up fast pathway
C. Repetitive activation down slow pathway
D. Repetitive activation down fast pathway

*Repetitive activation down the slow and up the fast pathway results in typical AV nodal reentrant tachycardia.*

### 554. Atrioventricular nodal reentrant tachycardia is caused by a reentrant loop that involves atrioventricular node and?
*N Engl J Med. 2012;367:1438-48*

A. Atrial tissue
B. Ventricular tissue
C. Bundle of His
D. Fascicles

*Atrioventricular nodal reentrant tachycardia is caused by a reentrant loop that involves the atrioventricular node and the atrial tissue.*

### 555. P waves immediately precede the QRS complex in all except?
*N Engl J Med. 2012;367:1438-48*

A. Atrial tachycardia
B. Multifocal atrial tachycardia
C. Atrioventricular nodal reentrant tachycardia
D. Multiple atrial premature contractions

*P waves immediately precede the QRS complex in sinus tachycardia, atrial tachycardia, multifocal atrial tachycardia, and multiple atrial premature contractions. P waves follow the QRS complex in atrioventricular nodal reentrant tachycardia and atrioventricular reciprocating tachycardia.*

**556. Junctional ectopic tachycardia (JET) is due to automaticity within the?**
*Harrison's 20th Ed. Chapter 244 Page 1739*

A. AV node
B. Bundle of His
C. Bundle branch
D. Purkinje fibers

*Junctional ectopic tachycardia (JET) is due to automaticity within the AV node.*

**557. Which of the following about junctional ectopic tachycardia (JET) is false?**
*Harrison's 20th Ed. Chapter 244 Page 1739*

A. Narrow QRS tachycardia
B. Often with ventriculoatrial (VA) block
C. May be seen after administration of isoproterenol
D. None of the above

**558. What is the heart rate in accelerated junctional rhythm?**
*Harrison's 20th Ed. Chapter 244 Page 1739*

A. 40 to 60 beats / minute
B. 50 to 100 beats / minute
C. 100 to 120 beats / minute
D. 120 to 160 beats / minute

*Accelerated junctional rhythm is a junctional automatic rhythm between 50 and 100 beats/minute.*

**559. Which of the followig resembles AVNRT at a slow rate?**
*Harrison's 20th Ed. Chapter 244 Page 1739*

A. First degree heart block
B. Torsade de pointes
C. Multifocal atrial tachycardia
D. Accelerated junctional rhythm

**560. Which of the following is false about automatic atrial tachycardias?**
*Harrison's 19th Ed. 1479*

A. Respond to adenosine
B. Provoked by isoproterenol infusion
C. First P wave of AT has same morphology as remaining waves
D. None of the above

*Automatic ATs start with a "warm-up" period over the first 3 - 10 complexes and slow in rate before termination. They may respond to adenosine. Initiation of automatic ATs frequently can be provoked by isoproterenol infusion. First P wave of tachycardia has same morphology as remaining waves.*

**561. Which of the following is false about focal reentrant atrial tachycardias?**
*Harrison's 19th Ed. 1479*

A. Initiate with spontaneous premature beats
B. P wave initiating tachycardia has different morphology than P wave during sustained AT
C. Do not slow and/or terminate with adenosine
D. None of the above

*Focal reentrant AT initiate with programmed atrial stimulation or spontaneous premature beats. P wave initiating tachycardia has a different morphology than P wave during sustained AT. P wave in AT is characteristically distinct from the sinus P-wave morphology. With adenosine, reentrant ATs will produce AV block but typically do not slow and/or terminate.*

**562. Which of the following arrhythmia may be a manifestation of digoxin toxicity?**
*Harrison's 18th Ed. 1888*

A. Multifocal atrial tachycardia
B. Focal atrial tachycardias
C. AV junctional tachycardias
D. AV nodal reentrant tachycardia

**563. Junctional tachycardia due to abnormal automaticity can be treated pharmacologically with?**
*Harrison's 18th Ed. 1888*

A. Digitalis
B. Beta blockers
C. Calcium channel blockers
D. All of the above

*Junctional tachycardia due to abnormal automaticity can be treated with beta blockers.*

**564. AV bypass tracts are associated with which of the following?**
*Harrison's 20th Ed. Chapter 244 Page 1739*

A. Narrow-complex PSVT
B. Wide-complex tachycardias
C. Sudden death
D. All of the above

**565. Accessory pathways (APs) are associated with which of the following?**
*Harrison's 20th Ed. Chapter 244 Page 1739*

A. Ebstein's anomaly of the tricuspid valve
B. Forms of HCM including PRKAG2 mutations
C. Danon's disease
D. All of the above

**566. AV bypass tracts are associated with which of the following congenital abnormalities?**
*Harrison's 20th Ed. Chapter 244 Page 1739*

A. ASD
B. VSD
C. TOF
D. Ebstein's anomaly

*Accessory pathways (APs) are associated with Ebstein's anomaly of the tricuspid valve and forms of hypertrophic cardiomyopathy including PRKA G2 mutations, Danon's disease and Fabry's disease.*

**567. Which of the following statements about accessory pathways (APs) is false?**
*Harrison's 20th Ed. Chapter 244 Page 1739*

A. Abnormal connections
B. Allow conduction between atrium & ventricles across AV ring
C. Present from birth
D. None of the above

**568. The most common accessory pathway (AP) connects which of the following?**
*Harrison's 20th Ed. Chapter 244 Page 1740*

A. Left atrium to left ventricle
B. Right atrium to right ventricle
C. Left atrium to right ventricle
D. Right atrium to left ventricle

*The most common AP connects the left atrium to the left ventricle, followed by posterior septal, right free wall, and anterior septal APs.*

569. Accessory pathways (APs) occur most frequently between?
*Harrison's 20th Ed. Chapter 244 Page 1740*
   A. Left atrium and free wall of left ventricle
   B. Left atrium and posteroseptal
   C. Left atrium and anteroseptal
   D. Left atrium and right free wall

*APs are abnormal connections that allow conduction between the atrium and ventricles across the AV ring. They are present from birth and are due to failure of complete partitioning of atrium and ventricle by the fibrous AV rings. APs occur across either an AV valve annulus or septum, most frequently between the left atrium and free wall of left ventricle, followed by posteroseptal, right free wall and anteroseptal locations.*

570. Which of the following occurs when ventricles are "preexcited" during sinus rhythm?
*Harrison's 20th Ed. Chapter 244 Page 1740*
   A. Short P-R interval (<0.12 second)
   B. Slurred initial portion of the QRS (delta wave)
   C. Prolonged QRS duration
   D. All of the above

*If the impulse from sinus node conducts through AP to ventricle (antegrade) before the impulse conducts through AV node & His bundle, the ventricles are "preexcited" during sinus rhythm, and ECG shows a short P-R interval (<0.12 second), slurred initial portion of QRS (delta wave), and prolonged QRS duration produced by slow conduction through direct activation of ventricular myocardium over the AP.*

571. The morphology of the QRS and delta wave is determined by?
*Harrison's 20th Ed. Chapter 244 Page 1740*
   A. Thickness of accessory pathway
   B. Length of accessory pathway
   C. Location of accessory pathway
   D. All of the above

*The morphology of the QRS and delta wave is determined by the AP location and the degree of fusion between the excitation wave fronts from conduction over the AV node and conduction over the AP.*

572. Which of the following is false about right-sided accessory pathways?
*Harrison's 20th Ed. Chapter 244 Page 1740*
   A. Create marked preexcitation
   B. Preexcite the right ventricle
   C. Produce an LBBB like configuration in lead V1
   D. None of the above

*Right-sided pathways preexcite right ventricle, produce a left bundle branch block–like configuration in lead V1, and often create marked preexcitation because of relatively close proximity of the AP to sinus node.*

573. Which of the following is false about left-sided accessory pathways?
*Harrison's 20th Ed. Chapter 244 Page 1740*
   A. Produce a right bundle branch like configuration in lead $V_1$
   B. Produce a negative delta wave in aVL
   C. Preexcitation may be minimal or absent
   D. None of the above

*Left-sided pathways preexcite left ventricle & produce a right bundle branch–like configuration in lead V1 and a negative delta wave in aVL, due to initial depolarization of lateral portion of left ventricle. Due to a relatively large distance between sinus node & left free wall APs, preexcitation may be minimal or absent on 12-lead ECG.*

574. Delta waves may be negative in leads III and aVF when preexcitation due to an AP is at?
*Harrison's 20th Ed. Chapter 244 Page 1740*
   A. Left lateral wall
   B. Right lateral wall
   C. Diaphragmatic surface
   D. All of the above

*Preexcitation due to an AP at the diaphragmatic surface of heart produces delta waves that are negative in leads III & aVF, mimicking q waves of inferior wall infarction.*

575. Preexcitation can be intermittent and disappear during?
*Harrison's 20th Ed. Chapter 244 Page 1740*
   A. Sleep
   B. Hyperventilation
   C. Exercise
   D. All of the above

*Preexcitation can be intermittent & disappear during exercise as conduction over AV node accelerates and may take over ventricular activation completely.*

576. Which of the following rhythms is associated with WPW syndrome?
*Harrison's 20th Ed. Chapter 244 Page 1741 Figure 244-3*
   A. Sinus rhythm - antegrade AP conduction
   B. Orthodromic AV reentry - retrograde AP conduction
   C. Antidromic AV reentry - antegrade AP conduction
   D. All of the above

*Most common rhythms associated with WPW syndrome are sinus rhythm with antegrade conduction over AP & AV node, orthodromic AVRT using retrograde conduction over AP and antegrade conduction over AV node and antidromic AVRT using retrograde conduction over AV node and antegrade conduction over AP.*

577. Which of the following about concealed accessory pathways is false?
*Harrison's 20th Ed. Chapter 244 Page 1740*
   A. Allow only retrograde conduction, from ventricle to atrium
   B. No preexcitation is present during sinus rhythm
   C. SVT can occur
   D. None of the above

578. Which of the following statements about accessory pathways (APs) is correct?
*Harrison's 20th Ed. Chapter 244 Page 1740*
   A. APs connect the atria with the ventricles
   B. There may be no delta wave in the ECG of concealed APs
   C. More than 50% of APs are located at the left free wall
   D. All of the above

579. Pseudopreexcitation syndrome is related to which of the following?
*Cleveland Clinic J of Medicine 2018;85(7):508*
   A. Hypoplastic left heart syndrome
   B. Atrioventricular canal defect
   C. Ebstein anomaly
   D. All of the above

*A short PR interval with or without delta waves can also be seen in the absence of an accessory pathway, e.g. in hypoplastic left heart syndrome, atrioventricular canal defect, and Ebstein anomaly. These conditions are termed pseudopreexcitation syndrome.*

580. Wolff-Parkinson-White (WPW) syndrome is defined as?
*Harrison's 20th Ed. Chapter 244 Page 1740*
   A. A preexcited QRS
   B. During sinus rhythm
   C. Episodes of PSVT
   D. All of the above

### 581. WPW pattern is defined by preexcitation findings on ECG without?
*Cleveland Clinic J of Medicine. 2018;85(7):508*

A. Family history
B. Genetic predisposition
C. Symptomatic arrhythmias
D. All of the above

*WPW pattern is defined only by preexcitation findings on ECG without symptomatic arrhythmias. Patients with WPW syndrome can present with palpitation, dizziness, and syncope resulting from underlying arrhythmia. This is not seen in patients with WPW pattern.*

### 582. WPW pattern can be unmasked by?
*Cleveland Clinic J of Medicine. 2018;85(7):508*

A. Anesthesia
B. Sympathomimetic drugs
C. Postoperatively
D. All of the above

*WPW pattern can be unmasked by anesthesia, sympathomimetic drugs, and postoperatively.*

### 583. Which of the following about atriofascicular accessory pathways is false?
*Harrison's 20th Ed. Chapter 244 Page 1740*

A. Originate from the right atrium
B. Conduct more slowly
C. Has decremental antegrade conduction
D. None of the above

### 584. Which of the following is an accessory pathway?
*Circulation. 2016;133(14):e506-74*

A. Nodo-fascicular
B. Nodo-ventricular
C. Fasciculoventricular
D. All of the above

*Accessory pathways include atriofascicular, nodo-fascicular, nodo-ventricular, and fasciculoventricular pathways.*

### 585. Which of the following accessory pathway do not cause arrhythmia?
*Harrison's 20th Ed. Chapter 244 Page 1740*

A. Atriofascicular
B. Fasciculoventricular
C. Atrioventricular
D. None of the above

*Fasciculoventricular connections between the His bundle and ventricular septum produce preexcitation but do not cause arrhythmia, probably because the circuit is too short to promote reentry.*

### 586. Which of the following best relates to connection between right atrium to fascicles of the right bundle branch?
*Harrison's 20th Ed. Chapter 244 Page 1740*

A. James fibers
B. Bundle of Kent
C. Mahaim fibers
D. Brechenmacher fibers

*There are several types of accessory pathways. The classic accessory pathway is the AV bypass tract or bundle of Kent in WPW that directly connects atrial and ventricular myocardium, bypassing the AV node/His-Purkinje system. James fibers or atrionodal tracts, connect atrium to distal or compact AV node. Brechenmacher fibers (atrio-Hisian tracts) connect the atrium to His bundle. Atriofascicular pathways, also known as Mahaim fibers, probably represent a duplicate AV node and His-Purkinje system that connect the right atrium to fascicles of the right bundle branch and conduct slowly only in the anterograde direction.*

### 587. Wolff-Parkinson-White syndrome is best related to?
*N Engl J Med. 1987; 317:109-111*

A. James fibers
B. Bundle of Kent
C. Mahaim fibers
D. Brechenmacher fibers

*Preexcitation through an AV bypass tract, the bundle of Kent, produces the ECG pattern described by Wolff, Parkinson, and White in 1930. Bundle of Kent in WPW directly connects atrial & ventricular myocardium, bypassing the AV node/His-Purkinje system. AV conduction is nondecremental and more rapid through the accessory pathway than through the AV node, a difference that is increased at fast heart rates. Decremental conduction means increase in conduction time of the impulse propagating through the AV node as the cycle length shortens (heart rate increased).*

### 588. Classic electrocardiographic triad in WPW syndrome includes all except?
*N Engl J Med. 2003;349:1787*

A. Short PR interval
B. Slurred QRS upstroke (delta wave)
C. Prolonged QRS complex
D. Prolonged QT interval

*In WPW syndrome, classic electrocardiographic triad is a short PR interval, a slurred QRS upstroke (delta wave), and a prolonged QRS complex.*

### 589. Most common arrhythmia associated with WPW syndrome is?
*N Engl J Med. 2003;349:1787*

A. Atrioventricular reciprocating tachycardia
B. Atrioventricular nodal reentrant tachycardia
C. Atrial tachycardia
D. Multifocal atrial tachycardia

*Most common arrhythmia associated with WPW syndrome is atrioventricular reciprocating tachycardia.*

### 590. The following are ECG features of WPW syndrome except?
*Harrison's 20th Ed. Chapter 244 Page 1740*

A. Presence of delta wave
B. Shortened PR interval of < 0.12 seconds
C. PR depression
D. Prolonged QRS interval of > 0.12 seconds

### 591. Which of the following are known conditions associated with WPW syndrome?
*Harrison's 20th Ed. Chapter 244 Page 1740*

A. ST elevation myocardial infarction
B. Ebstein anomaly
C. Acute pericarditis
D. Marfan's syndrome

### 592. The WPW ECG may mimic the following?
*Harrison's 20th Ed. Chapter 244 Page 1740*

A. Left ventricular hypertrophy
B. Right ventricular hypertrophy
C. Bundle branch block
D. All of the above

**593. AV bypass tract in ventricular preexcitation are composed of?**
*Harrison's 20th Ed. Chapter 244 Page 1740*

A. Atrial-like muscle
B. Ventricular-like muscle
C. Specialized conduction tissue
D. All of the above

**594. Which of the following is not a feature of Wolff-Parkinson-White (WPW) syndrome?**
*Harrison's 20th Ed. Chapter 244 Page 1740*

A. Short PR interval (< 0.12 sec.)
B. Slurred upstroke of QRS complex (delta wave)
C. Wide QRS complex
D. Prolonged QT interval

**595. Which of the following is not true regarding Wolff-Parkinson-White syndrome?**
*Harrison's 20th Ed. Chapter 244 Page 1740*

A. During PSVT in WPW, impulse is conducted antegradely over normal AV system and retrogradely through bypass tract
B. Atrial flutter and AF are common
C. Ventricular responses during atrial flutter or fibrillation is unusually rapid and may cause VF
D. Quinidine or flecainide slow conduction and increase refractoriness primarily of the AV node

**596. In AV reentry tachycardia, relation between P wave and QRS complex is?**
*Harrison's 20th Ed. Chapter 244 Page 1740*

A. P waves are simultaneous with a narrow QRS complex
B. P waves always precede the QRS
C. P waves always follow the QRS
D. Any of the above

*Unlike typical AVNRT, in AVRT, P waves always follow QRS & are never simultaneous with QRS complex because ventricles must be activated before reentry wavefront reaches AP and conducts back to atrium.*

**597. Most common tachycardia caused by an accessory pathway is?**
*Harrison's 20th Ed. Chapter 244 Page 1740*

A. Macroreentrant atrial tachycardia
B. Antidromic AV reentry
C. Orthodromic AV reentry
D. Permanent junctional reciprocating tachycardia (PJRT)

*The most common tachycardia caused by an AP is the PSVT designated orthodromic AV reentry. The circulating reentry wavefront propagates from the atrium anterogradely over the AV node and His-Purkinje system to the ventricles and then reenters the atria via retrograde conduction over the AP.*

**598. Which of the following about permanent junctional reciprocating tachycardia (PJRT) is false?**
*Harrison's 20th Ed. Chapter 244 Page 1741*

A. Slow AP conduction
B. Incessant tachycardia
C. Tachycardia-induced cardiomyopathy
D. None of the above

**599. Which of the following about permanent junctional reciprocating tachycardia (PJRT) is false?**
*Circulation. 2016;134:1655-1663*

A. Incessant orthodromic AVRT
B. Involves a slowly conducting, concealed, usually posteroseptal accessory pathway
C. Produces delayed atrial activation & a long RP interval
D. None of the above

**600. Which of the following is the most common mechanism in preexcited tachycardia?**
*Harrison's 20th Ed. Chapter 244 Page 1741*

A. Macrorerentrant atrial tachycardia
B. Antidromic AV reentry
C. Orthodromic AV reentry
D. Paroxysmal junctional reciprocating tachycardia (PJRT)

**601. Which of the following tachycardia is indistinguishable from monomorphic ventricular tachycardia?**
*Harrison's 20th Ed. Chapter 244 Page 1741*

A. Macrorerentrant atrial tachycardia
B. Antidromic AV reentry
C. Orthodromic AV reentry
D. Paroxysmal junctional reciprocating tachycardia (PJRT)

*Preexcitated tachycardia occurs when the ventricles are activated by antegrade conduction over the AP. The most common is antidromic AV reentry in which activation propagates from atrium to ventricle via the AP and then conducts retrogradely to the atria via the His-Purkinje system and the AV node.*

**602. Which of the following is false about preexcited tachycardia?**
*Harrison's 20th Ed. Chapter 244 Page 1741*

A. Presence of preexcitation in sinus rhythm
B. Atrium to ventricle activation via the AP
C. Ventricle to atrium activation via the AV node
D. None of the above

**603. Preexcited tachycardia occurs if an AP allows antegrade conduction to ventricles during?**
*Harrison's 20th Ed. Chapter 244 Page 1741*

A. AT
B. Atrial flutter
C. Atrial fibrillation
D. All of the above

**604. Which of the following is contraindicated during preexcited AF?**
*Harrison's 20th Ed. Chapter 244 Page 1741*

A. Diltiazem
B. Intravenous adenosine
C. Intravenous amiodarone
D. All of the above

*Administration of AV nodal blocking agents like oral or intravenous verapamil, diltiazem, beta blockers, intravenous adenosine, and intravenous amiodarone are contraindicated during preexcited AF.*

**605. Rapid preexcited tachycardia should be treated with?**
*Harrison's 20th Ed. Chapter 244 Page 1741*

A. Electrical cardioversion
B. Intravenous procainamide
C. Intravenous ibutilide
D. Any of the above

*Rapid preexcited tachycardia should be treated with electrical cardioversion or intravenous procainamide or ibutilide, which may terminate the arrhythmia or slow the ventricular rate.*

**606. In preexcited atrial fibrillation, what duration of shortest R-R interval indicate a risk of sudden death?**

*Harrison's 20th Ed. Chapter 244 Page 1741*

A. < 250 ms
B. < 300 ms
C. < 350 ms
D. < 400 ms

*In preexcited atrial fibrillation, shortest R-R intervals between preexcited QRS complexes of <250 ms indicate a risk of sudden death.*

**607. Patients with WPW syndrome may have wide-complex tachycardia due to?**

*Harrison's 20th Ed. Chapter 244 Page 1741*

A. Antidromic AV reentry
B. Orthodromic AV with bundle branch block
C. Preexcited tachycardia
D. Any of the above

*Patients with WPW syndrome may have wide-complex tachycardia due to antidromic AV reentry, orthodromic AV with bundle branch block, or a preexcited tachycardia, and treatment depends on the underlying rhythm.*

**608. Which of the following is a complication of catheter ablation?**

*Harrison's 20th Ed. Chapter 244 Page 1742*

A. AV block
B. Cardiac tamponade
C. Thromboemboli
D. All of the above

*Serious complications of catheter ablation occur in <3% of patients and include AV block, cardiac tamponade, thromboemboli, coronary artery injury, and vascular access complications. Procedure mortality is <1 in 1000 patients.*

**609. Which of the following rhythms is associated with WPW syndrome?**

*Harrison's 20th Ed. Chapter 244 Page 1741 Figure 244-3*

A. Sinus rhythm demonstrating antegrade conduction over the AP and AV node
B. Orthodromic AVRT using retrograde conduction over the AP and antegrade conduction over the AV node
C. Antidromic AVRT using retrograde conduction over the AV node and antegrade conduction over the AP
D. All of the above

*Three most common rhythms associated with WPW syndrome: sinus rhythm demonstrating antegrade conduction over the AP and AV node; orthodromic AVRT using retrograde conduction over the AP and antegrade conduction over the AV node; and antidromic AVRT using retrograde conduction over the AV node and antegrade conduction over the AP.*

**610. Which of the following can cause Wide–QRS Complex Tachycardia?**

*Circulation. 2016;134:1655-1663*

A. SVT with aberrant conduction
B. SVT with pre-existing bundle-branch block
C. Paced rhythm
D. All of the above

*Causes of Wide–QRS Complex Tachycardia are Ventricular tachycardia, SVT with pre-existing bundle-branch block or intraventricular conduction defect, SVT with aberrant conduction due to tachycardia (normal QRS when in sinus rhythm), SVT with wide QRS related to electrolyte or metabolic disorder, SVT with conduction over an accessory pathway (pre-excitation), Paced rhythm, Artifact.*

**611. Wide-complex tachycardia includes which of the following?**

*Harrison's 20th Ed. Chapter 244 Page 1742*

A. Ventricular tachycardia
B. PSVT with bundle branch block aberrancy
C. Preexcited tachycardia
D. All of the above

*Wide-complex tachycardia includes ventricular tachycardia, PSVT with bundle branch block aberrancy and preexcited tachycardia.*

**612. Very irregular wide-complex tachycardia should be managed with?**

*Harrison's 20th Ed. Chapter 244 Page 1742*

A. Cardioversion
B. Intravenous procainamide
C. Intravenous ibutilide
D. Any of the above

*Very irregular wide-complex tachycardia should be managed with cardioversion, intravenous procainamide or ibutilide, which presumes preexcited atrial fibrillation or flutter.*

**613. Intravenous adenosine terminates PSVT episodes by transiently blocking conduction in?**

*Harrison's 20th Ed. Chapter 244 Page 1742*

A. AV node
B. Accessory pathway
C. AV node + accessory pathway
D. None of the above

*Intravenous adenosine terminates PSVT episodes by transiently blocking conduction in the AV node.*

# Common Atrial Flutter, Macroreentrant, and Multifocal Atrial Tachycardias

**614. Which of the following statements is false about macroreentrant arrhythmias?**
*Harrison's 20th Ed. Chapter 245 Page 1743*

A. Macroreentrant arrhythmias involving atrial myocardium are called AFL
B. Nonfocal source of an atrial arrhythmia
C. AFL is poorly tolerated than AF
D. None of the above

*Macroreentrant nonfocal arrhythmias involving the atrial myocardium are referred to collectively as AFL.*

**615. Cavotricuspid isthmus-dependent atrial flutter is known as?**
*Harrison's 20th Ed. Chapter 245 Page 1743*

A. Common right atrial flutter
B. Left atrial flutter
C. Perimitral left atrial flutter
D. None of the above

*Common right atrial flutter is also known as sub-Eustachian or cavotricuspid isthmus flutter. Macroreentrant atrial tachycardia is due to a large reentry circuit, often associated with areas of scar in the atria. Common or typical right atrial flutter is due to a circuit that revolves around the tricuspid valve annulus, bounded anteriorly by the annulus and posteriorly by functional conduction block in the crista terminalis. The wavefront passes through an isthmus between the inferior vena cava and the tricuspid valve annulus, known as the sub-Eustachian or cavotricuspid isthmus.*

**616. Atrial flutter is a form of atrial reentry localized to the?**
*Harrison's 20th Ed. Chapter 245 Page 1743*

A. Right atrium
B. Left atrium
C. Both atria
D. Both atria and AV node

**617. Typical AFL circuit rotates around?**
*Harrison's 20th Ed. Chapter 245 Page 1743*

A. Mitral valve annulus
B. Tricuspid valve annulus
C. Aortic valve annulus
D. Pulmonary valve annulus

**618. In ECG, flutter waves of atrial flutter are most prominent in?**
*Harrison's 20th Ed. Chapter 245 Page 1743*

A. Inferior leads
B. Anterior leads
C. Posterior leads
D. Lateral leads

*Typical AFL circuit rotates in right atrium around tricuspid valve annulus. Counterclockwise right AFL with superiorly directed activation of interatrial septum produces saw-toothed appearance of P waves in ECG leads II, III and aVF. Clockwise rotation of right atrial circuit produces predominantly positive P waves in leads II, III, and aVF.*

**619. In atrial flutter, the atrial rate is?**
*Harrison's 20th Ed. Chapter 245 Page 1743*

A. 150 and 240 bpm
B. 240 and 300 bpm
C. 300 and 400 bpm
D. 400 and 550 bpm

*Classic or typical right AFL has an atrial rate of 240 - 300 beats/minute with a ventricular response at 2:1 or 120 - 150 beats/minute.*

**620. Which of the following is not an ECG feature of common right atrial flutter?**
*Harrison's 20th Ed. Chapter 245 Page 1744 Figure 245-1*

A. Atrial rate 240–300 beats/minute
B. Positive P waves in lead $V_1$
C. Negative "sawtooth" pattern in lead II
D. QRS duration > 0.12 seconds

*Common right atrial flutter or cavotricuspid isthmus flutter, shows on ECG positive P waves in lead V1 & negative "sawtooth" pattern in lead II, typical of counterclockwise rotation relative to the tricuspid valve annulus.*

**621. Which of the following is false about atypical atrial flutter?**
*Harrison's 20th Ed. Chapter 245 Page 1743*

A. Not dependent on conduction through cavotricuspid isthmus
B. Can occur in either atrium
C. Almost always associated with areas of atrial scar
D. None of the above

**622. Atypical atrial flutter can be difficult to distinguish from?**
*Harrison's 20th Ed. Chapter 245 Page 1743*

A. Atrial fibrillation
B. Focal AT
C. Paroxysmal supraventricular tachycardia
D. AV Nodal reentrant tachycardia

**623. Which of the following drugs is particularly effective for conversion of atrial flutter to sinus rhythm?**
*Harrison's 20th Ed. Chapter 245 Page 1743*

A. Ibutilide
B. Beta blocker
C. Calcium antagonist
D. Digitalis

*In AFL, rate control with calcium antagonists (diltiazem, verapamil), beta blockers, and/or digoxin is difficult. In patients with high anesthetic risk, pharmacologic cardioversion with procainamide, amiodarone or ibutilide is appropriate. Antiarrhythmic drug therapy may enhance efficacy of direct current cardioversion & maintenance of sinus rhythm after cardioversion.*

**624. Which of the following drugs is useful in preventing recurrences of atrial flutter?**
*Harrison's 20th Ed. Chapter 245 Page 1743*

A. Dofetilide
B. Sotalol
C. Amiodarone
D. All of the above

*For recurrent episodes, antiarrhythmic drug therapy with sotalol, dofetilide, disopyramide and amiodarone is effective.*

625. Which of the following statements about multifocal atrial tachycardia (MAT) is false?
*Harrison's 20th Ed. Chapter 245 Page 1745*

   A. Defined as ≥ 3 consecutive P waves of different morphologies at rates >100 beats/minute
   B. Common following theophylline administration
   C. Irregular ventricular rate
   D. High incidence of VF

*There is a high incidence of AF in patients with MAT.*

626. Which of the following is the signature tachycardia of significant pulmonary disease?
*Harrison's 20th Ed. Chapter 245 Page 1745*

   A. Atrial flutter
   B. Atrial fibrillation
   C. Multifocal atrial tachycardia
   D. AV Nodal reentrant tachycardia

*Multifocal AT (MAT) is the signature tachycardia of patients with significant pulmonary disease.*

627. Which of the following about multifocal atrial tachycardia is false?
*Harrison's 20th Ed. Chapter 245 Page 1745*

   A. Signature tachycardia of significant pulmonary disease
   B. Clear isoelectric intervals between P waves on ECG
   C. Absence of any intervening sinus rhythm
   D. None of the above

*Macroreentrant ATs represent continuous atrial activation and isoelectric baseline between P waves is frequently absent.*

628. Electrical cardioversion has no effect in which of the following?
*Harrison's 20th Ed. Chapter 245 Page 1745*

   A. Atrial flutter
   B. Atrial fibrillation
   C. Multifocal atrial tachycardia
   D. Paroxysmal supraventricular tachycardia

## Atrial Fibrillation

**629. Which of the following is characteristic of Atrial fibrillation?**
*Harrison's 20th Ed. Chapter 246 Page 1746*

A. Disorganized, rapid, and irregular atrial activation
B. Loss of atrial contraction
C. Irregular ventricular rate determined by AV nodal conduction
D. All of the above

Atrial fibrillation (AF) is characterized by disorganized, rapid, and irregular atrial activation with loss of atrial contraction and an irregular ventricular rate that is determined by AV nodal conduction. Patients with high vagal tone or AV nodal conduction disease have slow ventricular rates.

**630. Which of the following is characteristic of Atrial fibrillation?**
*Harrison's 20th Ed. Chapter 246 Page 1746 Figure 246-1*

A. Paroxysmal AF is initiated by premature beats
B. Persistent AF is associated with atrial structural and electrophysiologic remodeling
C. Triggering foci are an important cause of AF
D. All of the above

**631. In atrial fibrillation, the ventricular rate is usually?**
*Harrison's 20th Ed. Chapter 246 Page 1746*

A. 120 and 160 bpm
B. 150 and 180 bpm
C. 200 and 260 bpm
D. 250 and 280 bpm

AF produces disorganized, rapid & irregular atrial activation with irregular ventricular response. Depending on conduction properties of AV junction, rate varies between 120 & 160 beats/minute.

**632. Which of the following is the most common sustained arrhythmia?**
*Harrison's 20th Ed. Chapter 246 Page 1746*

A. Atrial flutter
B. Atrial fibrillation
C. AV nodal reentrant tachycardia (AVNRT)
D. None of the above

AF is the most common sustained arrhythmia.

**633. Which of the following about AF is false?**
*Harrison's 20th Ed. Chapter 246 Page 1746*

A. ~95% of AF patients are older than 60 years
B. Prevalence by age 80 years is ~10%
C. Lifetime risk of developing AF over 40 years is ~25%
D. None of the above

**634. Risk factor for developing AF is?**
*Harrison's 20th Ed. Chapter 246 Page 1746*

A. Hypertension
B. Diabetes mellitus
C. Sleep apnea
D. All of the above

AF is a marker for heart disease. Risk factors for developing AF are age, hypertension, diabetes mellitus, cardiac disease, obesity and sleep apnea.

**635. AF is associated with increased risk of?**
*Harrison's 20th Ed. Chapter 246 Page 1746*

A. Heart failure
B. Stroke
C. Dementia
D. All of the above

AF is associated with increased risk of mortality, heart failure, stroke and dementia.

**636. AF is associated with?**
*Harrison's 20th Ed. Chapter 246 Page 1746*

A. Hyperthyroidism
B. Acute alcohol intoxication
C. Pulmonary embolism
D. All of the above

AF is associated with an acute precipitating factor such as hyperthyroidism, acute alcohol intoxication or an acute illness including myocardial infarction or pulmonary embolism.

**637. Paroxysmal AF is defined by episodes that start spontaneously & stop within?**
*Harrison's 20th Ed. Chapter 246 Page 1746*

A. 24 hours of onset
B. 3 days of onset
C. 7 days of onset
D. 14 days of onset

Paroxysmal AF is defined by episodes that start spontaneously and stop within 7 days of onset.

**638. Long-standing persistent AF is defined as?**
*Harrison's 20th Ed. Chapter 246 Page 1746*

A. AF > 7 days
B. AF > 1 month
C. AF > 3 months
D. AF > 1 year

Long-standing persistent AF (>1 year), significant fibrosis is usually present and it is difficult to restore and maintain sinus rhythm.

**639. Paroxysmal AF is triggered by automatic foci located in?**
*Harrison's 20th Ed. Chapter 246 Page 1746*

A. Left atrium
B. Right atrium
C. Pulmonary veins
D. Left atrial appendage

**640. Which of the following relates best to AF initiation & maintenance?**
*Harrison's 20th Ed. Chapter 246 Page 1746*

A. Atrial scarring
B. Atrialized musculature that enters pulmonary veins
C. Accessory atrio-ventricular tracts
D. All of the above

Drivers responsible for initiation and maintenance of AF originate from atrialized musculature that enters the pulmonary veins.

### 641. AF, episodes are often initiated by rapidly firing foci within?
*Harrison's 20th Ed. Chapter 246 Page 1746*

A. Pulmonary veins
B. Myocardial sleeves around superior vena cava (SVC)
C. Myocardial sleeves around coronary sinus
D. All of the above

### 642. Persistent AF is associated with?
*Harrison's 20th Ed. Chapter 246 Page 1746*

A. Atrial structural remodeling
B. Atrial electrophysiologic remodeling
C. Triggering foci in many patients
D. All of the above

*Persistent AF is associated with atrial structural, electrophysiologic remodeling and triggering foci in many patients.*

### 643. It is difficult to convert AF to sinus rhythm and/or maintain it, despite therapy, when the left atrial diameter exceeds?
*Harrison's 19th Ed. 1487*

A. 2.5 cm
B. 3.5 cm
C. 4.5 cm
D. 5.5 cm

### 644. Clinical consequences of AF are related to?
*Harrison's 20th Ed. Chapter 246 Page 1746*

A. Rapid ventricular rates
B. Loss of atrial contribution to ventricular filling
C. Predisposition to thrombus formation in left atrial appendage
D. All of the above

*Clinical consequences of AF are related to rapid ventricular rates, loss of atrial contribution to ventricular filling, and predisposition to thrombus formation in the left atrial appendage with potential embolization.*

### 645. Treatment for AF is primarily guided by?
*Harrison's 20th Ed. Chapter 246 Page 1746*

A. Patients' symptoms
B. Hemodynamic effect of AF
C. Duration of AF
D. All of the above

*Treatment for AF is primarily guided by patients' symptoms, the hemodynamic effect of AF, the duration of AF, the risk of stroke and the underlying heart disease.*

### 646. Electric cardioversion is done in patients of new-onset AF who have?
*Harrison's 20th Ed. Chapter 246 Page 1746*

A. Severe hypotension
B. Pulmonary edema
C. Angina
D. All of the above

### 647. In AF, if a patient's clinical status is severely compromised, which of the following is the treatment of choice?
*Harrison's 20th Ed. Chapter 246 Page 1746*

A. β adrenergic blocker
B. Calcium channel antagonist
C. Digitalis
D. Electrical cardioversion

### 648. Electrical cardioversion for new-onset AF is accomplished through delivery of?
*Harrison's 20th Ed. Chapter 246 Page 1746*

A. 40 J
B. 100 J
C. 200 J
D. 400 J

*New-onset AF that produces severe hypotension, pulmonary edema, or angina should be electrically cardioverted starting with a QRS synchronous shock of 200 J, ideally after sedation or anesthesia. Anticoagulation strategies for new-onset AF are debated.*

### 649. In AF, pretreatment with which of the following drugs facilitates cardioversion?
*Harrison's 20th Ed. Chapter 246 Page 1746*

A. Ibutilide
B. Beta blocker
C. Calcium antagonist
D. Digitalis

*IV ibutilide may be used in selected patients to facilitate termination with direct current (DC) cardioversion. It should not be used in patients with prolonged QT interval or severe LV dysfunction because of a significant risk of torsades de Pointes.*

### 650. Anticoagulation must be commenced before cardioversion, if the duration of AF is?
*Harrison's 20th Ed. Chapter 246 Page 1747*

A. > 3 hours
B. > 6 hours
C. > 12 hours
D. > 48 hours

*If the duration of AF is unclear or is known to be >48 hours, anticoagulation must be commenced before cardioversion.*

### 651. The major source of thromboembolism & stroke in AF is formation of thrombus in?
*Harrison's 20th Ed. Chapter 246 Page 1747*

A. Left atrial appendage
B. Left atrium
C. Left ventricle
D. All of the above

*The major source of thromboembolism & stroke in AF is formation of thrombus in the left atrial appendage where flow is relatively stagnant.*

### 652. Which of the following patients undergoing cardioversion to restore sinus rhythm are at high risk for stroke?
*Harrison's 20th Ed. Chapter 246 Page 1747*

A. Rheumatic mitral stenosis
B. Hypertrophic cardiomyopathy
C. Marked left atrial enlargement
D. All of the above

*Patients with a prior history of embolic events, rheumatic mitral stenosis, or hypertrophic cardiomyopathy with marked left atrial enlargement are at high risk for stroke when undergoing cardioversion to restore sinus rhythm.*

**653. In AF, conversion to sinus rhythm by cardioversion should be done after proper anticoagulation for?**
*Harrison's 20th Ed. Chapter 246 Page 1747*

A. 1 week
B. 2 weeks
C. 3 weeks
D. 4 weeks

**654. In AF, following cardioversion, anticoagulation must be maintained for?**
*Harrison's 20th Ed. Chapter 246 Page 1747*

A. 1 week
B. 2 weeks
C. 3 weeks
D. 4 weeks

For patients who do not warrant early cardioversion of AF, anticoagulation should be maintained for at least 3 weeks with the INR confirmed to be >1.8 on at least two separate occasions prior to attempts at cardioversion and maintained for a minimum of 4 weeks after cardioversion.

**655. Ventricular rate control for acute AF is best established with?**
*Harrison's 20th Ed. Chapter 246 Page 1747*

A. Adenosine
B. Beta blockers
C. Amiodarone
D. All of the above

Ventricular rate control for acute AF is best established with beta blockers and/or calcium channel blocking agents, verapamil or diltiazem. Digoxin may add to the rate-controlling benefit of other agents but is uncommonly used as a stand-alone agent, especially in acute AF.

**656. Goal of acute rate control in AF is to reduce ventricular rate to?**
*Harrison's 20th Ed. Chapter 246 Page 1747*

A. < 70 / minute
B. < 80 / minute
C. < 90 / minute
D. < 100 / minute

The goal of acute rate control in AF is to reduce the ventricular rate to <100/minute.

**657. 'Tachycardia-induced cardiomyopathy' is caused by?**
*Harrison's 20th Ed. Chapter 246 Page 1747*

A. Digitalis
B. Atrial Fibrillation
C. Thyrotoxicosis
D. Acute alcoholic intoxication

**658. In $CHA_2DS_2$-VASc Score, 2 refers to?**
*Harrison's 20th Ed. Chapter 246 Page 1748 Table 246-1*

A. Age and angina
B. Stroke and sex
C. Two points for age and stroke
D. Half points for age and stroke

**659. In AF, anticoagulation is recommended for a $CHA_2DS_2$-VASc score of?**
*Harrison's 20th Ed. Chapter 246 Page 1748*

A. ≥ 1
B. ≥ 2
C. ≥ 3
D. ≥ 4

Anticoagulation is recommended for a $CHA_2DS_2$-VASc score of ≥2.

**660. In high-risk patients with AF, which of the following is not advised?**
*Harrison's 20th Ed. Chapter 246 Page 1748*

A. Dabigatran
B. Aspirin and clopidogrel
C. Rivaroxaban
D. Apixaban

Antiplatelet agents (aspirin and clopidogrel) are not given in high-risk patients with AF because they have substantially less effect. Major options for anticoagulation are antithrombin inhibitor dabigatran, factor Xa inhibitors rivaroxaban, apixaban, and edoxaban, vitamin K antagonist warfarin.

**661. Which of the following anticoagulant is preferred for patients with rheumatic mitral stenosis or mechanical heart valves?**
*Harrison's 20th Ed. Chapter 246 Page 1748*

A. Dabigatran
B. Warfarin
C. Rivaroxaban
D. Apixaban

Warfarin is the agent required for patients with rheumatic mitral stenosis or mechanical heart valves.

**662. Which of the following newer oral anticoagulants have renal excretion?**
*Harrison's 20th Ed. Chapter 246 Page 1748*

A. Dabigatran
B. Rivaroxaban
C. Apixaban
D. All of the above

Dabigatran, rivaroxaban and apixaban have renal excretion and cannot be used with severe renal insufficiency.

**663. Which of the following is a thrombin inhibitor?**
*Harrison's 20th Ed. Chapter 246 Page 1749*

A. Warfarin
B. Dabigatran
C. Rivaroxaban
D. Apixaban

**664. Which of the following oral anticoagulants has no reversal agent for bleeding?**
*Harrison's 20th Ed. Chapter 246 Page 1749*

A. Dabigatran
B. Rivaroxaban
C. Apixaban
D. All of the above

**665. Which of the following is a reversal agent of anticoagulants?**
*Harrison's 20th Ed. Chapter 246 Page 1749*

A. Idarucizumab
B. Andexanet alfa
C. Ciraparantag
D. All of the above

A reversal agent, idarucizumab, is available for dabigatran and reversal agents for the Xa inhibitors like andexanet alfa and ciraparantag are being evaluated.

666. **Risk factors for bleeding in patients on chronic anticoagulation include?**
*Harrison's 20th Ed. Chapter 246 Page 1749*

   A. Heart failure
   B. Renal insufficiency
   C. Excessive alcohol consumption
   D. All of the above

Risk factors for bleeding in patients on chronic anticoagulation include age >65-75 years, heart failure, renal insufficiency, excessive alcohol or nonsteroidal anti-inflammatory, aspirin and a thienopyridine drug use.

667. **AF is associated with?**
*Harrison's 20th Ed. Chapter 246 Page 1749*

   A. Obesity
   B. Hypertension
   C. Sleep apnea
   D. All of the above

AF is associated with obesity, hypertension, excessive alcohol use and sleep apnea.

668. **Which of the following is false about rhythm control strategy with antiarrhythmic medications?**
*Harrison's 20th Ed. Chapter 246 Page 1749*

   A. Did not improve survival or symptoms
   B. Drug therapy group had more hospitalizations
   C. More likely to be beneficial in younger patients
   D. None of the above

669. **A rhythm control strategy is usually selected for patients with?**
*Harrison's 20th Ed. Chapter 246 Page 1749*

   A. Symptomatic paroxysmal AF
   B. Recurrent episodes of symptomatic persistent AF
   C. AF with difficult rate control
   D. All of the above

A rhythm control strategy is usually selected for patients with symptomatic paroxysmal AF, recurrent episodes of symptomatic persistent AF, AF with difficult rate control, and AF that has resulted in depressed ventricular function or that aggravates heart failure.

670. **Which drug is preferred in AF to maintain sinus rhythm in patients without evidence of structural heart disease?**
*Harrison's 20th Ed. Chapter 246 Page 1749*

   A. Sotalol
   B. Flecainide
   C. Amiodarone
   D. Dofetilide

In AF patients without evidence of structural heart disease, use of flecainide, disopyramide or propafenone (class I sodium channel-blocking agents) is well tolerated and does not have significant proarrhythmia risk.

671. **Which drug is preferred in AF to maintain sinus rhythm in patients with evidence of structural heart disease?**
*Harrison's 20th Ed. Chapter 246 Page 1749*

   A. Disopyramide
   B. Flecainide
   C. Propafenone
   D. Dofetilide

Class III agents sotalol and dofetilide can be given to patients with coronary artery disease or structural heart disease but have a ~3% risk of inducing excessive QT prolongation and torsades des pointes.

672. **The Cox-MAZE procedure is a surgical approach to cure?**
*Harrison's 20th Ed. Chapter 246 Page 1749*

   A. AF
   B. VT
   C. PSVT
   D. All of the above

Most ablation strategies isolate atrial muscle sleeves entering the pulmonary veins which are a source of triggers responsible for initiation of AF. Risks include pulmonary vein stenosis, atrioesophageal fistula, systemic embolic events & perforation/tamponade. The Cox-Maze procedure is designed to interrupt all macroreentrant circuits that might potentially develop in the atria, thereby precluding the ability of the atria to fibrillate.

673. **Exogenous digoxin-like immunoreactive substances include?**
*N Engl J Med. 2018;378:1931-8*

   A. Spironolactone
   B. Canrenone
   C. Chinese herbal medications
   D. All of the above

Exogenous digoxin-like immunoreactive substances include spironolactone, canrenone and Chinese herbal medications.

674. **Which of the following is related to digoxin toxicity?**
*N Engl J Med. 2018;378:1931-8*

   A. Chloropsia
   B. Erythropsia
   C. Cyanopsia
   D. Xanthopsia

Xanthopsia refers to yellow vision.

675. **Adverse events associated with use of digoxin immune Fab include?**
*N Engl J Med. 2018;378:1931-8*

   A. Heart failure
   B. Hypokalemia
   C. Hypersensitivity to ovine Fab epitopes
   D. All of the above

Adverse events associated with the use of digoxin immune Fab include heart failure, hypokalemia, and hypersensitivity to ovine Fab epitopes.

676. **Vortex keratopathy is an ocular side effect of which of the following?**
*S Afr Fam Pract. 2014;56(1):8-14*

   A. Amiodarone
   B. Corticosteroids
   C. Chloroquine
   D. Acetazolamide

Vortex keratopathy refers to innocuous corneal deposits.

677. **Toxic optic neuropathy, with loss of central and colour vision is an ocular side effect of?**
*S Afr Fam Pract. 2014;56(1):8-14*

   A. Streptomycin
   B. Ethambutol
   C. Isoniazid
   D. All of the above

**678. Which of the following is not an ocular finding in Marfan's syndrome?**
*S Afr Fam Pract. 2014;56(1):8-14*

A. Myopia
B. Retinal haemorrhage
C. Dislocated lens
D. Retinal detachment

**679. Which of the following is an ocular manifestation of ankylosing spondylitis?**
*S Afr Fam Pract. 2014;56(1):8-14*

A. Uveitis
B. Scleritis, episcleritis
C. Keratitis
D. All of the above

**680. Electrical cardioversion for atrial flutter is accomplished through delivery of?**
*Harrison's 19th Ed. 1487*

A. 20 - 40 J
B. 50 - 100 J
C. 100 - 150 J
D. 150 - 300 J

*Organized atrial flutter activity can frequently be terminated with low-energy external cardioversion of 50 - 100 J.*

**681. Electrical cardioversion for atrioventricular nodal reentrant tachycardia (AVNRT) is accomplished through delivery of?**
*Harrison's 19th Ed. 1487*

A. 20 - 40 J
B. 50 - 100 J
C. 100 - 200 J
D. 200 - 300 J

*R wave synchronous DC cardioversion using 100 - 200 J can terminate atrioventricular nodal reentrant tachycardia (AVNRT).*

**682. Which of the following statements is false?**
*Harrison's 19th Ed. 1486*

A. Pacing does not provoke automatic rhythms
B. Pacing provoke tachycardias due to triggered activity
C. Abnormal automaticity is responsible for APCs & VPCs
D. None of the above

**683. Abnormal impulse formation due to triggered activity is related to?**
*Harrison's 18th Ed. 1879*

A. Reentry
B. Extra pathways
C. Myocardial ion channel abnormalities
D. Cellular afterdepolarizations

*Abnormal impulse formation is due to the development of triggered activity. Triggered activity is related to cellular afterdepolarizations that occur at the end of the action potential, during phase 3 (early afterdepolarizations), or after the action potential, during phase 4 (late afterdepolarizations).*

**684. Afterdepolarizations are due to an increase in?**
*Harrison's 18th Ed. 1879*

A. Intracellular calcium accumulation
B. Altered sodium transport
C. Altered potassium transport
D. Intracellular potassium deficiency

*Afterdepolarizations are attributable to an increase in intracellular calcium accumulation.*

**685. Early afterdepolarizations are responsible for?**
*Harrison's 18th Ed. 1879*

A. Catecholamine-sensitive VT
B. Atrial tachyarrhythmias caused by digoxin toxicity
C. Torsades des pointes
D. All of the above

*Early afterdepolarizations may be responsible for VPCs that trigger torsades des pointes (TDP). Late afterdepolarizations are responsible for atrial, junctional & fascicular tachyarrhythmias caused by digoxin toxicity and for catecholamine-sensitive VT originating in the outflow tract.*

**686. Late afterdepolarizations in digoxin toxicity may lead to?**
*Harrison's 18th Ed. 1879*

A. Atrial tachyarrhythmias
B. Junctional tachyarrhythmias
C. Fascicular tachyarrhythmias
D. All of the above

*Late afterdepolarizations caused by digoxin toxicity may lead to atrial, junctional, and fascicular tachyarrhythmias.*

**687. Inhomogeneities in myocardial conduction and/or recovery leading to reentry is exaggerated by?**
*Harrison's 18th Ed. 1879*

A. Presence of extra pathways
B. Myocardial ion channel abnormalities
C. Myocardial fibrosis
D. All of the above

*Reentry is due to inhomogeneities in myocardial conduction and/or recovery properties. Inhomogeneities can be exaggerated by the presence of extra pathways (WPW syndrome), generalized genetically determined myocardial ion channel abnormalities (long QT syndrome) or by the interruption of normal myocardial patterns of activation due to the development of fibrosis.*

**688. Which of the following is a genetically determined ion channel abnormality?**
*Harrison's 18th Ed. 1879*

A. Brugada syndrome
B. LQTS
C. Catecholaminergic polymorphic VT
D. All of the above

**689. Which of the following statements about mechanism of sustained paroxysmal tachyarrhythmia is false?**
*Harrison's 19th Ed. 1486*

A. Electrophysiologic inhomogeneity
B. Unidirectional block in one pathway
C. Fast conduction over an alternative pathway
D. Reexcitation of the initially blocked pathway

690. **Which of the following statements about mechanism of tachyarrhythmia is false?**
   *Harrison's 19th Ed. 1486*
   
   A. Reentrant arrhythmias can be reproducibly initiated and terminated by premature complexes and rapid stimulation
   B. Myocardial cells do not possess pacemaker activity
   C. Tachycardia caused by automaticity cannot be started or stopped by pacing
   D. Triggered activity is caused by early afterdepolarizations only

691. **Which of the following statements about atrial premature complexes (APCs) is false?**
   *Harrison's 16th Ed. 1342*
   
   A. Can be found in over 90% of normal adults
   B. May originate from any location in either atrium
   C. P wave of APC differs from sinus P wave morphology
   D. Conduct to ventricles when they occur late in cardiac cycle

692. **Which of the following statements about atrial premature complexes (APCs) is false?**
   *Harrison's 16th Ed. 1342*
   
   A. Sum of pre and postextrasystolic PP intervals is less than the sum of two sinus PP intervals
   B. QRS complex following most APCs is normal
   C. Alcohol, tobacco or adrenergic stimulants precipitate APCs
   D. None of the above

693. **Which of the following about APCs is false?**
   *Harrison's 18th Ed. 1880*
   
   A. Most common arrhythmia
   B. Frequently increases with age & structural heart disease
   C. Asymptomatic
   D. None of the above

694. **APCs from which of the following may mimic the sinus P wave morphology?**
   *Harrison's 18th Ed. 1880*
   
   A. Right atrial appendage
   B. Superior vena cava (SVC)
   C. Superior aspect of crista terminalis
   D. All of the above

*P wave contour differs from that seen during sinus rhythm. APCs from right atrial appendage, superior vena cava (SVC) and superior aspect of the crista terminalis in the region of sinus node may mimic sinus P wave morphology.*

695. **Which of the following about APCs is false?**
   *Harrison's 18th Ed. 1880*
   
   A. APCs characteristically reset the sinus node
   B. Sum of pre- & post-APC RR is < 2 sinus PP intervals
   C. Class IC antiarrhythmic agents may eliminate APCs
   D. None of the above

*APCs characteristically reset the sinus node. The resulting sum of the pre- and post-APC RR interval is less than two sinus PP intervals. Class IC antiarrhythmic agents may eliminate the APCs but should be avoided if structural heart disease is present.*

696. **Which of the following about junctional premature complexes is false?**
   *Harrison's 18th Ed. 1880*
   
   A. Extremely uncommon
   B. Originate from AV node & His bundle region
   C. Produce retrograde atrial activation
   D. None of the above

*JPCs are extremely uncommon. Complexes originate from AV node & His bundle region & may produce retrograde atrial activation with P wave distorting the initial or terminal portions of QRS complex producing pseudo Q or S waves in leads II, III, and aVF.*

697. **Incidence of supraventricular tachycardia (SVT) is about?**
   *N Engl J Med. 2006;354:1039-51*
   
   A. 35 cases per 100,000 persons per year
   B. 70 cases per 100,000 persons per year
   C. 100 cases per 100,000 persons per year
   D. 150 cases per 100,000 persons per year

698. **Prevalence of supraventricular tachycardia is about?**
   *N Engl J Med. 2006;354:1039-51*
   
   A. 2.25 per 1000
   B. 5 per 1000
   C. 10 per 1000
   D. 20 per 1000

699. **Which of the following symptoms is uncommon in supraventricular tachycardia?**
   *N Engl J Med. 2006;354:1039-51*
   
   A. Palpitations
   B. Dyspnea
   C. Light-headedness
   D. Syncope

700. **Which of the following statements about SVT is false?**
   *N Engl J Med. 2006;354:1039-51*
   
   A. Most have a reentry mechanism
   B. Classified according to location of reentry circuit
   C. ~ 60% are due to AV nodal reentry circuit
   D. SVT is usually associated with structural heart disease

701. **In SVT, adenosine is contraindicated in patients with?**
   *N Engl J Med. 2006;354:1039-51*
   
   A. In heart-transplant recipients
   B. In patients with severe obstructive lung disease
   C. In patients with tachycardia with a wide QRS complex
   D. All of the above

702. **Which of the following drugs are used in treatment of SVT?**
   *N Engl J Med. 2006;354:1039-51*
   
   A. Adenosine
   B. Intravenous verapamil
   C. Intravenous beta-blocker
   D. All of the above

703. Which of the following drugs are used in treatment of SVT?
*N Engl J Med. 2006;354:1039-51*

   A. Intravenous Procainamide
   B. Intravenous Ibutilide
   C. Intravenous Propafenone
   D. All of the above

704. Danger of radiofrequency catheter ablation of accessory pathway in SVT is?
*N Engl J Med. 2006;354:1039-51*

   A. Atrioventricular block that requires pacemaker therapy
   B. Damage to an artery, bleeding, arteriovenous fistula
   C. Coronary venous thrombosis
   D. All of the above

705. Danger of radiofrequency catheter ablation of accessory pathway in SVT is?
*N Engl J Med. 2006;354:1039-51*

   A. Pulmonary embolism
   B. Myocardial perforation
   C. Valvular damage
   D. All of the above

706. Characteristic of radiofrequency current used for catheter ablation of accessory pathways in SVT is?
*N Engl J Med. 2006;354:1039-51*

   A. Low-voltage, high-frequency form of electrical energy
   B. High-voltage, low-frequency form of electrical energy
   C. High-voltage, high-frequency form of electrical energy
   D. Low-voltage, low-frequency form of electrical energy

*Catheter ablation, directed at elimination or modification of slow pathway conduction, is very effective in permanently eliminating AVNRT.*

707. Which of the following statements about SVT is false?
*Harrison's 19th Ed. 1486*

   A. Most common cause is AV nodal reentrant tachycardia
   B. More commonly observed in women
   C. Presents as regular narrow QRS complex tachycardia @ 120 to 250 bpm
   D. APCs that initiate the SVT has a normal PR interval

*APC initiating AVNRT is characteristically followed by a long PR interval consistent with conduction via the slow pathway.*

708. Which of the following about sinus tachycardia is false?
*N Engl J Med. 2012;367:1438-48*

   A. Sudden in onset and recession
   B. Regular
   C. Rate < 220 bpm minus the patient's age
   D. P waves precede the QRS complex

*Sinus tachycardia is gradual in onset and recession. The heart rate is regular and classically does not exceed 220 beats per minute minus the patient's age. In sinus tachycardia, P waves precede the QRS complex.*

709. Atrial flutter results from a reentrant circuit around?
*N Engl J Med. 2012;367:1438-48*

   A. Mitral valve
   B. Tricuspid valve
   C. Aortic valve
   D. Pulmonary valve

*Atrial flutter, the second most common pathologic supraventricular tachycardia, results from a reentrant circuit around the tricuspid valve in the right atrium.*

710. Which of the following parameter helps distinguish atrial flutter from other supraventricular tachycardias?
*N Engl J Med. 2012;367:1438-48*

   A. Regularity
   B. Rate
   C. Blood pressure
   D. Jugular venous pulsations

*Atrial flutter is an organized regular rhythm that is characterized by an atrial rate of 280 to 300 beats per minute and with 2:1 conduction in AV node results in a ventricular rate of 140 to 150 beats per minute. Flutter waves are usually obscured by T waves, making the surface ECG tracing for this tachycardia difficult to distinguish from that of other supraventricular tachycardias. However, a heart rate of 150 beats per minute is highly suggestive of this tachyarrhythmia.*

711. Which of the following occurs more frequently in the pediatric population?
*N Engl J Med. 2012;367:1438-48*

   A. Atrioventricular nodal reentrant tachycardia
   B. Atrioventricular reciprocating tachycardia
   C. Atrial tachycardia
   D. Atrial flutter

*Atrioventricular nodal reentrant tachycardia is most common in persons >20 years of age, whereas atrioventricular reciprocating tachycardia occurs more frequently in pediatric population.*

712. Regular supraventricular tachycardias include all except?
*N Engl J Med. 2012;367:1438-48*

   A. Atrial tachycardia (AT)
   B. Atrioventricular nodal reentrant tachycardia (AVNRT)
   C. Atrioventricular reciprocating tachycardia (AVRT)
   D. Multifocal atrial tachycardia (MAT)

*Regular supraventricular tachycardias include sinus tachycardia, atrial flutter (AFL), atrioventricular nodal reentrant tachycardia (AVNRT), atrioventricular reciprocating tachycardia (AVRT), and atrial tachycardia (AT). Orthodromic AVRT is more common than antidromic AVRT. Irregular supraventricular tachycardias include atrial fibrillation (AF), AFL when it occurs in a patient with variable AV block, multifocal atrial tachycardia (MAT) & sinus rhythm with multiple atrial premature beats.*

713. Which of the following arrhythmias are seen with bypass tracts?
*N Engl J Med. 2012;367:1438-48*

   A. Orthodromic AV reentry
   B. Antidromic AV reentry
   C. Wide irregular QRS complex (atrial fibrillation)
   D. All of the above

*Three arrhythmias are seen with bypass tracts: a narrow regular QRS complex (orthodromic; conduction down the atrioventricular node and retrograde conduction through the bypass tract), a wide regular QRS complex (antidromic; conduction down the bypass tract and retrograde conduction through the atrioventricular node), and a wide irregular QRS complex (atrial fibrillation).*

714. **Heart rate regularity is defined as beat-to-beat timing variation of less than?**
*N Engl J Med. 2012;367:1438-48*

A. 5%
B. 10%
C. 15%
D. 20%

Regularity is defined as variation of less than 10% in beat-to-beat timing, but most regular tachycardias actually vary by less than 5%.

715. **Which of the following is a wide-complex tachycardia?**
*N Engl J Med. 2012;367:1438-48*

A. Ventricular tachycardia
B. Ventricular fibrillation
C. Torsades de pointes
D. All of the above

Wide-complex tachycardias are caused by ventricular arrhythmia (ventricular tachycardia, ventricular fibrillation, and torsades de pointes or polymorphic ventricular tachycardia) or supraventricular tachycardias with aberrant conduction resulting from disease in His–Purkinje system (left or right bundle-branch block), a bypass tract (Wolff–Parkinson–White syndrome), with depolarization of ventricle from bypass tract; and a ventricular paced rhythm from a pacemaker.

716. **Vagomimetic maneuvers include?**
*N Engl J Med. 2012;367:1438-48*

A. Carotid sinus massage
B. Valsalva maneuver
C. Immersion of face in cold water (dive response)
D. All of the above

Vagal maneuvers include Valsalva maneuver, carotid sinus massage, bearing down, and immersion of the face in ice water They increase vagal tone and block the atrioventricular node.

717. **Adenosine terminates which of the following?**
*N Engl J Med. 2012;367:1438-48*

A. Atrioventricular nodal reentrant tachycardias
B. Atrioventricular reciprocating tachycardias
C. Atrial tachycardias
D. All of the above

Adenosine, a very short-acting endogenous nucleotide that blocks atrioventricular nodal conduction, terminates nearly all atrioventricular nodal reentrant tachycardias and atrioventricular reciprocating tachycardias as well as up to 80% of atrial tachycardias.

718. **Adenosine should not be given in?**
*N Engl J Med. 2012;367:1438-48*

A. Regular wide-complex tachycardias
B. Irregular wide-complex tachycardias
C. Atrioventricular nodal reentrant tachycardias
D. Atrioventricular reciprocating tachycardias

Adenosine is also useful in the differential diagnosis and treatment of wide-complex tachycardias, but it should be given only when these tachycardias are regular, since irregular wide-complex tachycardias may be rendered unstable after the administration of adenosine.

719. **Arrhythmias that cause which of the following require urgent electrical cardioversion?**
*N Engl J Med. 2012;367:1438-48*

A. Hypotension
B. Heart failure
C. Coronary ischemia
D. All of the above

Arrhythmias causing hemodynamic instability (hypotension, heart failure, or coronary ischemia) require urgent electrical cardioversion.

720. **If hemodynamic compromise is present, which of the following is preferred to terminate atrioventricular nodal reentrant tachycardia?**
*Harrison's 19th Ed. 1486*

A. Intravenous adenosine
B. Intravenous beta blockade
C. Intravenous calcium channel therapy
D. R-wave synchronous DC cardioversion (100 - 200 J)

If hemodynamic compromise is present, R-wave synchronous DC cardioversion using 100–200 J can terminate atrioventricular nodal reentrant tachycardia.

721. **Which of the following drugs slow conduction in the antegrade slow pathway in atrioventricular nodal reentrant tachycardia?**
*Harrison's 19th Ed. 1486*

A. Digitalis
B. Beta blockers
C. Calcium channel blockers
D. All of the above

AVNRT prevention may be achieved with drugs that slow conduction in the antegrade slow pathway, such as digitalis, beta blockers, and calcium channel blockers.

722. **Which of the following drugs is useful in preventing exercise-precipitated atrioventricular nodal reentrant tachycardia?**
*Harrison's 19th Ed. 1486*

A. Digitalis
B. Beta blockers
C. Calcium channel blockers
D. All of the above

In patients who have a history of exercise-precipitated AVNRT, use of beta blockers frequently eliminates symptoms.

723. **Which of the following drugs slow conduction in the antegrade slow pathway in atrioventricular nodal reentrant tachycardia?**
*Harrison's 19th Ed. 1486*

A. Digitalis
B. Beta blockers
C. Calcium channel blockers
D. Flecainide

In patients who do not respond to drug therapy directed at antegrade slow pathway, treatment with class IA or IC agents directed at altering conduction of the fast pathway may be considered.

724. **Which of the following is false for carotid sinus massage?**
*Harrison's 19th Ed. 1486*

A. Not performed in patients with carotid arterial bruits
B. Massage one carotid bulb at a time
C. Performed by applying firm pressure just underneath the angle of jaw for up to 10 seconds
D. Patient should be supine with neck extended

## Approach to Ventricular Arrhythmias

**725. Ventricular arrhythmias originate from?**
*Harrison's 20th Ed. Chapter 247 Page 1750*

A. A focus of myocardial cells
B. A focus of Purkinje cells
C. Reentry through areas of scar
D. All of the above

*Ventricular arrhythmias originate from a focus of myocardial or Purkinje cells capable of automaticity, or triggered automaticity, or from reentry through areas of scar or a diseased Purkinje system.*

**726. Which of the following statements is false?**
*Harrison's 20th Ed. Chapter 247 Page 1750*

A. QRS complex during ventricular arrhythmias is wide (>0.12 s)
B. Two consecutive ventricular beats are ventricular couplets
C. Arterial pressure following premature beats is attenuated
D. None of the above

**727. VT is defined as ≥3 consecutive ventricular beats @?**
*Harrison's 20th Ed. Chapter 247 Page 1750*

A. ≥ 90 beats/minute
B. ≥ 100 beats/minute
C. ≥ 120 beats/minute
D. ≥ 150 beats/minute

**728. Which of the following statements is false?**
*Harrison's 20th Ed. Chapter 247 Page 1750*

A. Idioventricular rhythm is ≥3 consecutive ventricular beats @ <100 beats/minute
B. Non-sustained VT terminates spontaneously within 30 sec.
C. Sustained VT persists >30 sec. or is terminated by an active intervention
D. None of the above

**729. Which of the following is false about ventricular tachycardia (VT) of right ventricular outflow tract origin?**
*Harrison's 20th Ed. Chapter 247 Page 1751 Figure 247-2*

A. Has a left bundle branch block pattern
B. Inferior axis
C. Tall QRS complexes in inferior leads
D. None of the above

**730. Which of the following about monomorphic VT is false?**
*Harrison's 20th Ed. Chapter 247 Page 1750*

A. VT that originate from right ventricle produce LBBB like configuration
B. VT that originate from septum produce LBBB like configuration
C. VT that originate from free wall of left ventricle produce RBBB like configuration
D. None of the above

**731. Very rapid monomorphic VT is also called?**
*Harrison's 20th Ed. Chapter 247 Page 1750*

A. Ventricular flutter
B. Ventricular fibrillation
C. Idioventricular rhythm
D. Torsade de Pointes

*Very rapid monomorphic VT has a sinusoidal appearance and is also called ventricular flutter, because it is not possible to distinguish the QRS complex from the T wave.*

**732. Relatively slow sinusoidal VTs with wide QRS can be caused by?**
*Harrison's 20th Ed. Chapter 247 Page 1750*

A. Hyperkalemia
B. Toxicity from sodium channel blockers
C. Severe global myocardial ischemia
D. All of the above

*Relatively slow sinusoidal VTs with wide QRS indicate slowed ventricular conduction. It can be caused by hyperkalemia, toxicity from sodium channel blockers (flecainide, propafenone, or tricyclic antidepressants) and severe global myocardial ischemia.*

**733. Polymorphic VT is also called?**
*Harrison's 20th Ed. Chapter 247 Page 1750*

A. Ventricular flutter
B. Ventricular fibrillation
C. Idioventricular rhythm
D. Torsade de Pointes

**734. Which of the following about ventricular fibrillation is false?**
*Harrison's 20th Ed. Chapter 247 Page 1750*

A. Continuous irregular activation
B. No discrete QRS complexes
C. Monomorphic or polymorphic VT may transition to VF
D. None of the above

**735. Which of the following about idiopathic ventricular arrhythmias is false?**
*Harrison's 20th Ed. Chapter 247 Page 1750*

A. PVCs / VT that occurs without structural heart disease
B. Not associated with a genetic syndrome
C. Not associated with a risk of sudden death
D. None of the above

**736. Which of the following can cause syncope?**
*Harrison's 20th Ed. Chapter 247 Page 1750*

A. An episode of VT
B. Neuro-cardiogenic (vasovagal) reflex
C. Orthostatic hypotension
D. All of the above

737. Medications that prolong the QT interval predispose to?
*Harrison's 20th Ed. Chapter 247 Page 1752*

   A. Monomorphic VT
   B. Polymorphic VT
   C. Idioventricular rhythm
   D. All of the above

Medications that prolong the QT interval predispose to polymorphic VT.

738. Which of the following suggests a genetic arrhythmia syndrome?
*Harrison's 20th Ed. Chapter 247 Page 1752*

   A. Dysbiotic features
   B. Biochemical features
   C. Dysmorphic features
   D. Systemic features

Stigmata of neuromuscular disease or dysmorphic features may suggest a genetic arrhythmia syndrome.

739. Which of the following is a genetic arrhythmia syndrome?
*Harrison's 20th Ed. Chapter 247 Page 1752*

   A. Long QT syndrome
   B. Brugada syndrome
   C. Short QT syndrome
   D. All of the above

740. Which of the following is the first choice of therapy for most ventricular arrhythmias?
*Harrison's 20th Ed. Chapter 247 Page 1753*

   A. Beta-adrenergic Blockers
   B. Calcium Channel Blockers
   C. Sodium Channel Blocking Agents
   D. Potassium Channel Blocking Agents

741. Which of the following is a sodium channel blocker?
*Harrison's 20th Ed. Chapter 247 Page 1753*

   A. Quinidine
   B. Disopyramide
   C. Propafenone
   D. All of the above

742. Which of the following is a sodium channel blocker?
*Harrison's 20th Ed. Chapter 247 Page 1753*

   A. Mexiletine
   B. Flecainide
   C. Propafenone
   D. All of the above

743. Which of the following sodium channel blocking agents has a potassium channel blocking effect?
*Harrison's 20th Ed. Chapter 247 Page 1753*

   A. Quinidine
   B. Disopyramide
   C. Procainamide
   D. All of the above

744. Which of the following is false about Dronedarone?
*Harrison's 20th Ed. Chapter 247 Page 1754*

   A. No iodine moiety
   B. Efficacy for ventricular arrhythmias is poor
   C. Increases mortality in patients with heart failure
   D. None of the above

745. Which of the following is a toxicity of amiodarone?
*Harrison's 20th Ed. Chapter 247 Page 1754*

   A. Hyper or hypothyroidism
   B. Pneumonitis or pulmonary fibrosis
   C. Neuropathy and ocular toxicity
   D. All of the above

# Premature Ventricular Beats, Non-Sustained Ventricular Tachycardia, and Idioventricular Rhythm

**746.** Which of the following statements about premature ventricular contractions (PVCs) is false?
*Harrison's 20th Ed. Chapter 248 Page 1755*
- A. Can be due to automaticity or reentry
- B. Can be a sign of increased sympathetic tone
- C. Can be a harbinger of sustained VT or VF
- D. None of the above

**747.** Which of the following statements about PVCs is false?
*Harrison's 20th Ed. Chapter 248 Page 1755*
- A. Smooth uninterrupted contours & sharp QRS deflections suggest an ectopic focus in relatively normal myocardium
- B. Broad notching & slurred QRS deflections suggest a diseased myocardial substrate
- C. Those with RBBB configuration are more likely to be associated with structural heart disease
- D. None of the above

**748.** Most ventricular arrhythmias that are not associated with structural heart disease have?
*Harrison's 20th Ed. Chapter 248 Page 1756*
- A. Left bundle branch block like configuration
- B. Right bundle branch block like configuration
- C. Left anterior hemiblock like configuration
- D. Left posterior hemiblock like configuration

*Most ventricular arrhythmias that are not associated with structural heart disease have a left bundle branch block like configuration.*

**749.** Which of the following about nonsustained VT is false?
*Harrison's 20th Ed. Chapter 248 Page 1756*
- A. Usually monomorphic
- B. Rate < 200 beats / minute
- C. Lasts less than 8 beats
- D. None of the above

*Nonsustained VT is usually monomorphic with rates < 200 beats/minute and typically lasts < 8 beats.*

**750.** Which of the following features of nonsustained VT has ominous prognosis?
*Harrison's 20th Ed. Chapter 248 Page 1756*
- A. Very rapid
- B. Polymorphic
- C. First beat that occurs prior to peak of T-wave ("short-coupled")
- D. All of the above

*Nonsustained VT that is very rapid, polymorphic, or with a first beat that occurs prior to the peak of the T-wave ("short-coupled") should prompt careful evaluation for underlying disease or genetic syndromes associated with sudden death.*

**751.** Genetic syndromes associated with sudden death include?
*Harrison's 20th Ed. Chapter 248 Page 1756*
- A. Cardiomyopathy
- B. Long QT syndrome
- C. Arrhythmogenic right ventricular cardiomyopathy
- D. All of the above

*Genetic syndromes associated with sudden death include cardiomyopathy, long QT syndrome, and arrhythmogenic right ventricular cardiomyopathy.*

**752.** Which of the following is included in 'Genetically determined arrhythmia syndrome'?
*Harrison's 20th Ed. Chapter 248 Page 1756*
- A. Long QT syndrome
- B. Brugada syndrome
- C. Hypertrophic cardiomyopathy
- D. All of the above

**753.** Which of the following 'Genetically determined arrhythmia syndromes' have autosomal dominant inheritance?
*Harrison's 20th Ed. Chapter 248 Page 1756*
- A. Long QT syndrome
- B. Brugada syndrome
- C. Hypertrophic cardiomyopathy
- D. All of the above

**754.** Repolarization abnormalities are seen in which of the following genetically determined syndromes?
*Harrison's 20th Ed. Chapter 248 Page 1756*
- A. Long QT syndrome
- B. Brugada syndrome
- C. Arrhythmogenic right ventricular cardiomyopathy (ARVC)
- D. All of the above

*Repolarization abnormalities are seen in genetically determined syndromes associated with sudden death. These include long QT syndrome, Brugada syndrome, arrhythmogenic right ventricular cardiomyopathy (ARVC) and hypertrophic cardiomyopathy.*

**755.** Following recovery from acute MI, which of the following is a marker for depressed ventricular function and increased mortality?
*Harrison's 20th Ed. Chapter 248 Page 1756*
- A. > 10 PVCs per hour
- B. Repetitive PVCs with couplets
- C. Nonsustained VT
- D. All of the above

*Following recovery from acute MI, frequent PVCs (> 10 PVCs per hour), repetitive PVCs with couplets and nonsustained VT are markers for depressed ventricular function and increased mortality, but routine antiarrhythmic drug therapy to suppress these arrhythmias is not warranted.*

**756.** Which of the following is a potassium channel blocker?
*Harrison's 20th Ed. Chapter 248 Page 1757*
- A. Mexiletine
- B. Quinidine
- C. Disopyramide
- D. Dofetilide

*Antiarrhythmic drugs that block cardiac sodium channel are flecainide, propafenone, mexiletine, quinidine and disopyramide. Antiarrhythmic drug that block cardiac potassium channel blocker is dofetilide.*

**757. Depression of ventricular function occurs when PVCs account for?**
*Harrison's 20th Ed. Chapter 248 Page 1757*

A. > 1– 2% of total beats over a 24-hour period
B. > 2 – 5% of total beats over a 24-hour period
C. > 5 – 10% of total beats over a 24-hour period
D. > 15 – 20% of total beats over a 24-hour period

*Depression of ventricular function rarely occurs unless PVCs account for more than 15–20% of total beats over a 24-hour period.*

**758. Idioventricular rhythms are commonly associated with?**
*Harrison's 20th Ed. Chapter 248 Page 1757*

A. Acute MI
B. Cardiomyopathies
C. Sleep apnea
D. All of the above

## Sustained Ventricular Tachycardia

**759. Which of the following is a feature of sustained monomorphic ventricular tachycardia (VT)?**
*Harrison's 20th Ed. Chapter 249 Page 1757*

A. Wide QRS tachycardia
B. Same QRS configuration from beat to beat
C. Originates from a stable focus or reentry circuit
D. All of the above

**760. Clinical presentation of sustained ventricular tachycardia depends on?**
*Harrison's 20th Ed. Chapter 249 Page 1757*

A. Rate of arrhythmia
B. Underlying cardiac function
C. Autonomic adaptation in response to arrhythmia
D. All of the above

**761. Sustained monomorphic VT can mimic which of the following?**
*Harrison's 20th Ed. Chapter 249 Page 1757*

A. SVT with left / right bundle branch block aberrant conduction
B. SVT conducted to ventricles over an accessory pathway
C. Rapid cardiac pacing in patient with ICD
D. All of the above

*Sustained monomorphic VT has to be distinguished from other causes of uniform wide QRS tachycardia. These include supraventricular tachycardia with left or right bundle branch block aberrant conduction, supraventricular tachycardias conducted to ventricles over an accessory pathway and rapid cardiac pacing in a patient with a pacemaker or defibrillator.*

**762. Which of the following favor the diagnosis of sustained monomorphic VT?**
*Harrison's 20th Ed. Chapter 249 Page 1757*

A. Presence of AV dissociation
B. Monophasic R wave or Rs complex in AVR
C. Concordance from V1 to V6 of monophasic R or S waves
D. All of the above

**763. Which of the following is rarely a cause of sustained monomorphic VT?**
*Harrison's 20th Ed. Chapter 249 Page 1758*

A. Nonischemic cardiomyopathy
B. Acute MI
C. Arrhythmogenic right ventricular cardiomyopathy
D. Long QT syndrome

*Acute MI is rarely a cause of sustained monomorphic VT.*

**764. Scars in myocardium is suggested by?**
*Harrison's 20th Ed. Chapter 249 Page 1758*

A. Pathologic Q-waves on ECG
B. Segmental LV or RV wall motion abnormalities on 2D echo
C. Areas of delayed gadolinium enhancement in MR imaging
D. All of the above

**765. Scars that cause VT are often located adjacent to?**
*Harrison's 20th Ed. Chapter 249 Page 1758*

A. Apex
B. Papillary muscle
C. Valve annulus
D. Interventricular septum

*Scars that cause VT are often located adjacent to a valve annulus and can occur in either ventricle.*

**766. Which of the following is associated with monomorphic VT?**
*Harrison's 20th Ed. Chapter 249 Page 1758*

A. Chagas' disease
B. Leishmaniasis
C. Babesiosis
D. All of the above

*Cardiac sarcoidosis, Chagas' disease and cardiomyopathy due to Lamin A/C genetic cardiomyopathy are particularly associated with monomorphic VT due to intramural or sub-epicardial scars.*

**767. VT in the absence of structural heart disease is called?**
*Harrison's 20th Ed. Chapter 249 Page 1758 Table 249-1*

A. Functional VT
B. Idiopathic VT
C. Casual VT
D. Benign VT

*VT in the absence of structural heart disease is called idiopathic VT.*

**768. Long QT syndrome is complicated by?**
*Harrison's 20th Ed. Chapter 249 Page 1758 Table 249-1*

A. Torsade de Pointes VT
B. Polymorphic VT or bidirectional VT
C. Ventricular fibrillation
D. All of the above

**769. Brugada syndrome is complicated by?**
*Harrison's 20th Ed. Chapter 249 Page 1758 Table 249-1*

A. Torsade de Pointes VT
B. Polymorphic VT or bidirectional VT
C. Ventricular fibrillation
D. All of the above

**770. Which of the following is due to mutation in genes encoding for cardiac desmosomal proteins?**
*Harrison's 20th Ed. Chapter 249 Page 1758*

A. Arrhythmogenic right ventricular cardiomyopathy (ARVC)
B. Naxos disease
C. Carvajal syndrome
D. All of the above

**771. Epsilon wave is an ECG feature of?**
*Harrison's 20th Ed. Chapter 249 Page 1758*

A. Arrhythmogenic right ventricular cardiomyopathy (ARVC)
B. Naxos disease
C. Carvajal syndrome
D. All of the above

772. **Location of epsilon wave in ECG is?**
   *Harrison's 20th Ed. Chapter 249 Page 1758*
   A. Deflection at the beginning of QRS
   B. Deflection at the end of QRS
   C. Deflection at the beginning of T
   D. Deflection at the end of T

773. **Which of the following is related to arrhythmogenic RV cardiomyopathy (ARVC)?**
   *Harrison's 20th Ed. Chapter 249 Page 1758*
   A. Genetically determined
   B. After viral myocarditis
   C. Sporadic
   D. Any of the above

ARVCM/D due to a genetically determined dysplastic process or after a suspected viral myocarditis is also associated with VT/VF. Sporadic nonfamilial/nondysplastic form of RV cardiomyopathy is also seen.

774. **Epsilon wave is characteristic ECG finding of?**
   *Harrison's 20th Ed. Chapter 249 Page 1758*
   A. Arrhythmogenic RV cardiomyopathy
   B. Brugada syndrome
   C. Long QT syndrome (LQTS)
   D. Digoxin toxicity

Epsilon wave is the terminal notching of QRS complex & is separated from the QRS complex. It is seen in ARVCM/D. Epsilon waves are due to marked delay in ventricular activation in RV free wall near the base of tricuspid & pulmonic valves which undergo extensive fibrosis.

775. **In arrhythmogenic RV cardiomyopathy (ARVC), ventricles have an excess of?**
   *Harrison's 20th Ed. Chapter 249 Page 1758*
   A. Fat
   B. Glycogen
   C. Mucopolysaccharide
   D. All of the above

MRI in arrhythmogenic RV cardiomyopathy/dysplasia (ARVCM/D) shows fibrosis and fibro-fatty replacement of the ventricle, thinning of the RV free wall with increased fibrosis, and associated wall motion abnormalities.

776. **Echocardiographic finding in arrhythmogenic RV cardiomyopathy (ARVC) is?**
   *Harrison's 20th Ed. Chapter 249 Page 1758*
   A. RV enlargement
   B. RV wall motion abnormalities
   C. RV apical aneurysm formation
   D. All of the above

In patients with ARVCM/D, echocardiography shows RV enlargement with RV wall motion abnormalities and RV apical aneurysm formation.

777. **Which of the following about Naxos disease is false?**
   *Harrison's 20th Ed. Chapter 254 Page 1781 Table 254-3*
   A. Arrhythmogenic RV dysplasia
   B. Palmar-plantar keratosis
   C. Autosomal dominant inheritance
   D. Woolly hair

Naxos disease, an autosomal recessive cardio-cutaneous syndrome, consists of arrhythmogenic RV dysplasia with palmar-plantar keratosis & woolly hair with a high risk of SCD in adolescents & young adults.

778. **Which of the following is false about bundle branch reentry VT?**
   *Harrison's 20th Ed. Chapter 249 Page 1759*
   A. Reentry circuit revolves retrograde via left bundle
   B. Reentry circuit revolves anterograde via right bundle
   C. Usually associated with severe underlying heart disease
   D. None of the above

Reentry through the Purkinje system occurs in ~5% of patients with monomorphic VT in the presence of structural heart disease. Catheter ablation of the right bundle branch abolishes this VT.

779. **In ECG, bundle branch reentrant VT presents as?**
   *Harrison's 20th Ed. Chapter 249 Page 1759*
   A. Right bundle block
   B. Left bundle block
   C. Complete heart block
   D. Any of the above

In sinus rhythm, bundle branch reentrant VT presents as left bundle block.

780. **Sudden death due to VT is rare in which of the following conditions?**
   *Harrison's 20th Ed. Chapter 249 Page 1759*
   A. Premature ventricular beats and nonsustained VT
   B. Idiopathic VT
   C. Genetically determined syndromes
   D. Depressed ventricular function

781. **Which of the following about idiopathic outflow tract VTs is false?**
   *Harrison's 20th Ed. Chapter 249 Page 1759*
   A. Produces monophasic R waves in leads II, III & aVF
   B. Occur as repeated bursts of nonsustained bursts of VT
   C. Provoked by exercise or emotional upset
   D. Most originate in the left ventricular outflow tract

Acute medical therapy for idiopathic outflow tract VT is rarely required because the VT is hemodynamically tolerated and is typically nonsustained. Most originate in the right ventricular outflow tract.

782. **Which of the following can be induced by exercise?**
   *Harrison's 20th Ed. Chapter 249 Page 1759*
   A. Anaphylaxis
   B. Asthma
   C. Arrhythmia
   D. All of the above

783. **Which of the following can terminate the idiopathic outflow tract ventricular tachycardia?**
   *Harrison's 20th Ed. Chapter 249 Page 1759*
   A. IV lidocaine
   B. IV procainamide
   C. IV amiodarone
   D. IV beta blockers

Intravenous beta blockers frequently terminate idiopathic outflow tract ventricular tachycardia.

784. **Which of the following VT can be terminated by intravenous verapamil?**

*Harrison's 20th Ed. Chapter 249 Page 1759*

A. Idiopathic VT
B. Bundle branch reentry VT
C. LV intrafascicular VT
D. All of the above

785. **Which of the following about LV intrafascicular VT is false?**

*Harrison's 20th Ed. Chapter 249 Page 1759*

A. Right bundle branch block-like configuration
B. Exercise-induced
C. Reentry in or near septal ramifications of LV Purkinje system
D. None of the above

*LV intrafascicular VT presents with sustained VT that has a right bundle branch block-like configuration. It is often exercise-induced and occurs more often in men than women. The mechanism is reentry in or near the septal ramifications of the LV Purkinje system. This VT can be terminated by intravenous administration of verapamil.*

# Polymorphic Ventricular Tachycardia and Ventricular Fibrillation

**786.** Which of the following is a potential mechanism for polymorphic ventricular tachycardia?
*Harrison's 20th Ed. Chapter 250 Page 1759*

- A. Reentry with continually changing reentrant paths
- B. Spiral wave reentry
- C. Multiple automatic foci
- D. All of the above

Sustained polymorphic VT is seen with any form of structural heart disease, but does not always indicate a structural abnormality or focus of automaticity. Potential mechanisms include reentry with continually changing reentrant paths, spiral wave reentry and multiple automatic foci.

**787.** Polymorphic VT is typically seen in association with?
*Harrison's 20th Ed. Chapter 250 Page 1759*

- A. Acute myocardial infarction or ischemia
- B. Ventricular hypertrophy
- C. Genetic mutations that affect cardiac ion channels
- D. All of the above

**788.** What percentage of patients with acute MI develop VT that degenerates to VF?
*Harrison's 20th Ed. Chapter 250 Page 1759*

- A. 1%
- B. 3%
- C. 5%
- D. 10%

Approximately 10% of patients with acute MI develop VT that degenerates to VF, related to reentry through the infarct border zone. The risk is greatest in the first hour of acute MI.

**789.** Patients who survive primary VF within first 48 hours of onset of acute infarction have?
*Harrison's 20th Ed. Chapter 250 Page 1759*

- A. Good short-term prognosis
- B. Good long-term prognosis
- C. Poor long-term prognosis
- D. None of the above

Polymorphic VT & VF that occur within the first 48 h of acute MI are associated with greater in-hospital mortality but those who survive past hospital discharge are not at increased risk for arrhythmic sudden death.

**790.** "Pause-dependent" phrase best relates to?
*Harrison's 20th Ed. Chapter 250 Page 1760*

- A. Short QT syndrome
- B. Brugada syndrome
- C. Torsade de pointes
- D. Early repolarization syndrome

Polymorphic VT Torsade de pointes has a characteristic initiation sequence of a premature ventricular beat that induces a pause, followed by a sinus beat that has a longer QT interval and interruption of the T wave by the PVC that is the first beat of the polymorphic VT. This characteristic initiation is termed "pause-dependent".

**791.** Bazett's formula for the calculation of QTc is?
*N Engl J Med. 1993;328:287*

- A. QT / Square root of PR
- B. QT / Square root of RR
- C. QT x Square root of PR
- D. QT x Square root of RR

QT interval is from the onset of QRS complex to the end of the T wave. Bazett's formula (QT interval is adjusted for heart rate) for the calculation of QTc is QT interval (in seconds) divided by the square root of the RR interval (in seconds). Bazett's formula, however, overcorrects QT interval at fast heart rates & undercorrects it at low heart rates. Fridericia, Hodges or Framingham formula can be used instead.

**792.** Which of the following about congenital long QT syndromes is false?
*Harrison's 20th Ed. Chapter 250 Page 1760*

- A. Type 1 has reduced repolarizing current $I_{Ks}$
- B. Type 2 has reduced repolarizing current $I_{Kr}$
- C. Type 3 has delayed inactivation of the $I_{Na}$
- D. None of the above

**793.** Which of the following do not cause QT prolongation?
*Harrison's 20th Ed. Chapter 250 Page 1761 Table 250-3*

- A. Ibutilide
- B. Sotalol
- C. Lidocaine
- D. Disopyramide

Class IB antiarrhythmic agents (lidocaine) do not cause QT prolongation. Class IA (Quinidine, Disopyramide and Procainamide) and Class III antiarrhythmic agents (Sotalol, Dofetilide, Ibutilide and almokalant) prolong QT interval and may precipitate torsades de pointes.

**794.** Which of the following prolong QT interval?
*Harrison's 20th Ed. Chapter 250 Page 1761 Table 250-3*

- A. Hypocalcemia
- B. Hypomagnesemia
- C. Hypokalemia
- D. All of the above

**795.** Which of the following prolong QT interval?
*Harrison's 20th Ed. Chapter 250 Page 1761 Table 250-3*

- A. Hyperparathyroidism
- B. Pheochromocytoma
- C. Hyperaldosteronism
- D. All of the above

**796.** Which of the following intracranial disorders prolong QT interval?
*Harrison's 20th Ed. Chapter 250 Page 1761 Table 250-3*

- A. Subarachnoid hemorrhage
- B. Thalamic hematoma
- C. Encephalitis
- D. All of the above

**797. Long QT syndrome (LQTS) was first described by?**
*Circulation. 2006;113:783-790*

- A. Romano and Ward
- B. Levine and Woodworth
- C. Jervell and Lange-Nielsen
- D. Moss and Schwartz

In 1957, Anton Jervell and Fred Lange-Nielsen first described a family with long QT syndrome (LQTS). The family consisted of unrelated parents and their six children, four of whom were deaf with frequent fainting attacks precipitated by acute emotional arousal and exercise. Three of the four deaf children died suddenly while playing at the ages of 4, 5, and 9 years. In 1963 and 1964, Romano and Ward respectively, reported separate families with QT prolongation in one parent and several children, all of whom possessed normal hearing but experienced recurrent syncope and sudden death (autosomal dominant mode of inheritance). In 1979 Moss and Schwartz established the prospective International LQTS Registry for enrollment and follow-up of proband-identified LQTS families.

**798. Syncope in long-QT syndrome is attributed to?**
*N Engl J Med. 2008;358:169-76*

- A. Emotional or physical stress
- B. Electrolyte disturbances
- C. Torsades de pointes
- D. Lack of sleep

Syncope in patients with the long-QT syndrome is generally attributed to the form of polymorphic ventricular tachycardia called torsades de pointes. Death is usually due to ventricular fibrillation.

**799. LQT1-specific trigger is?**
*N Engl J Med. 2008;358:169-76*

- A. Emotional stress
- B. Physical stress
- C. Diving and swimming
- D. All of the above

**800. Schwartz scoring system for diagnosis of LQTS includes all except?**
*N Engl J Med. 2008;358:169-76*

- A. Genetic information
- B. ECG features
- C. Personal history
- D. Family history

Schwartz scoring system for LQTS includes ECG features, personal & family history, but does not take into account genetic information.

**801. Which of the following is not useful in diagnosis of LQTS?**
*N Engl J Med. 2008;358:169-76*

- A. Echocardiography
- B. Holter monitoring
- C. Electrophysiological testing
- D. All of the above

Physical examination, echocardiography, MRI, Holter monitoring and electrophysiological testing show no abnormalities in LQTS.

**802. Most powerful predictor of risk in LQTS is?**
*N Engl J Med. 2008;358:169-76, Harrison's 17th Ed. 1441*

- A. QTc duration
- B. Family history
- C. History of syncope
- D. Gender

The most powerful predictor of risk is the QTc duration. Marked lengthening of the QT interval to > 500 ms is clearly associated with a greater arrhythmia risk in patients with the LQTS. In LQT2, females fared worse than their males, while opposite was true in LQT3, and no sex bias occurs in LQT1. Syncope and sudden death are most frequent in childhood and adolescence. The risk of cardiac events is higher in males before puberty and higher in females during adulthood.

**803. Which of the following is false about LQT1?**
*Harrison's 20th Ed. Chapter 250 Page 1760*

- A. Most common genotypic abnormality in LQTS
- B. QT interval fails to shorten with exercise
- C. T wave is broad
- D. None of the above

**804. Which of the following is false about LQT1?**
*Harrison's 20th Ed. Chapter 250 Page 1760*

- A. Exercise is the most common trigger for arrhythmias
- B. Respond to beta blocker therapy
- C. Due to mutation in potassium-channel gene (KCNQ1) on chromosome 11
- D. None of the above

**805. Which of the following is false about LQT2?**
*Harrison's 20th Ed. Chapter 250 Page 1760*

- A. T wave is low amplitude, notched and bifid
- B. Emotional stress /startle triggers arrhythmias
- C. Sleep or auditory stimulation triggers arrhythmias
- D. None of the above

**806. Which of the following is false about LQT2?**
*Harrison's 20th Ed. Chapter 250 Page 1760*

- A. Risk of syncope & sudden death increased in postpartum period
- B. Respond to beta blocker therapy
- C. Due to a mutation in a potassium-channel gene on chromosome 7 (KCNH2 or HERG)
- D. None of the above

**807. Which of the following is false about LQT3?**
*Harrison's 20th Ed. Chapter 250 Page 1760*

- A. Due to a mutation in cardiac sodium channel gene on chromosome 3
- B. Late-onset peaked biphasic/asymmetric T waves
- C. Prognosis for LQT3 is the poorest of all LQTs
- D. None of the above

**808. Which of the following is false about LQT3?**
*Harrison's 20th Ed. Chapter 250 Page 1760*

- A. Beta blockers are not recommended
- B. Exercise is not restricted in LQT3
- C. QT shortening occurs with mexiletine
- D. None of the above

**809. Which of the following is false about LQT3?**
*Harrison's 20th Ed. Chapter 250 Page 1760*

- A. Most events in LQT3 patients occur during sleep
- B. LQT3 is caused by a mutation in sodium channel gene on chromosome 3 (SCN5A)
- C. Male patients have worst prognosis in LQT3
- D. None of the above

**810. In short QT syndrome, QT interval is?**
*Harrison's 20th Ed. Chapter 250 Page 1760*

A. < 300 ms
B. < 340 ms
C. < 360 ms
D. < 380 ms

Usually, a QT interval < 300 ms is required to establish the diagnosis of Short QT syndrome.

**811. Mutations in which of the following gene is the cause of short QT syndrome?**
*Harrison's 20th Ed. Chapter 250 Page 1760*

A. HERG
B. KvLQT1
C. KCNJ2
D. Any of the above

Mutations in the HERG, KvLQT1 & KCNJ2 genes cause of Short QT syndrome due to a gain of function of the potassium channel (IK) or reduced inward depolarizing currents.

**812. Which of the following is a feature of short QT syndrome?**
*Harrison's 20th Ed. Chapter 250 Page 1760*

A. Short PR interval
B. Flat P waves
C. Tall and peaked T waves
D. Prominent U waves

In Short QT syndrome, T waves tends to be tall and peaked especially in leads V2 to V4 and may be interpreted as R waves by an implantable cardioverter-defibrillator. Patients with the syndrome are predisposed to both AF and VF.

**813. Which of the following can shorten QT interval?**

A. Hypercalcemia
B. Hyperkalemia
C. Acidosis
D. All of the above

Conditions that can shorten QT interval include hypercalcemia (with an accompanying prolonged PR interval and a wide QRS complex), hyperkalemia, acidosis, increased vagal tone, after ventricular fibrillation (due to increased intracellular calcium), digitalis use, androgen use. Interestingly, a shorter-than-expected QT interval was noted in patients with chronic fatigue syndrome. Quinidine is helpful.

**814. Which of the following is a repolarization abnormality?**

A. Brugada syndrome
B. Arrhythmogenic right ventricular cardiomyopathy
C. Short QT syndrome
D. All of the above

Besides LQTS, other repolarization abnormalities are Brugada syndrome (opposite of LQT3), arrhythmogenic right ventricular cardiomyopathy, & short QT syndrome.

**815. In Brugada syndrome, ST segment elevation in V1 - V3 may be?**
*Harrison's 19th Ed. 1497*

A. Manifest
B. Transient
C. Concealed
D. Any of the above

**816. ECG manifestations of Brugada syndrome are provoked with?**
*Harrison's 19th Ed. 1497*

A. Ajmaline
B. Flecainide
C. Procainamide
D. All of the above

The major clinical features of autosomal dominant Brugada syndrome include manifest, transient, or concealed ST segment elevation in V1 to V3 that can typically be provoked with sodium channel-blocking drugs ajmaline, flecainide & procainamide & a risk of polymorphic ventricular arrhythmias.

**817. Which of the following is false about Brugada syndrome?**
*Harrison's 19th Ed. 1497*

A. Left bundle branch block pattern
B. ST elevation leads $V_1 - V_3$
C. Terminal T-wave inversion in leads $V_1 - V_3$
D. Due to mutation in cardiac sodium channel SCN5A

In ECG, right bundle-branch block (rSR') and downsloping ST-segment elevation in lead V1 is typical of Brugada syndrome. It is syndrome of RBBB & nonischemic ST-segment elevations.

**818. Which of the following is false about Brugada syndrome?**
*Harrison's 19th Ed. 1497*

A. Most common in young Asian male
B. Affected region is RV outflow tract epicardium
C. Patients do not benefit from beta blocker therapy
D. Procainamide & flecainide are beneficial

Procainamide & flecainide exacerbate Brugada syndrome. Quinidine is successful in suppressing frequent episodes of VT.

**819. Which of the following statements about PVCs is false?**
*Harrison's 20th Ed. Chapter 248 Page 1755*

A. May occur in up to 80% of patients with previous MI
B. On ECG show wide (usually > 0.12 s), bizarre QRS complexes not preceded by P waves
C. When they arise in specialized conduction system (fascicles), they may be < 0.12 s in duration
D. They result in a fully compensatory pause

PVCs are associated with a "fully compensatory pause" i.e. duration between last QRS before PVC and next QRS complex is equal to twice the sinus rate. PVC produces slow ventricular activation and a wide QRS complex that is typically >140 ms in duration.

**820. Which of the following statements about PVCs is false?**
*Harrison's 19th Ed. 1490*

A. When fixed coupling is not present and interval between PVCs has a common denominator, ventricular parasystole is said to be present
B. Trigeminy means two sinus beats followed by a PVC
C. Two successive PVCs are termed pairs or couplets
D. ≥3 consecutive PVCs are termed ventricular tachycardia when the rate exceeds 160 beats/minute

PVCs may occur in patterns of bigeminy, in which every sinus beat is followed by a PVC, or trigeminy, in which two sinus beats are followed by a PVC. PVCs may have different morphologies and are thus referred to as multiformed. Two successive PVCs are termed pairs or couplets. Three or more consecutive PVCs are termed VT when the rate is >100 beats/minute.

**821. Which of the following statements about PVCs is false?**
*Harrison's 19th Ed. 1490*

A. Ventricular impulses are never conducted retrogradely to atrium
B. PVC that does not produce retrograde concealed conduction and fails to influence oncoming sinus impulse is termed interpolated PVC
C. Antiarrhythmic agents can produce lethal arrhythmias
D. Prophylactic antiarrhythmic therapy is recommended only for young patients with complicated MI

*PVC typically does not conduct to the atrium. Occasionally PVC can occur early enough & conduct retrograde to atrium to reset the sinus node. Pause that results will be less than compensatory. PVCs that fail to influence the oncoming sinus impulse are termed interpolated PVCs.*

**822. QRS duration of a premature ventricular complex (PVC) is?**
*Harrison's 19th Ed. 1490*

A. > 110 ms
B. > 120 ms
C. > 130 ms
D. > 140 ms

*A PVC has a wide QRS complex that is typically >140 ms in duration.*

**823. Sustained ventricular tachycardia is defined as VT that persists for?**
*Harrison's 19th Ed. 1490*

A. > 10 seconds
B. > 15 seconds
C. > 20 seconds
D. > 30 seconds

*A time duration of 30 seconds is frequently used to distinguish sustained from nonsustained VT. Hemodynamically unstable VT that requires termination before 30 seconds or VT that is terminated by therapy from an implantable defibrillator is also typically classified as sustained.*

**824. Which of the following is not true for sustained VT?**
*Harrison's 19th Ed. 1490*

A. Almost always symptomatic
B. Mostly associated with marked hemodynamic compromise
C. Almost always leads to development of myocardial ischemia
D. Acute ischemia is responsible for most recurrent episodes of sustained uniform VT

**825. The heart rate in ventricular flutter usually is?**
*Harrison's 19th Ed. 1490*

A. 100 to 150 beats/minute
B. 150 to 300 beats/minute
C. 300 to 450 beats/minute
D. 450 to 600 beats/minute

*Ventricular flutter appears as a sine wave on the ECG and has a rate of >250 beats/minute.*

**826. It is not possible to assign a specific morphology to which of the following arrhythmia?**
*Harrison's 19th Ed. 1490*

A. Atrial flutter
B. Ventricular flutter
C. Torsades de pointes
D. WPW syndrome with AF

*A rapid rate with sine wave oscillations of ventricular flutter make it impossible to assign it a specific morphology and in some cases to distinguish it from rapid VT.*

**827. VT that shows an alternation in QRS axis is called?**
*Harrison's 19th Ed. 1491*

A. Monomorphic VT
B. Polymorphic VT
C. Bidirectional tachycardia
D. Torsades de pointes

**828. Torsades de pointes occurs most often in the setting of?**
*Harrison's 19th Ed. 1491*

A. Slow heart rate
B. QT prolongation
C. Hypokalemia
D. All of the above

*TDP occurs most often with slow heart rates, QT prolongation & hypokalemia or hypomagnesemia and at the time of conversion from atrial fibrillation to sinus rhythm.*

**829. Characteristics ECG findings that suggest VT are all except?**
*Harrison's 19th Ed. 1491, Figure 233-10, Table 233–6*

A. QRS complex > 0.20 seconds
B. AV dissociation
C. Inferior QRS frontal plane axis
D. Concordance of QRS pattern in all precordial leads

*Ventricular tachycardia on ECG shows AV dissociation, wide QRS >200 ms, superior frontal plane axis, slurring of initial portion of QRS, and large S wave in V6.*

**830. Which of the following always produce hemodynamic collapse if allowed to continue?**
*Harrison's 19th Ed. 1491*

A. Polymorphic ventricular arrhythmias
B. Ventricular flutter
C. Ventricular fibrillation
D. All of the above

*Polymorphic ventricular arrhythmias, ventricular flutter, and VF always produce hemodynamic collapse if allowed to continue.*

**831. Characteristics ECG findings that suggest VT are all except?**
*Harrison's 19th Ed. 1491*

A. Superior and rightward QRS frontal plane axis
B. Bizarre QRS complex mimiking LBBB or RBBB
C. Slurring of the initial portion of QRS
D. AV dissociation

*VT on ECG is suggested by presence of QRS duration >140 ms in the absence of drug therapy, superior & rightward QRS frontal plane axis, bizarre QRS complex that does not mimic the characteristic QRS pattern associated with LBBB or RBBB, and slurring of initial portion of QRS.*

**832. Which of the following about idiopathic ventricular arrhythmias is false?**
*Harrison's 20th Ed. Chapter 248 Page 1756*

A. ~80% of outflow tract VTs originate in LV
B. Not associated with SCD
C. Vagal maneuvers terminate them
D. Adenosine & beta blockers terminate them

*~80% of outflow tract VTs originate in RV & ~20% in LV outflow tract regions.*

### 833. Idioventricular rhythm is defined as?
*Harrison's 20th Ed. Chapter 248 Page 1757*

- A. 2 or more ventricular beats at a rate <100 beats/minute
- B. 3 or more ventricular beats at a rate <100 beats/minute
- C. 4 or more ventricular beats at a rate <100 beats/minute
- D. 5 or more ventricular beats at a rate <100 beats/minute

Three or more ventricular beats at a rate slower than 100 beats/minute are termed idioventricular rhythm. Automaticity is the likely mechanism.

### 834. Accelerated idioventricular rhythm (AIVR) has overlap features with?
*Harrison's 19th Ed. 1490*

- A. Monomorphic VT
- B. Polymorphic VT
- C. Slow VT
- D. None of the above

By definition there is an overlap between AIVR and "slow" VT.

### 835. Which of the following about AIVR is false?
*Harrison's 19th Ed. 1490*

- A. Heart rate ranges from 60 to 120 beats/min
- B. Occurs in acute MI
- C. Usually transient
- D. Treatment consists of b blockers

AIVR refers to a ventricular rhythm that is characterized by three or more complexes at a rate >40 and <120 beats/minute due to abnormal automaticity. Transient AIVR is frequently seen in acute myocardial infarction, cocaine intoxication, acute myocarditis, digoxin intoxication & postoperative cardiac surgery. Sustained AIVR is seen in acute MI & postoperatively. Treatment consists of atropine and atrial pacing.

### 836. Which of the following is the cause of ST-segment elevation?
*N Engl J Med. 2003;349:2128-35*

- A. Acute pericarditis
- B. Hyperkalemia
- C. Pulmonary embolism
- D. All of the above

### 837. ST-segment elevation in normal healthy young men (male pattern) is seen in?
*N Engl J Med. 2003;349:2128-35*

- A. V1
- B. V2
- C. V3
- D. V4

Concave ST-segment elevation of 1–3 mm seen in ~90% of healthy young men (male pattern) is most marked in V2.

### 838. ST-segment elevation in early repolarization is seen in?
*N Engl J Med. 2003;349:2128-35*

- A. V1
- B. V2
- C. V3
- D. V4

ST-segment elevation due to early repolarization is most marked in V4, with notching at J point, tall, upright T waves, reciprocal ST depression in aVR, not in aVL, when limb leads are involved.

### 839. Which of the following is an ECG marker of abnormality in repolarization?
*N Engl J Med. 2001;345:1476*

- A. PR-interval dispersion
- B. QT-interval dispersion
- C. J-point dispersion
- D. All of the above

Two ECG markers of abnormalities in repolarization are QT-interval dispersion & T-wave alternans. They identify patients who are at risk for sudden death from arrhythmia. QT-interval dispersion refers to difference between maximal & minimal QT intervals from various leads on standard ECG. T-wave alternans is defined as alternating T-wave amplitude from beat to beat on special ECG recording techniques.

### 840. Catecholaminergic polymorphic VT is best related to?
*Harrison's 19th Ed. 1498*

- A. Ang II type I receptor
- B. B2-Bradykinin receptor
- C. Ryanodine receptor
- D. All of the above

In catecholaminergic polymorphic VT there occurs a mutation of myocardial ryanodine release channel, which creates a "leak" in calcium from sarcoplasmic reticulum (SR). Accumulation of intracellular calcium potentiates delayed afterdepolarizations and triggered activity. $Ca^{2+}$ is released from SR through a $Ca^{2+}$ release channel-ryanodine receptor (RyR2), which controls intracytoplasmic $[Ca^{2+}]$ and leads to local changes in intracellular $[Ca^{2+}]$ called calcium sparks. Regulatory protein, calsequestin 2 inhibit RyR2 and thereby release of $Ca^{2+}$ from SR. PKA dissociates calstabin from RyR2, enhancing $Ca^{2+}$ release and thereby myocardial contractility. Excessive plasma catecholamine levels and cardiac sympathetic neuronal release of norepinephrine cause hyperphosphorylation of PKA, leading to calstabin 2 depleted RyR2. The latter depletes SR $Ca^{2+}$ stores and thereby impairs cardiac contraction, leading to heart failure, and also triggers ventricular arrhythmias.

### 841. Patients of catecholaminergic polymorphic VT may present with?
*Harrison's 19th Ed. 1498*

- A. Bidirectional VT
- B. Precipitated by exercise & emotional stress
- C. Polymorphic VT resembles that seen with digitalis toxicity
- D. Any of the above

Patients of catecholaminergic polymorphic VT can manifest bidirectional VT, nonsustained polymorphic VT, or recurrent VF resembling that seen with digitalis toxicity. The arrhythmias are precipitated by exercise & emotional stress. Treatment with beta blockers & ICD implantation is recommended.

## Electrical Storm and Incessant VT

**842.** Electrical storm refers to the occurrence of ≥3 episodes of VT or ventricular fibrillation (VF) within?
*Harrison's 20th Ed. Chapter 251 Page 1762*

A. 1 hour
B. 3 hours
C. 12 hours
D. 24 hours

*Electrical storm or ventricular tachycardia (VT) storm refers to the occurrence of three or more episodes of VT or ventricular fibrillation (VF) within 24 hours.*

**843.** Repeated VT episodes requiring defibrillation is called?
*Harrison's 20th Ed. Chapter 251 Page 1762*

A. VT storm
B. VT paroxysm
C. VT battle
D. VT flow

**844.** "VT storm" or "electrical storm" is most commonly encountered in patients with?
*Harrison's 20th Ed. Chapter 251 Page 1762*

A. ICDs
B. Myocardial infarction
C. Cardiomyopathy
D. Cardiac surgery

*Repeated VT episodes requiring external cardioversion/defibrillation or repeated appropriate ICD shock therapy are referred to as VT storm. "VT storm" or "electrical storm" refers to three or more separate episodes of VT within 24 hours most commonly encountered in patients with ICDs.*

**845.** If QT prolongation causes torsades de pointes, which of the following is useful?
*Harrison's 20th Ed. Chapter 251 Page 1762*

A. Intravenous magnesium
B. Intravenous beta blocker
C. Intravenous amiodarone
D. Intravenous quinidine

*If QT prolongation causing torsades de pointes is possible intravenous magnesium should be administered and bradycardia treated.*

**846.** In Brugada syndrome, polymorphic VT/VF episode is managed with?
*Harrison's 20th Ed. Chapter 251 Page 1762*

A. Intravenous lidocaine
B. Intravenous beta blocker
C. Intravenous amiodarone
D. Intravenous quinidine

*If QT interval is not prolonged & Brugada syndrome is possible, administration of quinidine and/or isoproterenol may abolish recurrent polymorphic VT/VF episodes.*

**847.** VT is designated incessant when VT continues to recur shortly after?
*Harrison's 20th Ed. Chapter 251 Page 1762*

A. Electrical conversion to sinus rhythm
B. Pharmacologic conversion to sinus rhythm
C. Spontaneous conversion to sinus rhythm
D. Any of the above

*VT is designated incessant when VT continues to recur shortly after electrical, pharmacologic, or spontaneous conversion to sinus rhythm.*

**848.** Which of the following about sotalol is false?
*Harrison's 20th Ed. Chapter 251 Page 1762*

A. Class III antiarrhythmic drug, non-selective β-blocker
B. Blocks repolarizing potassium currents, prolongs QT
C. Excreted via the kidneys
D. None of the above

**849.** Which of the following should be considered for polymorphic VT storm?
*Harrison's 19th Ed. 1498*

A. Intravenous beta blocker
B. Intravenous calcium channel blocker
C. Intravenous nitroglycerine
D. Intravenous digoxin

*Intravenous beta blockade therapy should be considered for polymorphic VT storm.*

**850.** Which of the following is available as intravenous formulation?
*Harrison's 19th Ed. 1498*

A. Lidocaine
B. Quinidine
C. Procainamide
D. All of the above

*Lidocaine, quinidine and procainamide are available as intravenous formulations.*

**851.** Which of the following can prevent recurrences in patients with recurrent monomorphic VT?
*Harrison's 19th Ed. 1491*

A. IV lidocaine
B. IV procainamide
C. IV amiodarone
D. Any of the above

*In patients with recurrent monomorphic VT, acute IV administration of lidocaine, procainamide, or amiodarone can prevent recurrences.*

**852.** Verapamil is least effective / contraindicated in which of the following?
*Harrison's 19th Ed. 1498*

A. Idiopathic LV septal VT
B. Ventricular tachycardia
C. Accessory pathway mediated tachycardias
D. Atrial fibrillation

*Most VTs do not respond to carotid sinus massage, Valsalva maneuver or adenosine administration. IV administration of verapamil and/or adenosine is not recommended as a diagnostic test. Verapamil is associated with hemodynamic collapse when administered to patients with structural heart disease and VT.*

853. Which of the following is unique in its suppression with verapamil?
*Harrison's 19th Ed. 1498*

A. Idiopathic LV septal VT
B. VT associated with LV dilated cardiomyopathy
C. Bundle branch reentrant VT
D. All of the above

*Idiopathic LV septal VT responds uniquely to IV verapamil.*

854. Which of the following drug exhibits properties consistent with multiple classes in Vaughan-Williams classification?
*Harrison's 19th Ed. 1498*

A. Quinidine
B. Amiodarone
C. Mexiletine
D. Propafenone

*Amiodarone is consistent with multiple classes.*

855. Which of the following antiarrhythmic drugs is used to treat painful sensory neuropathy?
*Harrison's 19th Ed. 2682*

A. Mexiletine
B. Flecainide
C. Propafenone
D. Amiodarone

856. Which of the following antiarrhythmic drugs is used to treat myotonia?
*Harrison's 19th Ed. 462e-18*

A. Mexiletine
B. Flecainide
C. Propafenone
D. Amiodarone

*Mexiletine is helpful in patients with significant myotonia in paramyotonia congenita (PC).*

857. Which of the following antiarrhythmic drugs is least likely to produce bradycardia?
*Harrison's 19th Ed. 1498*

A. Mexiletine
B. Flecainide
C. Propafenone
D. Amiodarone

858. Which of the following is not an adverse effect of amiodarone?
*Harrison's 19th Ed. 1498*

A. Pulmonary infiltrates
B. Hepatitis
C. Photosensitivity
D. Bronchospasm

859. Which of the following is an adverse effect of amiodarone?
*Harrison's 19th Ed. 1498*

A. Photosensitivity
B. Neuropathy
C. Ocular toxicity
D. All of the above

860. Vaughan-Williams classification is used to classify?
*Harrison's 19th Ed. 273e-5*

A. Cardiotonic drugs
B. Antiarrhythmic drugs
C. Vasodilator drugs
D. Vasopressor drugs

*Antiarrhythmic agents classification scheme was proposed in 1970 by Vaughan-Williams and later modified by Singh and Harrison. The classes of antiarrhythmic action are class I - local anesthetic effect due to blockade of Na+ current; class II - interference with the action of catecholamines at the β-adrenergic receptor; class III - delay of repolarization due to inhibition of K+ current or activation of depolarizing current; and class IV - interference with calcium conductance. Class I antiarrhythmics have been further subdivided based on the kinetics and potency of Na+ channel binding. Class Ia agents (quinidine, procainamide) have moderate potency and intermediate kinetics; class Ib agents (lidocaine, mexiletine) have low potency and rapid kinetics; and class Ic drugs (flecainide, propafenone) have high potency and the slowest kinetics.*

861. Which of the following drug does not fit in Vaughan-Williams classification of antiarrhythmic drugs?
*Harrison's 19th Ed. 1480, Table 276-3*

A. Ibutilide
B. Adenosine
C. Bretylium
D. Propafenone

*Adenosine does not fit into VW classification.*

862. Class III antiarrhythmics exert their action through?
*Harrison's 19th Ed. 1480, Table 276-4*

A. Cardiac cellular excitatory current
B. Action potential duration
C. Automaticity
D. All of the above

863. Class I and IV antiarrhythmics exert their action through?
*Harrison's 19th Ed. 1480, Table 276-4*

A. Cardiac cellular excitatory current
B. Action potential duration
C. Automaticity
D. All of the above

864. Which of the following antiarrhythmic drugs can cause 'Lupus erythematosus like syndrome'?
*Harrison's 19th Ed. 1480 Table 276-5*

A. Procainamide
B. Bretylium
C. Lidocaine
D. Mexiletine

865. Which of the following antiarrhythmic drugs can cause 'Lupus erythematosus like syndrome'?
*Harrison's 19th Ed. 2134*

A. Procainamide
B. Disopyramide
C. Propafenone
D. All of the above

866. Which of the following antiarrhythmic drugs can cause true myositis?

*Harrison's 19th Ed. 2199*

A. Procainamide
B. Ibutilide
C. Propafenone
D. Bretylium

*D-Penicillamine, procainamide and statins may produce a true myositis resembling PM or necrotizing myositis.*

867. Which of the following antiarrhythmic drugs can cause seizures?

*Harrison's 19th Ed. 1480 Table 276-5*

A. Procainamide
B. Disopyramide
C. Lidocaine
D. Mexiletine

868. Which of the following antiarrhythmic drugs can cause congestive heart failure?

*Harrison's 19th Ed. 1480 Table 276-5*

A. Procainamide
B. Disopyramide
C. Lidocaine
D. Mexiletine

869. Which of the following antiarrhythmic drugs can cause taste disturbance?

*Harrison's 19th Ed. 1480 Table 276-5*

A. Procainamide
B. Disopyramide
C. Propafenone
D. Sotalol

870. Which of the following antiarrhythmic drugs can cause bronchospasm?

*Harrison's 19th Ed. 1480 Table 276-5*

A. Procainamide
B. Disopyramide
C. Propafenone
D. Sotalol

871. Most uniform sustained VT associated with LV dilated cardiomyopathy can be mapped to?

*Harrison's 18th Ed. 1895*

A. Mitral valvular region
B. Tricuspid valvular region
C. Pulmonary valvular region
D. All of the above

*VT associated with LV dilated cardiomyopathy may be mono- or polymorphic. Myopathic process has a predilection for fibrosis around mitral & aortic valvular regions. Most uniform sustained VT are mapped to these regions.*

872. WPW syndrome is observed in patients with hypertrophic cardiomyopathy associated with which mutation?

*Harrison's 19th Ed. 433e-2, Table 433e-1*

A. ACTN2
B. S135L mutation
C. PRKAG2 mutation
D. CRYAB

*WPW syndrome is seen in patients with hypertrophic cardiomyopathy associated with PRKAG2 mutations.*

873. Infiltrative / Inflammatory & neuromuscular disorders associated with increased ventricular arrhythmia risk include?

*Harrison's 18th Ed. 1896, Table 233-7*

A. Sarcoidosis
B. Myotonic muscular dystrophy
C. Kearn-Sayre syndrome
D. All of the above

874. Infiltrative / Inflammatory & disorders associated with increased ventricular arrhythmia risk include?

*Harrison's 18th Ed. 1896, Table 233-7*

A. Chagas disease
B. Fabry disease
C. Amyloidosis
D. All of the above

875. Infiltrative / Inflammatory & neuromuscular disorders associated with increased ventricular arrhythmia risk include?

*Harrison's 18th Ed. 1896, Table 233-7*

A. Becker's muscular dystrophy
B. Hemochromatosis
C. Friedreich's ataxia
D. All of the above

876. Neuromuscular disorders associated with increased ventricular arrhythmia risk include all except?

*Harrison's 18th Ed. 1896, Table 233-7*

A. Facioscapulohumeral muscular dystrophy
B. Emery-Dreyfuss muscular dystrophy
C. Limb-girdle muscular dystrophy
D. Duchenne's muscular dystrophy

*Characteristically, FSH muscular dystrophy does not involve other organ systems. Labile hypertension & nerve deafness is common. Coats' disease (telangiectasia, exudation & retinal detachment) also occurs.*

877. Ventricular fibrillation can occur due to?

*N Engl J Med. 2003;349:2128-35*

A. Antiarrhythmic drugs
B. Torsades de pointes
C. WPW syndrome with AF
D. All of the above

*IHD is mostly responsible for VF which also occur with antiarrhythmic drugs, TDP and WPW syndrome who develop AF with an extremely rapid ventricular response.*

**878. Which of the following about digoxin toxicity is false?**
*N Engl J Med. 2003;349:2128-35*

A. Myocardial cell calcium overload
B. Bidirectional VT from left anterior & posterior fascicles
C. Narrow QRS right bundle branch configuration
D. None of the above

The signature VT associated with digoxin toxicity is bidirectional VT due to triggered activity associated with calcium overload resulting from inhibition of Na⁺/K⁺ ATPase by digoxin. Bidirectional VT originates from left anterior & posterior fascicles creating a relatively narrow QRS right bundle branch configuration with beat-to-beat alternating right & left frontal plane QRS axis.

**879. Which of the following is an ECG feature of acute pericarditis?**
*N Engl J Med. 2003;349:2128-35*

A. Diffuse ST-segment elevation
B. Reciprocal ST-segment depression in aVR, not in aVL
C. PR-segment depression
D. All of the above

In acute pericarditis, ECG shows diffuse ST-segment elevation (seldom >5 mm), reciprocal ST-segment depression in aVR, not in aVL and PR-segment depression.

**880. Which of the following is not an ECG feature of hyperkalemia?**
*N Engl J Med. 2003;349:2128-35*

A. Widened QRS
B. Tall, peaked, tented T waves
C. Low-amplitude or absent P waves
D. ST segment usually upsloping

In Hyperkalemia, ECG shows widened QRS, tall, peaked, tented T waves, low-amplitude or absent P waves, with ST segment usually downsloping.

**881. Which of the following "Channelopathies" can cause Ventricular Fibrillation–Induced Cardiac Arrest?**
*N Engl J Med. 2005;353:2492-501*

A. Long-QT syndrome
B. Short-QT syndrome
C. Brugada syndrome
D. All of the above

**882. Noncardiac causes of Ventricular Fibrillation Induced Cardiac Arrest include?**
*N Engl J Med. 2005;353:2492-501*

A. Bronchospasm
B. Sleep apnea
C. Seizure
D. All of the above

Noncardiac causes of Ventricular Fibrillation Induced Cardiac Arrest are Respiratory (Bronchospasm, Aspiration, Sleep apnea, Primary pulmonary hypertension, Pulmonary embolism), Metabolic or toxic (Electrolyte disturbances, Medications or drug ingestion, Environmental poisoning, Sepsis) and Neurologic (Seizure, Cerebrovascular accident: intracranial hemorrhage, or ischemic stroke).

**883. Who, from the following, was one of the inventors of cardiac defibrillator?**
*N Engl J Med. 2001;344:1311*

A. Mickey Isenberg
B. Bardy GH
C. Claude Beck
D. Terry Mengert

Claude Beck is one of the inventors of cardiac defibrillation.

**884. The first intervention in the "chain of survival" is?**
*N Engl J Med. 2001;344:1311*

A. Rapid access
B. Rapid cardiopulmonary resuscitation
C. Rapid defibrillation
D. Rapid advanced care

The sequence of rapid access, rapid cardiopulmonary resuscitation, rapid defibrillation, and rapid advanced care is termed the chain of survival.

**885. In cardiopulmonary resuscitation, chest compression should be administered in the center of the chest on the?**
*N Engl J Med. 2001;344:1311*

A. Upper half of the sternum
B. Middle of the sternum
C. Lower half of the sternum
D. Any of the above

In cardiopulmonary resuscitation, chest compression should be administered in the center of the chest on the lower half of the sternum.

**886. In cardiopulmonary resuscitation in adults, the depth of chest compression should be?**
*N Engl J Med. 2001;344:1311*

A. 2 to 3 cm
B. 3 to 4 cm
C. 4 to 5 cm
D. 5 to 6 cm

In CPR in adults, the depth of chest compression should be 4 to 5 cm in adults.

**887. In cardiopulmonary resuscitation in adults, the rate of chest compression should be approximately?**
*N Engl J Med. 2001;344:1311*

A. 30 per minute
B. 50 per minute
C. 75 per minute
D. 100 per minute

**888. In cardiopulmonary resuscitation performed by two persons, the ratio of compressions to breaths is?**
*N Engl J Med. 2001;344:1311*

A. 10 : 1
B. 10 : 2
C. 15 : 1
D. 15 : 2

When cardiopulmonary resuscitation is performed by two persons, the ratio of chest compressions to breaths remains 15:2 with pause during ventilations. After endotracheal intubation, the ratio should be five compressions to one ventilation, and there should be no pause in chest compressions for the ventilatory breath.

**889. In ventricular fibrillation, initial shock with a monophasic wave-form defibrillator should be?**
*N Engl J Med. 2001;344:1311*

A. 100 J
B. 200 J
C. 300 J
D. 360 J

When a monophasic wave-form defibrillator is used for ventricular fibrillation, the initial shock should be 200 J. If the arrhythmia persists, a second shock of 200 to 300 J should be given, followed by a third shock of 360 J if still necessary. All three shocks should be given in quick succession.

890. What energy should be used for initial attempts at terminating VF?
*N Engl J Med. 2001;344:1311*

   A. At least 100 W
   B. At least 200 W
   C. At least 300 W
   D. At least 400 W

891. Paddle diameter for external cardioversion is?
*N Engl J Med. 2001;344:1311*

   A. 10 cm
   B. 12 cm
   C. 18 cm
   D. 24 cm

892. One paddle during external cardioversion is placed at?
*N Engl J Med. 2001;344:1311*

   A. Fourth ICS, midclavicular line
   B. Fifth ICS, midclavicular line
   C. Fourth ICS, left anterior axillary line
   D. Fifth ICS, left anterior axillary line

893. One paddle during external cardioversion is placed at?
*N Engl J Med. 2001;344:1311*

   A. Right parasternally at the level of first rib
   B. Right parasternally at the level of second rib
   C. Right parasternally at the level of third rib
   D. Right parasternally at the level of fourth rib

# Heart Failure: Pathophysiology and Diagnosis

**894. Which of the following is false about heart failure (HF)?**
*Harrison's 20th Ed. Chapter 252 Page 1763*

- A. Cardinal clinical symptoms are dyspnea & fatigue
- B. Cardinal clinical signs are edema and rales
- C. Term "congestive heart failure" is preferred over HF
- D. None of the above

*Because many patients present without signs or symptoms of volume overload, term "heart failure" is preferred over the older term "congestive heart failure".*

**895. Which of the following is false about heart failure (HF)?**
*Harrison's 20th Ed. Chapter 252 Page 1763*

- A. Complex clinical syndrome
- B. Due to structural or functional impairment of ventricular filling
- C. Due to structural or functional impairment of ejection of blood
- D. None of the above

**896. Overall prevalence of HF in adult population in developed countries is?**
*Harrison's 20th Ed. Chapter 252 Page 1763*

- A. 0.3%
- B. 0.5%
- C. 1%
- D. 2%

*Overall prevalence of HF in the adult population in developed countries is 2%.*

**897. Prevalence of HF in people aged > 65 years is?**
*Harrison's 20th Ed. Chapter 252 Page 1763*

- A. 2 - 4%
- B. 4 - 6%
- C. 6 - 10%
- D. 10 - 13%

*Prevalence of HF in people aged > 65 years is 6 - 10%.*

**898. What percentage of patients who develop Heart failure (HF) have normal or preserved EF?**
*Harrison's 20th Ed. Chapter 252 Page 1763*

- A. ≥ 10%
- B. ≥ 20%
- C. ≥ 35%
- D. ≥ 50%

*Epidemiologic studies show that approximately one-half of patients who develop HF have a normal or preserved EF (EF ≥ 50%) i.e. diastolic failure.*

**899. Which of the following is a category of HF?**
*Harrison's 20th Ed. Chapter 252 Page 1763*

- A. HF with a reduced EF (HFrEF)
- B. HF with a preserved EF (HRpEF)
- C. Borderline or mid-range EF
- D. All of the above

**900. LV ejection fraction is considered depressed if it is?**
*Harrison's 20th Ed. Chapter 252 Page 1763 Table 252-1*

- A. < 60%
- B. < 50%
- C. < 40%
- D. < 30%

**901. Which of the following is a cadiac cytoskeletal protein?**
*Harrison's 20th Ed. Chapter 252 Page 1763*

- A. Desmin
- B. Myosin
- C. Vinculin
- D. All of the above

**902. Which of the following is not a cadiac cytoskeletal protein?**
*Harrison's 20th Ed. Chapter 252 Page 1763*

- A. Desmin
- B. Myosin
- C. Vinculin
- D. Laminin

*Cytoskeletal proteins include desmin, cardiac myosin & vinculin. Laminin is a nuclear membrane protein.*

**903. Which of the following condition does not lead to HF in a normal heart?**
*Harrison's 20th Ed. Chapter 252 Page 1763*

- A. Hypertension
- B. Infiltrative disorders
- C. Chagas' disease
- D. Arteriovenous fistula

*Conditions that lead to a high cardiac output like arteriovenous fistula and anemia seldom lead to HF in a normal heart.*

**904. Dilated cardiomyopathy is associated with which of the following muscular dystrophies?**
*Harrison's 20th Ed. Chapter 252 Page 1764*

- A. Duchenne's
- B. Becker's
- C. Limb-girdle
- D. All of the above

*Dilated cardiomyopathy is associated with Duchenne's, Becker's and limb-girdle muscular dystrophies.*

**905. Chagas' disease is a major cause of HF in?**
*Harrison's 20th Ed. Chapter 252 Page 1764*

- A. Africa
- B. South America
- C. Western Europe
- D. South east Asia

### 906. Which of the following is the single most common cause of HF?
*Harrison's 20th Ed. Chapter 252 Page 1764*

A. Hypertension
B. Diabetes mellitus
C. CAD
D. Anemia

*CAD is the single most common cause of HF.*

### 907. New York Heart Association (NYHA) classification was introduced in which year?
*Harrison's 20th Ed. Chapter 252 Page 1764 Table 252-2*

A. 1960
B. 1964
C. 1968
D. 1972

*New York Heart Association Inc., Diseases of the Heart and Blood Vessels: Nomenclature and Criteria for Diagnosis, 6th ed. Boston, Little Brown, 1964, p. 114.*

### 908. In heart failure, which of the following compensatory mechanisms is activated after an index event?
*Harrison's 20th Ed. Chapter 252 Page 1764 Figure 252-1*

A. Adrenergic nervous system
B. Renin-angiotensin-aldosterone system
C. Cytokine system
D. All of the above

*Heart failure begins after an index event produces an initial decline in the heart's pumping capacity. After this initial decline in pumping capacity, a compensatory mechanisms are activated that includes adrenergic nervous system, renin-angiotensin-aldosterone system and cytokine system.*

### 909. Which of the following is a vasodilatory molecule?
*Harrison's 20th Ed. Chapter 252 Page 1764*

A. Atrial and brain natriuretic peptides (ANP & BNP)
B. Prostaglandins ($PGE_2$ & $PGI_2$)
C. Nitric oxide (NO)
D. All of the above

*In HF, there is activation of a family of compensatory vasodilatory molecules like atrial & brain natriuretic peptides (ANP & BNP), prostaglandins ($PGE_2$ & $PGI_2$) and nitric oxide (NO), that oppose excessive peripheral vascular vasoconstriction.*

### 910. Which of the following is false about neprilysin?
*Harrison's 20th Ed. Chapter 252 Page 1764*

A. Membrane-bound peptidase
B. Degrades natriuretic peptides
C. Degrades bradykinin
D. None of the above

### 911. Which of the following clinical trials studied neprilysin inhibition in HF?
*Heart 2016;102:1342-1347*

A. Consensus
B. Titration
C. Paradigm-HF
D. Overture

### 912. Neprilysin is found in high concentrations in?
*Heart 2016;102:1342-1347*

A. Kidney
B. Lungs
C. Heart
D. Liver

*Neprilysin is found in a number of tissues but in especially high concentrations in the kidney.*

### 913. Which of the following are cleaved & inactivated by neprilysin?
*Heart 2016;102:1342-1347*

A. ANP
B. BNP
C. CNP
D. All of the above

*ANP, BNP, CNP and urodilatin are cleaved & inactivated by a membrane bound endopeptidase, neprilysin. Natriuretic peptides are also cleared via the natriuretic peptide clearance receptor (NPRC & NPRC3).*

### 914. Neprilysin breaks down which of the following?
*Heart 2016;102:1342-1347*

A. Angiotensin II
B. Vasopressin
C. Bradykinin
D. All of the above

### 915. Carperitide is related to which of the following?
*Heart 2016;102:1342-1347*

A. ANP
B. BNP
C. CNP
D. All of the above

*Carperitide is a recombinant ANP.*

### 916. Nesiritide is related to which of the following?
*Heart 2016;102:1342-1347*

A. ANP
B. BNP
C. CNP
D. All of the above

*Nesiritide is a recombinant human BNP.*

### 917. Urodilatin is related to which of the following?
*Heart 2016;102:1342-1347*

A. ANP
B. BNP
C. CNP
D. All of the above

*Urodilatin is structurally related to ANP, and is derived from kidneys.*

### 918. Which of the following is a combined ACE and neprilysin inhibitor?
*Heart 2016;102:1342-1347*

A. Racecodotril
B. Omapatrilat
C. Candoxatrilat
D. Ecadotril

*The combined ACE and neprilysin inhibitor omapatrilat was studied in the Omapatrilat Versus Enalapril Randomized Trial of Utility in Reducing Events (OVERTURE) trial. Both ACE & neprilysin break down bradykinin and omapatrilat also inhibits aminopeptidase P which also catabolises bradykinin resulting in high rates of serious angio-oedema.*

919. Adaptive changes in the myocardium or LV remodeling is due to increasing activation of?
*Harrison's 20th Ed. Chapter 252 Page 1764*

   A. Neurohormonal system
   B. Adrenergic system
   C. Cytokine system
   D. All of the above

920. Baroreceptors are located in which of the following locations?
*Harrison's 20th Ed. Chapter 252 Page 1765 Figure 252-2*

   A. Left ventricle
   B. Carotid sinus
   C. Aortic arch
   D. All of the above

High-pressure baroreceptors are located in left ventricle, carotid sinus and aortic arch.

921. Which of the following mechanism may be responsible in the development of HF with preserved EF (HRpEF)?
*Harrison's 20th Ed. Chapter 252 Page 1764*

   A. Diastolic dysfunction
   B. Increased vascular stiffness
   C. Impaired renal function
   D. All of the above

922. Which of the following contribute to LV remodeling?
*Harrison's 20th Ed. Chapter 252 Page 1765*

   A. Myocyte hypertrophy
   B. Altered contractile properties of myocyte
   C. Progressive loss of myocytes
   D. All of the above

Adaptive changes within the myocardium is collectively referred to as LV remodeling. LV remodeling is a result of myocyte hypertrophy, altered contractile properties of myocyte, progressive loss of myocytes through necrosis, apoptosis, and autophagic cell death, beta-adrenergic desensitization, abnormal myocardial energetics and metabolism and reorganization of extracellular matrix (organized structural collagen around myocytes being replaced by interstitial collagen matrix that is unable to provide structural support to myocytes).

923. Activation of renin-angiotensin-aldosterone system causes?
*Harrison's 20th Ed. Chapter 252 Page 1765 Figure 252-2*

   A. Cardiomyocyte hypertrophy
   B. Cardiomyocyte cell death
   C. Myocardial fibrosis
   D. All of the above

Activation of the renin-angiotensin-aldosterone system promotes salt and water retention and leads to vasoconstriction of the peripheral vasculature, myocyte hypertrophy, myocyte cell death and myocardial fibrosis.

924. Which of the following act as a biologic stimuli in LV remodeling?
*Harrison's 20th Ed. Chapter 252 Page 1765*

   A. Mechanical stretch of myocyte
   B. Circulating neurohormones
   C. Circulating inflammatory cytokines
   D. All of the above

Biologic stimuli leading to LV remodeling include mechanical stretch of myocyte, circulating neurohormones (norepinephrine, angiotensin II), inflammatory cytokines (tumor necrosis factor), peptides and growth factors (endothelin) and reactive oxygen species (superoxide).

925. Which of the following is best related to a failing cardiac myocyte?
*Harrison's 20th Ed. Chapter 252 Page 1765*

   A. NCK-adaptor protein
   B. SERCA2A
   C. CD2-associated protein (CD2AP)
   D. Giant cell line-derived neutrophilic factor (GDNF)

Changes that regulate excitation-contraction include decreased function of sarcoplasmic reticulum $Ca^{2+}$ adenosine triphosphatase (SERCA2A), resulting in decreased calcium uptake into SR, and hyperphosphorylation of ryanodine receptor, leading to calcium leakage from SR.

926. In HF, which of the following changes occur in cross-bridges?
*Harrison's 20th Ed. Chapter 252 Page 1765*

   A. Decreased expression of α-myosin heavy chain
   B. Increased expression of β-myosin heavy chain
   C. Myocytolysis
   D. All of the above

927. Which of the following is false about myocardial relaxation?
*Harrison's 20th Ed. Chapter 252 Page 1765*

   A. Adenosine triphosphate (ATP)-dependent process
   B. Regulated by uptake of cytoplasmic calcium into the SR by SERCA2A
   C. Regulated by extrusion of calcium by sarcolemmal pumps
   D. None of the above

928. Left ventricular remodeling refers to changes in which of the following?
*Harrison's 20th Ed. Chapter 252 Page 1766*

   A. LV mass
   B. LV volume
   C. LV shape
   D. All of the above

Left ventricular remodeling refers to changes in LV mass, volume, and shape and the composition of heart that occur after cardiac injury and/or abnormal hemodynamic loading conditions. LV remodeling can be reversed following medical and device therapy.

929. In HF, which of the following changes occur in heart?
*Harrison's 20th Ed. Chapter 252 Page 1766*

   A. Increase in LV end-diastolic volume
   B. LV wall thinning
   C. Functional afterload mismatch
   D. All of the above

930. High end-diastolic wall stress leads to?
*Harrison's 20th Ed. Chapter 252 Page 1766*

   A. Hypoperfusion of the subendocardium
   B. Increased oxidative stress
   C. Sustained expression of hypertrophic signaling pathways
   D. All of the above

931. Dyspnea in HF is best related to?
*Harrison's 20th Ed. Chapter 252 Page 1766*

   A. Juxtacapillary J receptors
   B. Juxtacapillary K receptors
   C. Juxtacapillary L receptors
   D. Juxtacapillary M receptors

Most important mechanism of dyspnea in HF is pulmonary congestion with accumulation of interstitial or intra-alveolar fluid, which activates juxtacapillary J receptors, which in turn stimulate the rapid, shallow breathing characteristic of cardiac dyspnea.

### 932. Which of the following factors contribute to dyspnea on exertion in HF?
*Harrison's 20th Ed. Chapter 252 Page 1766*

A. Reductions in pulmonary compliance
B. Increased airway resistance
C. Respiratory muscle &/or diaphragm fatigue
D. All of the above

### 933. Dyspnea in HF may become less frequent with the onset of?
*Harrison's 20th Ed. Chapter 252 Page 1766*

A. Mitral regurgitation
B. Tricuspid regurgitation
C. Aortic regurgitation
D. Pulmonary regurgitation

*Dyspnea in HF may become less frequent with the onset of right ventricular (RV) failure and tricuspid regurgitation.*

### 934. Which of the following is a symptom of HF?
*Harrison's 20th Ed. Chapter 252 Page 1766*

A. Nocturia
B. Nocturnal cough
C. Early satiety
D. All of the above

### 935. Orthopnea is caused due to redistribution of fluid from?
*Harrison's 20th Ed. Chapter 252 Page 1766*

A. Coronary circulation
B. Pulmonary circulation
C. Splanchnic circulation
D. Cerebral circulation

*Orthopnea (dyspnea occurring in recumbent position), results from redistribution of fluid from splanchnic circulation and lower extremities into central circulation during recumbency, with a resultant increase in pulmonary capillary pressure.*

### 936. Orthopnea may occur in patients with?
*Harrison's 20th Ed. Chapter 252 Page 1766*

A. Heart failure
B. Abdominal obesity or ascites
C. Pulmonary disease
D. All of the above

### 937. Which of the following about orthopnea in HF is false?
*Harrison's 20th Ed. Chapter 252 Page 1766*

A. Later manifestation of HF
B. Relatively specific symptom of HF
C. Due to increase in pulmonary capillary pressure
D. None of the above

### 938. In HF, paroxysmal nocturnal dyspnea (PND) occurs how many hours after the patient retires?
*Harrison's 20th Ed. Chapter 252 Page 1766*

A. 15 - 30 minutes
B. 1 - 3 hours
C. 3 - 4 hours
D. 5 - 6 hours

*PND refers to acute episodes of severe shortness of breath and coughing that awaken the patient from sleep, usually 1 - 3 hours after the patient retires.*

### 939. Paroxysmal nocturnal dyspnea (PND) may manifest as?
*Harrison's 20th Ed. Chapter 252 Page 1766*

A. Severe shortness of breath
B. Persistent coughing even after assuming upright position
C. Persistent wheezing even after assuming upright position
D. All of the above

### 940. Paroxysmal nocturnal dyspnea (PND) is caused by?
*Harrison's 20th Ed. Chapter 252 Page 1766*

A. Increased pressure in bronchial arteries causing airway compression
B. Interstitial pulmonary edema
C. Increased airway resistance
D. All of the above

### 941. Which of the following is false for cardiac asthma?
*Harrison's 20th Ed. Chapter 252 Page 1766*

A. Closely related to PND
B. Wheezing
C. Bronchospasm
D. None of the above

*Cardiac asthma is closely related to PND & is characterized by wheezing secondary to bronchospasm.*

### 942. Cheyne-Stokes respiration is due to increased sensitivity of respiratory center to?
*Harrison's 20th Ed. Chapter 252 Page 1766*

A. Arterial $PCO_2$
B. Venous $PCO_2$
C. Arterial $PO_2$
D. Venous $PCO_2$

### 943. Cheyne-Stokes respiration is associated with?
*Harrison's 20th Ed. Chapter 252 Page 1766*

A. Increased intravascular volume
B. Low cardiac output
C. Cerebral vasoconstriction
D. All of the above

*In early 19th century, John Cheyne & William Stokes described cyclical episodes of apnea & hyperventilation. Cheyne-Stokes respiration (periodic respiration or cyclic respiration) is present in 40% of patients with advanced HF and usually is associated with low cardiac output. Cheyne-Stokes respiration is caused by an increased sensitivity of the respiratory center to arterial $PCO_2$. There is an apneic phase, during which arterial $PO_2$ falls and arterial $PCO_2$ rises. These changes in the arterial blood gas content stimulate the respiratory center, resulting in hyperventilation and hypocapnia, followed by recurrence of apnea. Ventilation length in Cheyne-Stokes respiration is >40 seconds compared to <40 seconds in central sleep apnea. Also, relative duration of hyperventilation is more than apnea duration.*

### 944. In HF, which of the following is caused by excessive adrenergic activity?
*Harrison's 20th Ed. Chapter 252 Page 1766*

A. Sinus tachycardia
B. Cool peripheral extremities
C. Cyanosis of lips and nail beds
D. All of the above

**945. Jugular venous pressure is quantified in which of the following units?**
*Harrison's 20th Ed. Chapter 252 Page 1766*

A. Centimeters of water
B. Centimeters of blood
C. Centimeters of mercury
D. Any of the above

Jugular venous pressure is quantified in centimeters of water (normal ≤8 cm) by estimating height of venous column of blood above the sternal angle in centimeters and then adding 5 cm.

**946. Which of the following is false about pleural effusions in HF?**
*Harrison's 20th Ed. Chapter 252 Page 1766*

A. Due to elevation of pleural capillary pressure
B. Due to transudation of fluid into the pleural cavities
C. Pleural veins drain into the systemic & pulmonary veins
D. None of the above

**947. Which of the following is false about pleural effusions in HF?**
*Harrison's 20th Ed. Chapter 252 Page 1766*

A. Occur most commonly with biventricular failure
B. Often bilateral in HF
C. If unilateral, more frequently in the right pleural space
D. None of the above

**948. Protodiastolic gallop best relates to?**
*Harrison's 20th Ed. Chapter 252 Page 1767*

A. S1
B. S2
C. S3
D. S4

S3 or protodiastolic gallop is mostly present in HF patients with volume overload who have tachycardia & tachypnea. It signifies severe hemodynamic compromise.

**949. In bedridden HF patients, edema may be found in?**
*Harrison's 20th Ed. Chapter 252 Page 1767*

A. Interscapular region
B. Scrotum
C. Nape of the neck
D. All of the above

In bedridden HF patients, edema may be found in sacral area (presacral edema) and scrotum.

**950. Which of the following is a late manifestation of HF?**
*Harrison's 20th Ed. Chapter 252 Page 1767*

A. Orthopnea
B. Ascites
C. Jaundice
D. All of the above

**951. Which of the following statements is false?**
*Harrison's 20th Ed. Chapter 252 Page 1767*

A. A normal ECG excludes LV systolic dysfunction
B. Majority of patients with chronic HF do not have evidence of pulmonary HT, interstitial edema, and/or pulmonary edema
C. Magnetic resonance imaging (MRI) is the gold standard for assessing LV mass & volumes
D. None of the above

Majority of patients with chronic HF do not have evidence of pulmonary hypertension, interstitial edema, and/or pulmonary edema due to increased capacity of the lymphatics to remove interstitial and/or pulmonary fluid.

**952. Which of the following denotes ejection fraction?**
*Harrison's 20th Ed. Chapter 252 Page 1767*

A. End-diastolic volume - End-systolic volume
B. End-diastolic volume / End-systolic volume
C. Stroke volume / End-diastolic volume
D. Stroke volume / End-systolic volume

**953. Which of the following is superior to EF as a measure of LV function?**
*Eur Heart J. 2016;37(15):1196-1207*

A. Global circumferential strain by speckle-tracking echocardiography
B. Global longitudinal strain by speckle-tracking echocardiography
C. Global diagonal strain by speckle-tracking echocardiography
D. All of the above

In echocardiography, the term 'strain' is used to describe local shortening, thickening & lengthening of the myocardium as a measure of regional LV function. Strain in myocardium can be measured by tissue Doppler imaging (TDI) or by speckle-tracking echocardiography (STE). Most laboratories record LV strain in long axis & use global longitudinal strain (GLS) calculated as average from all segments, as a measure of global LV function.

**954. Which of the following is useful in HF patients with a preserved EF?**
*Harrison's 20th Ed. Chapter 252 Page 1767*

A. B-type natriuretic peptide (BNP)
B. N-terminal pro-BNP
C. Left atrial dilation by 2D Echo
D. All of the above

By 2-D echocardiogram/Doppler, presence of left atrial dilation and LV hypertrophy, together with abnormalities of LV diastolic filling is useful for the assessment of HF with a preserved EF. B-type natriuretic peptide (BNP) and N-terminal pro-BNP are elevated in HF patients with a preserved EF, although to a lesser degree.

**955. Natriuretic peptide levels are more in?**
*Harrison's 20th Ed. Chapter 252 Page 1767*

A. Aged
B. Renal impairment
C. Women
D. All of the above

Natriuretic peptide levels increase with age & renal impairment, are more elevated in women, and can be elevated in right HF from any cause.

**956. Natriuretic peptide levels can be falsely low in?**
*Harrison's 20th Ed. Chapter 252 Page 1767*

A. Lean individuals
B. Obese individuals
C. Post meal
D. Fasting

Natriuretic peptide levels can be falsely low in obese patients.

**957. Which of the following is a biomarker used for determining the prognosis of HF patients?**
*Harrison's 20th Ed. Chapter 252 Page 1767*

- A. Galectin-1
- B. Galectin-2
- C. Galectin-3
- D. Galectin-4

*Newer biomarkers that can be used for determining the prognosis of HF patients are soluble ST-2 and galectin-3. Galectin-3 as a biomarker of fibrosis and inflammation has been implicated in the development and progression of HF, and may predict increased morbidity and mortality. Galectin-3 is a strong independent predictor of mortality in patients with chronic heart failure.*

**958. What level of peak oxygen uptake (vo2) is associated with a relatively poor prognosis in HF?**
*Harrison's 20th Ed. Chapter 252 Page 1767*

- A. <3 mL/kg per minute
- B. <7 mL/kg per minute
- C. <14 mL/kg per minute
- D. <21 mL/kg per minute

*A peak oxygen consumption (vo2) <14 mL/kg per minute is associated with a relatively poor prognosis in HF. They have better survival when transplanted than when treated medically.*

**959. Which of the following is known as pulmonary heart disease?**
*Harrison's 20th Ed. Chapter 252 Page 1767*

- A. Asthma
- B. Pulmonary hypertension
- C. Cor pulmonale
- D. Pulmonary thromboembolism

**960. Cor pulmonale is triggered by?**
*Harrison's 20th Ed. Chapter 252 Page 1768*

- A. Hypoxia
- B. Hypercarbia
- C. Pulmonary hypertension
- D. All of the above

*Cor pulmonale or pulmonary heart disease is defined as altered RV structure and/or function in the context of chronic lung disease and is triggered by the onset of pulmonary hypertension. Although RV dysfunction is also an important sequela of HFpEF and HFrEF, this is not considered as cor pulmonale.*

**961. Normally, mean pulmonary artery pressure is?**
*Harrison's 20th Ed. Chapter 252 Page 1768*

- A. ~ 5 mm Hg
- B. ~ 10 mm Hg
- C. ~ 15 mm Hg
- D. ~ 20 mm Hg

*Normally, mean pulmonary artery pressure is ~ 15 mm Hg.*

**962. Trigger for acute decompensation of previously compensated chronic cor pulmonale is?**
*Harrison's 20th Ed. Chapter 252 Page 1768*

- A. Acidemia
- B. Acute pulmonary embolus
- C. Atrial tachyarrhythmia
- D. All of the above

*Triggers for acute decompensation of previously compensated chronic cor pulmonale are worsening hypoxia (pneumonia), acidemia (exacerbation of COPD), acute pulmonary embolus, atrial tachyarrhythmia, hypervolemia and mechanical ventilation that leads to compressive forces on alveolar blood vessels.*

**963. Decompensation of chronic cor pulmonale is aggravated by?**
*Harrison's 20th Ed. Chapter 252 Page 1768*

- A. Obesity hypoventilation syndrome (OHS)
- B. Acute pulmonary emboli
- C. Positive-pressure (mechanical) ventilation
- D. All of the above

*Decompensation of chronic cor pulmonale can be aggravated by events that induce pulmonary vasoconstriction and RV afterload.*

**964. Which of the following is the most common symptom of chronic cor pulmonale?**
*Harrison's 20th Ed. Chapter 252 Page 1768*

- A. Dyspnea
- B. Orthopnea
- C. PND
- D. All of the above

*Orthopnea and PND are rarely symptoms of isolated right HF and usually point toward concurrent left heart dysfunction.*

**965. Which of the following about Tei index is false?**
*Harrison's 20th Ed. Chapter 252 Page 1769, J Cardiol. 1995; 26: 357-366*

- A. Ratio of time intervals
- B. Independent of ventricular geometry
- C. Independent of blood pressure, heart rate and age
- D. None of the above

**966. Formula for Tei index is?**
*J Cardiol. 1995; 26: 357-366*

- A. (IVCT + IVRT) / ET
- B. (IVCT + IVRT) x ET
- C. ET / (IVCT + IVRT)
- D. ET / (IVCT x IVRT)

*Isovolumic contraction time (IVCT), Isovolumic relaxation time (IVRT), Ejection time (ET).*

## Heart Failure: Management

**967. Which of the following is a syndrome of heart failure?**
*Harrison's 20th Ed. Chapter 253 Page 1769*

A. Heart failure with reduced ejection fraction (HFrEF)
B. Heart failure with preserved ejection fraction (HFpEF)
C. Acute decompensated heart failure (ADHF)
D. All of the above

Syndromes of heart failure include heart failure with reduced ejection fraction (HFrEF), heart failure with preserved ejection fraction (HFpEF), acute decompensated heart failure (ADHF) and advanced heart failure.

**968. Lusitropic effect best relates to?**
*Harrison's 20th Ed. Chapter 232 Page 1658 Figure 232-7*

A. Enhanced velocity
B. Enhanced rate
C. Enhanced relaxation
D. Enhanced contraction

**969. Which of the following trials were done on HFpEF patients?**
*Harrison's 20th Ed. Chapter 253 Page 1769*

A. Charm
B. Seniors
C. I-Preserve
D. All of the above

Candesartan in Heart Failure-Assessment of Mortality and Morbidity (CHARM) Preserved study, Irbesartan in Heart Failure with Preserved Systolic Function (I-PRESERVE) trial, Digitalis Investigation Group (DIG) trial, Study of the Effects of Nebivolol Intervention on Outcomes and Rehospitalization in Seniors with Heart Failure (SENIORS) trial, Phosphodiesterase-5 Inhibition to Improve Clinical Status and Exercise Capacity in Diastolic Heart Failure (RELAX), Aldosterone Antagonist Therapy in Adults with Preserved Ejection Fraction Congestive Heart Failure (TOPCAT) trial and Aldosterone Receptor Blockade in Diastolic Heart Failure (ALDO-DHF) study were done on HFpEF patients.

**970. Which of the following is an endopeptidase inhibitor?**
*Harrison's 20th Ed. Chapter 253 Page 1769*

A. LCZ596
B. LCZ696
C. LCZ796
D. LCZ896

A unique molecule that hybridizes an ARB with an endopeptidase inhibitor, LCZ696, increases the generation of myocardial cyclic guanosine 3'5'-monophosphate, enhances myocardial relaxation, and reduces ventricular hypertrophy. This dual blocker has been shown to reduce circulating natriuretic peptides and reduce left atrial size to a significantly greater extent than valsartan alone in patients with HFpEF.

**971. Which of the following is a precipitating cause of acute decompensated HF (ADHF)?**
*Harrison's 20th Ed. Chapter 253 Page 1770*

A. Infection
B. Pulmonary embolism
C. Occult myocardial ischemia
D. All of the above

Precipitating causes of acute decompensated HF (ADHF) include infection, arrhythmias, dietary indiscretion, pulmonary embolism, infective endocarditis, occult myocardial ischemia/infarction, and environmental and/or emotional stress.

**972. Which of the following is a component of heterogeneous clinical syndrome ADHF?**
*Harrison's 20th Ed. Chapter 253 Page 1770*

A. Decreased cardiac performance
B. Renal dysfunction
C. Alterations in vascular compliance
D. All of the above

ADHF is a heterogeneous clinical syndrome that increases need for hospitalization due to confluence of interrelated abnormalities of decreased cardiac performance, renal dysfunction, & alterations in vascular compliance.

**973. Which of the following is associated with worse outcomes in ADHF?**
*Harrison's 20th Ed. Chapter 253 Page 1770*

A. BUN level >43 mg/dL
B. Systolic blood pressure <115 mm Hg
C. Serum creatinine level >2.75 mg/dL
D. All of the above

**974. Which of the following provides a synergistic effect in patients receiving long-term therapy with loop diuretic agents?**
*Harrison's 20th Ed. Chapter 253 Page 1771*

A. Spironolactone
B. Eplerenone
C. Triamterene
D. Metolazone

Addition of a thiazide diuretic agent such as metolazone in combination provides a synergistic effect in patients receiving long-term therapy with loop diuretic agents.

**975. Which of the following is false about cardiorenal syndrome?**
*Harrison's 20th Ed. Chapter 253 Page 1771*

A. Complication of ADHF
B. Most patients have a preserved cardiac output
C. Due to complex interplay of neurohormonal factors
D. None of the above

**976. Which of the following trials pertain to cardiorenal syndrome?**
*Harrison's 20th Ed. Chapter 253 Page 1771*

A. Carress-HF trial
B. Relax-AHF trial
C. Revive II trial
D. Survive trial

**977. Which of the following is false about Ultrafiltration (UF)?**
*Harrison's 20th Ed. Chapter 253 Page 1771*

A. Controlled rates of fluid removal
B. Neutral effects on serum electrolytes
C. Decreased neurohormonal activity
D. None of the above

Ultrafiltration (UF) or aquapheresis is an invasive fluid removal technique.

**978. Which of the following drugs exerts dilating effect on arterial resistance and venous capacitance vessels?**
*Harrison's 20th Ed. Chapter 253 Page 1772*

A. Nitroglycerin
B. Nitroprusside
C. Nesiritide
D. All of the above

*By stimulating guanylyl cyclase within smooth-muscle cells, nitroglycerin, nitroprusside, and nesiritide exert dilating effects on arterial resistance and venous capacitance vessels.*

**979. Recombinant human relaxin-2 or serelaxin is upregulated in?**
*Harrison's 20th Ed. Chapter 253 Page 1772*

A. High altitude
B. Atheletes
C. Pregnancy
D. All of the above

*Recombinant human relaxin-2 or serelaxin is a peptide upregulated in pregnancy and examined in ADHF patients with a normal or elevated blood pressure.*

**980. Nesiritide is best related to?**
*Harrison's 20th Ed. Chapter 253 Page 1772*

A. Atrial-type natriuretic peptide
B. Brain-type natriuretic peptide
C. Phosphodiesterase III inhibitor
D. Endogenous catecholamine

*Nesiritide is a recombinant form of brain-type natriuretic peptide, which is an endogenous peptide secreted primarily from LV in response to an increase in wall stress.*

**981. Which of the following is an inotropic agent?**
*Harrison's 20th Ed. Chapter 253 Page 1772*

A. Dopamine
B. Dobutamine
C. Tolvaptan
D. All of the above

*Dobutamine is an inotropic agent for the treatment of acute HF. It exerts its effects by stimulating $\beta_1$ and $\beta_2$ receptors, with little effect on $\alpha_1$ receptors.*

**982. Which of the following is a phosphodiesterase III inhibitor?**
*Harrison's 20th Ed. Chapter 253 Page 1772*

A. Dopamine
B. Dobutamine
C. Tolvaptan
D. Milrinone

*Milrinone is a phosphodiesterase III inhibitor that leads to increased cyclic AMP by inhibiting its breakdown.*

**983. Dopamine stimulates which of the following?**
*Harrison's 20th Ed. Chapter 253 Page 1772*

A. $\alpha_1$ receptors
B. $\beta_1$ receptors
C. Dopaminergic receptors
D. All of the above

*Dopamine is an endogenous catecholamine that stimulates $\alpha_1$ and $\beta_1$ receptors and dopaminergic receptors ($DA_1$ and $DA_2$) in the heart and circulation.*

**984. Which of the following is administered orally?**
*Harrison's 20th Ed. Chapter 253 Page 1772*

A. Nesiritide
B. Nitroprusside
C. Tolvaptan
D. Milrinone

**985. TRUE-AHF trial evaluated which of the following in ADHF?**
*Harrison's 20th Ed. Chapter 253 Page 1772*

A. Nesiritide
B. Urodilatin
C. Serelaxin
D. Milrinone

**986. Which of the following is a calcium sensitizer that provides inotropic activity?**
*Harrison's 20th Ed. Chapter 253 Page 1772*

A. Serelaxin
B. Milrinone
C. Levosimendan
D. Nesiritide

*Levosimendan is a calcium sensitizer that provides inotropic activity and also possesses phosphodiesterase-3 inhibition properties that are vasodilators in action.*

**987. Which of the following is a selective myosin activator?**
*Harrison's 20th Ed. Chapter 253 Page 1772*

A. Serelaxin
B. Omecamtiv mecarbil
C. Tolvaptan
D. Rolofylline

*Omecamtiv mecarbil functions as a selective myosin activator. It prolongs ejection period and increases fractional shortening. Distinctively, the force of contraction is not increased and it does not increase myocardial oxygen demand.*

**988. Which of the following beta blockers is proven to improve survival in HFrEF clinical trials?**
*Harrison's 20th Ed. Chapter 253 Page 1773*

A. Carvedilol
B. Bisoprolol
C. Metoprolol succinate
D. All of the above

**989. Aldosterone antagonism reduces mortality in which symptomatic NYHA class of HFrEF?**
*Harrison's 20th Ed. Chapter 253 Page 1773*

A. Class II
B. Class III
C. Class IV
D. All of the above

*Aldosterone antagonism is associated with a reduction in mortality in all stages of symptomatic NYHA class II to IV HFrEF.*

**990. ASTRONAUT trial tested which of the following drug?**
*Harrison's 20th Ed. Chapter 253 Page 1773*

A. Aliskiren
B. Eplerenone
C. Spironolactone
D. Ivabradine

*Aliskiren Trial on Acute Heart Failure Outcomes (ASTRONAUT) tested the direct renin inhibitor, aliskiren, in addition to other heart failure medications, within a week after hospital discharge for decompensated HFrEF. No significant difference in cardiovascular death or hospitalization at 6 or 12 months was noted.*

**991. Bosentan is best related to?**
*Harrison's 20th Ed. Chapter 253 Page 1773*

A. Centrally acting sympatholytic agent
B. Endothelin antagonist
C. Endopeptidase inhibitor
D. Anticytokine agent

**992. Moxonidine is best related to?**
*Harrison's 20th Ed. Chapter 253 Page 1774*

A. Centrally acting sympatholytic agent
B. Endothelin antagonist
C. Endopeptidase inhibitor
D. Anticytokine agent

**993. Omapatrilat is best related to?**
*Harrison's 20th Ed. Chapter 253 Page 1774*

A. Centrally acting sympatholytic agent
B. Endothelin antagonist
C. Endopeptidase inhibitor
D. Anticytokine agent

*Omapatrilat hybridizes an ACEI with a neutral endopeptidase inhibitor.*

**994. Sacubitril-valsartan is best related to?**
*Harrison's 20th Ed. Chapter 253 Page 1774*

A. Centrally acting sympatholytic agent
B. Endothelin antagonist
C. Endopeptidase inhibitor
D. Angiotensin Receptor Neprilysin Inhibitor

**995. Which of the following is false about Ivabradine?**
*Harrison's 20th Ed. Chapter 253 Page 1774*

A. Inhibitor of the $I_f$ current in sinoatrial node
B. Slows heart rate
C. No negative inotropic effect
D. None of the above

*Ivabradine is an inhibitor of the $I_f$ current in the sinoatrial node. It slows the heart rate without a negative inotropic effect.*

**996. Which of the following is false about digitalis glycosides?**
*Harrison's 20th Ed. Chapter 253 Page 1775*

A. Inotropic
B. Attenuate carotid sinus baroreceptor activity
C. Sympatho-inhibitory
D. None of the above

*Digitalis glycosides exert a mild inotropic effect, attenuate carotid sinus baroreceptor activity and are sympathoinhibitory.*

**997. Digitalis glycosides decrease which of the following?**
*Harrison's 20th Ed. Chapter 253 Page 1775*

A. Serum norepinephrine levels
B. Plasma renin levels
C. Plasma aldosterone levels
D. All of the above

*Digitalis glycosides decrease serum norepinephrine levels, plasma renin levels and aldosterone levels.*

**998. Levels of which of the following may be elevated in HF?**
*Harrison's 20th Ed. Chapter 253 Page 1775*

A. C-reactive protein
B. TNF receptors
C. Uric acid
D. All of the above

*Levels of troponin T and I, C-reactive protein, TNF receptors, and uric acid, may be elevated in HF and provide important prognostic information.*

**999. Loop diuretics increase fractional excretion of sodium by?**
*J Clin Diagn Res. 2015;9(4):OC01-OC3*

A. 5 - 10%
B. 10 - 20%
C. 20 - 25%
D. 25 - 50%

*FENa, an indicator of diuretic resistance, is the fraction of the filtered sodium load that is reabsorbed by the tubules. FENa depends on sodium intake, effective intravascular volume, GFR, and intact tubular reabsorptive mechanisms. Loop diuretics increase the fractional excretion of sodium by 20 - 25%. Thiazide diuretics increase it by 5 - 10%.*

**1000. Which of the following diuretics lead to hyperkalemia?**
*Harrison's 20th Ed. Chapter 253 Page 1775*

A. Spironolactone
B. Eplerenone
C. Triamterene
D. All of the above

**1001. Which of the following can attenuate the effects of ACE inhibitors?**
*Harrison's 20th Ed. Chapter 253 Page 1775*

A. Anxiety
B. Physical exercise
C. Fluid retention
D. All of the above

*Fluid retention can attenuate the effects of ACE inhibitors. It is preferable to optimize the dose of diuretic before starting the ACE inhibitor.*

**1002. Nonproductive cough as a side effect of ACE inhibitors is related to?**
*Harrison's 20th Ed. Chapter 253 Page 1775*

A. Stimulating guanylyl cyclase
B. Interference with adrenergic nervous system
C. Kinin potentiation
D. All of the above

*The side effects of ACE inhibitors related to kinin potentiation include a nonproductive cough (10 - 15%) and angioedema (1%).*

**1003. Which of the following statements about beta blockers in HF is false?**
*Harrison's 20th Ed. Chapter 253 Page 1775*

A. Should be initiated in low doses
B. Upward titration at 2-week intervals
C. Maximum dose as reported effective in clinical trials
D. None of the above

**1004. Aldosterone antagonists are not recommended when?**
*Harrison's 20th Ed. Chapter 253 Page 1773*

A. Serum creatinine is > 2.5 mg/dL
B. Creatinine clearance is < 30 mL/minute
C. Serum potassium is > 5 mmol/L
D. Any of the above

**1005. Amiodarone increases the level of which of the following?**
*Harrison's 20th Ed. Chapter 63 Page 425*

A. Quinidine
B. Digoxin
C. Warfarin
D. All of the above

**1006. Most patients with acute pulmonary edema belong to which of the following profiles?**
*Int J Crit Care Emerg Med. 2017;3:023*

A. Profile A
B. Profile B
C. Profile C
D. Profile L

*Patients with acute HF present with one of four basic hemodynamic profiles. Profile A - normal LV filling pressure with normal perfusion, Profile B - elevated LV filling pressure with normal perfusion, Profile C - elevated LV filling pressures with decreased perfusion and Profile L - normal or low LV filling pressure with decreased tissue perfusion. Profile B includes most patients with acute pulmonary edema.*

**1007. Cyanide toxicity in nitroprusside therapy occurs at doses?**
*Ann Thorac Surg. 2015;99:1432-4*

A. > 150 μg / minute for over 24 hours
B. > 150 μg / minute for over 48 hours
C. > 250 μg / minute for over 24 hours
D. > 250 μg / minute for over 48 hours

*Cyanide toxicity (gastrointestinal & central nervous system) in nitroprusside therapy occurs at doses > 250 μg / minute for over 48 hours.*

**1008. Most common cause of right-heart failure is?**
*European Society of Cardiology. 2016;14(32)*

A. Pulmonary parenchymal disease
B. Pulmonary vascular disease
C. Left heart failure
D. Any of the above

*Most common cause of right-heart failure is not pulmonary parenchymal or vascular disease but left heart failure.*

## Cardiomyopathy and Myocarditis

**1009. Cardiomyopathy is disease of?**
*Harrison's 20th Ed. Chapter 254 Page 1779*

- A. Cardiac muscle
- B. Cardiac microvasculature
- C. Cardiac interstitium
- D. All of the above

*Cardiomyopathy is disease of the heart muscle. As of 2006, cardiomyopathies are defined as "a heterogeneous group of diseases of the myocardium associated with mechanical and/or electrical dysfunction that usually (but not invariably) exhibit inappropriate ventricular hypertrophy or dilatation and are due to a variety of causes that frequently are genetic".*

**1010. Cardiomyopathy can be a result of which of the following?**
*Harrison's 20th Ed. Chapter 254 Page 1779*

- A. Hypertension
- B. Congenital or acquired valvular abnormality
- C. Pericardial abnormalities
- D. None of the above

*Cardiomyopathies are a group of diseases that affect heart muscle itself & are not the result of hypertension or congenital or acquired valvular, coronary or pericardial abnormalities.*

**1011. In the diagnosis of restrictive cardiomyopathy, which of the following has most relevance?**
*Harrison's 20th Ed. Chapter 254 Page 1779*

- A. Atrial size
- B. Left ventricular diastolic dimension
- C. Left ventricular wall thickness
- D. Arrhythmia

*Prominent atrial enlargement is a distinguishing feature of restrictive cardiomyopathy.*

**1012. Which of the following is a cause of primary cardiomyopathy?**
*Harrison's 20th Ed. Chapter 254 Page 1779*

- A. Genetic
- B. Mixed genetic and acquired
- C. Acquired
- D. All of the above

*The primary cardiomyopathy causes are divided into genetic, mixed genetic and acquired, and acquired.*

**1013. All three types of cardiomyopathy can be associated with?**
*Harrison's 20th Ed. Chapter 254 Page 1779*

- A. Atrioventricular valve regurgitation
- B. Typical and atypical chest pain
- C. Atrial and ventricular tachyarrhythmias
- D. All of the above

*All three types of cardiomyopathy (dilated, restrictive and hypertrophic) can be associated with atrioventricular valve regurgitation, typical and atypical chest pain, atrial and ventricular tachyarrhythmias, and embolic events.*

**1014. Which of the following is the "right-sided symptom" in heart failure?**
*Harrison's 20th Ed. Chapter 254 Page 1780, Table 254-1*

- A. Dyspnea on exertion
- B. Discomfort on bending
- C. Orthopnea
- D. Paroxysmal nocturnal dyspnea

*Left-sided symptoms of pulmonary congestion are dyspnea on exertion, orthopnea, paroxysmal nocturnal dyspnea. Right-sided symptoms of systemic venous congestion are hepatic and abdominal distention, discomfort on bending and peripheral edema.*

**1015. What proportion of dilated cardiomyopathy are familial?**
*Harrison's 20th Ed. Chapter 254 Page 1779*

- A. 10%
- B. 20%
- C. 30%
- D. 40%

*Up to one-third of cases of dilated cardiomyopathy may be familial.*

**1016. Most familial cardiomyopathies are inherited in which of the following pattern?**
*Harrison's 20th Ed. Chapter 254 Page 1779*

- A. Autosomal dominant
- B. Autosomal recessive
- C. X-linked inheritance
- D. Any of the above

*Most familial cardiomyopathies are inherited in an autosomal dominant pattern, with occasional autosomal recessive and X-linked inheritance.*

**1017. Which of the following is most common in cardiomyopathy?**
*Harrison's 20th Ed. Chapter 254 Page 1779*

- A. Deletions of an entire exon or gene
- B. Duplications of an entire exon or gene
- C. Missense mutations with amino acid substitutions
- D. All of the above

*Missense mutations with amino acid substitutions are the most common in cardiomyopathy.*

**1018. Which of the following is false about cardiomyopathy?**
*Harrison's 20th Ed. Chapter 254 Page 1779*

- A. Defining phenotype of CMP is rarely present at birth
- B. Genetic CMP is characterized by age dependence
- C. Genetic CMP is characterized by incomplete penetrance
- D. None of the above

**1019. Most commonly recognized genetic causes of dilated cardiomyopathy are structural mutations of?**
*Harrison's 20th Ed. Chapter 254 Page 1780*

- A. Dystrophin
- B. Desmin
- C. Titin
- D. All of the above

*The most commonly recognized genetic causes of dilated cardiomyopathy are structural mutations of the giant protein titin, encoded TTN, which maintains sarcomere structure and acts as a key signaling molecule.*

**1020. Defects in sarcomeric proteins are mostly associated with?**
*Harrison's 20th Ed. Chapter 254 Page 1779*

A. Dilated cardiomyopathy
B. Restrictive cardiomyopathy
C. Hypertrophic cardiomyopathy
D. All of the above

*Defects in sarcomeric proteins of myosin, actin, and troponin are mostly associated with hypertrophic cardiomyopathy.*

**1021. The most commonly recognized genetic causes of DCM are truncating mutations of?**
*Harrison's 20th Ed. Chapter 254 Page 1780*

A. Actin
B. Myosin
C. Tropomyosin
D. Titin

*The most commonly recognized genetic causes of DCM are truncating mutations of titin, encoded by TTN, which maintains sarcomere structure and acts as a key signaling molecule.*

**1022. Most of the identified genetic defects in the Z-disk and cytoskeleton are associated with?**
*Harrison's 20th Ed. Chapter 254 Page 1780*

A. Dilated cardiomyopathy
B. Restrictive cardiomyopathy
C. Hypertrophic cardiomyopathy
D. All of the above

*Desmin forms intermediate filaments that connect the nuclear and plasma membranes, Z-lines, and the intercalated disks between muscle cells. Desmin mutations impair the transmission of force and signaling for both cardiac & skeletal muscle leading to a peripheral myopathy and a dilated cardiomyopathy. Most of the identified genetic defects in the Z-disk and cytoskeleton are associated with dilated cardiomyopathy.*

**1023. Which of the following is a sarcomeric protein?**
*Harrison's 20th Ed. Chapter 254 Page 1782 Figure 254-1*

A. Actin
B. Myosin
C. Tropomyosin
D. All of the above

**1024. Which of the following is related to "myocyte stabilizing and connecting the cell membrane to intracellular structures"?**
*Harrison's 20th Ed. Chapter 254 Page 1782 Figure 254-1*

A. Sarcomeric proteins
B. Dystrophin complex
C. Desmosome complex
D. All of the above

**1025. Which of the following is related to "cell-cell connections and myocyte stability"?**
*Harrison's 20th Ed. Chapter 254 Page 1782 Figure 254-1*

A. Sarcomeric proteins
B. Dystrophin complex
C. Desmosome complex
D. All of the above

*Sarcomeric proteins include actin, myosin, tropomyosin, and the associated regulatory proteins. Dystrophin complex stabilizes and connects the cell membrane to intracellular structures. Desmosome complexes are associated with cell-cell connections and stability.*

**1026. Abnormal dystrophin can be acquired during infection by?**
*Harrison's 20th Ed. Chapter 254 Page 1780*

A. Coxsackie virus
B. Varicella-zoster virus
C. Herpes simplex virus (HSV) type 1
D. Epstein-Barr virus

*Abnormal dystrophin can be acquired when Coxsackie virus cleaves dystrophin in viral myocarditis.*

**1027. Mutations in which of the following genes is associated with Brugada syndrome?**
*Harrison's 20th Ed. Chapter 254 Page 1780*

A. SCN5A
B. ACTN2
C. DES
D. TTN

*Mutations in SCN5A, distinct from those that cause the Brugada or long-QT syndromes, have been implicated in dilated cardiomyopathy with conduction disease.*

**1028. Which of the following about nuclear membrane protein defects in cardiac muscle is false?**
*Harrison's 20th Ed. Chapter 254 Page 1780*

A. Occurs in autosomal (lamin A/C) pattern
B. Occurs in X-linked (emerin) pattern
C. High prevalence of atrial arrhythmias & conduction system disease
D. None of the above

**1029. "Arrhythmogenic cardiomyopathy" is best related to?**
*Harrison's 20th Ed. Chapter 254 Page 1780*

A. Cellular metabolism
B. Nuclear membrane
C. Mitochondria
D. Desmosome

**1030. Which of the following diseases can affect heart without mutation of genes expressed in heart?**
*Harrison's 20th Ed. Chapter 254 Page 1780*

A. Fabry's disease
B. Familial amyloidosis
C. Becker's muscle dystrophy
D. Long QT syndrome

*Familial amyloidosis and hemochromatosis can affect heart without mutation of genes expressed in heart.*

**1031. Mostly, familial forms of DCM are due to mutations in?**
*Harrison's 20th Ed. Chapter 254 Page 1780*

A. Genes encoding nuclear envelope protein lamin A/C
B. Genes encoding sarcomeric proteins
C. Mitochondrial genes
D. None of the above

*Most commonly, familial forms of DCM are due to mutations in genes encoding sarcomeric proteins like alpha-cardiac actin, beta- & alpha-myosin, heavy chain alpha-tropomyosin & troponins T, I, and C. Mutations in gene encoding nuclear envelope protein lamin A/C are responsible for DCM associated with atrioventricular (AV) conduction disorder that may cause sudden cardiac death (SCD). Mutations in mitochondrial genes have also been reported in DCM.*

**1032. Upper limit of normal of the weight of human heart is?**
*Harrison's 20th Ed. Chapter 254 Page 1783 Figure 254-2*

A. 320 grams
B. 340 grams
C. 360 grams
D. 380 grams

Upper limit of normal of the weight of human heart is 360 grams.

**1033. Histopathological feature of a dilated cardiomyopathy specimen is?**
*Harrison's 20th Ed. Chapter 254 Page 1783 Figure 254-4*

A. Interstitial fibrosis
B. Increased myocyte size
C. Enlarged, irregular nuclei
D. All of the above

Microscopically, a dilated cardiomyopathy specimen would show nonspecific changes of interstitial fibrosis and myocyte hypertrophy characterized by increased myocyte size and enlarged, irregular nuclei.

**1034. What proportion of patients with new-onset cardiomyopathy have substantial spontaneous recovery?**
*Harrison's 20th Ed. Chapter 254 Page 1782*

A. 20%
B. 30%
C. 40%
D. 50%

Almost half of all patients with new-onset cardiomyopathy have substantial spontaneous recovery.

**1035. Which of the following is a feature of cardiac remodeling?**
*Circulation. 2000;102:Iv-14–Iv-23*

A. Impaired ventricular systolic pump function
B. Cardiac enlargement
C. Cardiac hypertrophy
D. All of the above

Left and/or right ventricular systolic pump function is impaired, leading to progressive cardiac enlargement and hypertrophy, a process called remodeling.

**1036. Myocardial damage leading to dilated cardiomyopathy can be produced by which of the following?**
*Circulation. 2000;102:Iv-14–Iv-23*

A. Toxic agents
B. Metabolic factors
C. Infectious agents
D. All of the above

DCM is either familial or the end result of myocardial damage produced by known or unknown infectious, metabolic, or toxic agents.

**1037. In which of the following conditions, dilated cardiomyopathy is reversible?**
*Circulation. 2000;102:Iv-14–Iv-23*

A. Alcohol abuse
B. Pregnancy
C. Thyroid disease
D. All of the above

Reversible form of dilated cardiomyopathy may be found with alcohol abuse, pregnancy, thyroid disease, cocaine use, and chronic uncontrolled tachycardia. Obesity & sleep apnea increases the risk of developing heart failure.

**1038. ECG of a DCM patient may show all of the following except?**
*Circulation. 2000;102:Iv-14–Iv-23*

A. Atrial fibrillation
B. Ventricular arrhythmias
C. High voltage
D. Intraventricular conduction defects

ECG in a case of DCM shows sinus tachycardia or atrial fibrillation, ventricular arrhythmias, left atrial abnormality, diffuse nonspecific ST-T-wave abnormalities & sometimes intraventricular conduction defects and low voltage.

**1039. Which of the following should be avoided in dilated cardiomyopathy?**
*Circulation. 2000;102:Iv-14–Iv-23*

A. Alcohol
B. Calcium channel blockers
C. Nonsteroidal anti-inflammatory drugs
D. All of the above

Alcohol, calcium channel blockers & NSAIDs should be avoided in DCM.

**1040. Which of the following drugs should be avoided in a patient of dilated cardiomyopathy?**
*Circulation. 2000;102:Iv-14–Iv-23*

A. Digitalis
B. Beta adrenergic blocker
C. Calcium channel blocker
D. Spironolactone

Standard therapy of heart failure with salt restriction, ACE inhibitors or angiotensin II receptor blocker, diuretics, and digitalis produces symptomatic improvement. Most patients should be treated with a beta adrenergic blocker. Spironolactone should be added for most patients with recent or current advanced heart failure.

**1041. Cardiac involvement is common in which of the following conditions?**
*Harrison's 20th Ed. Chapter 254 Page 1784*

A. Duchenne's progressive muscular dystrophy
B. Myotonic dystrophy
C. Friedreich's ataxia
D. All of the above

Cardiac involvement is common in Duchenne's progressive muscular dystrophy, Myotonic dystrophy and Friedreich's ataxia.

**1042. Cardiomyopathy-neutropenia syndrome is also called?**
*Am J Med Genet Part C Semin Med Genet 163C:198–205*

A. Pompe disease
B. Barth syndrome
C. Holt-Oram syndrome
D. Fraser syndrome

Barth syndrome (BTHS) is named after Dr. Peter Barth (Netherlands). It is found exclusively in males. It is also known as 3-Methylglutaconic aciduria type II and Cardiomyopathy-neutropenia syndrome. It is due to mutations in BTHS gene, tafazzin (TAZ) located at Xq28, the long arm of X chromosome and is associated with cardiolipin molecules in the electron transport chain & mitochondrial membrane structure. Syndrome consists of metabolism distortion, delayed motor skills, stamina deficiency, hypotonia, chronic fatigue, delayed growth, cardiomyopathy, and compromised immune system.

# Myocarditis

**1043. Infective agents injure myocardium through?**
*Harrison's 20th Ed. Chapter 254 Page 1783*

A. Direct invasion
B. Production of cardiotoxic substances
C. Chronic inflammation with or without persistent infection
D. All of the above

*Myocarditis is commonly attributed to infective agents that injure myocardium through direct invasion, production of cardiotoxic substances or chronic inflammation with or without persistent infection.*

**1044. Infectious myocarditis is most commonly associated with?**
*Harrison's 20th Ed. Chapter 254 Page 1783*

A. Borrelia burgdorferi
B. HIV
C. Trypanosoma cruzi
D. Diphtheria

*Infectious myocarditis is reported with almost all types of infective agents but is most commonly associated with viruses and the protozoan Trypanosoma cruzi.*

**1045. Which of the following receptor on heart cells has enhanced expression in viral-induced myocarditis?**
*Harrison's 20th Ed. Chapter 254 Page 1783*

A. Epidermal growth receptor 2
B. β-adrenergic receptor
C. Coxsackie-adenovirus receptor
D. All of the above

*Viral-induced myocarditis is due to abnormalities in cell surface receptors, such as coxsackie-adenovirus receptor, that bind viral proteins. Human coxsackievirus and adenovirus receptor (CAR) is a common receptor for two of the most common viral causes of myocarditis (coxsackieviruses B3 and B4, and adenoviruses 2 and 5). Increased expression of CAR has been reported in patients with DCM and myocarditis.*

**1046. Ventricular tachyarrhythmias may be a feature of?**
*Harrison's 20th Ed. Chapter 254 Page 1784*

A. Viral myocarditis
B. Sarcoidosis
C. Giant cell myocarditis
D. All of the above

*Ventricular tachyarrhythmias dominate the presentation in viral myocarditis, sarcoidosis and giant cell myocarditis.*

**1047. On auscultation in a case of myocarditis, which of the following murmur is frequently heard?**
*Harrison's 20th Ed. Chapter 254 Page 1784*

A. Mitral stenosis
B. Mitral regurgitation
C. Aortic stenosis
D. Aortic regurgitation

*Auscultatory findings in a case of myocarditis include muffled S1 with S3 & a murmur of mitral regurgitation. Pericardial rub may be heard in patients with associated pericarditis.*

**1048. Criteria used for myocarditis on endomyocardial biopsy is?**
*Harrison's 20th Ed. Chapter 254 Page 1784*

A. American
B. Boston
C. Chicago
D. Dallas

*Dallas Criteria for myocarditis on endomyocardial biopsy include lymphocytic infiltrate with evidence of myocyte necrosis.*

**1049. Which of the following viruses most often produces clinically significant acute myocarditis?**
*Harrison's 20th Ed. Chapter 254 Page 1785*

A. Influenza
B. Toxoplasma gondii
C. Coxsackievirus
D. HIV

*While almost every infectious agent is capable of producing myocarditis, clinically significant acute myocarditis in USA is caused by viruses, especially coxsackievirus B.*

**1050. Myocarditis can result from?**
*Harrison's 20th Ed. Chapter 254 Page 1785*

A. Infectious process
B. Hypersensitivity to drugs
C. Radiation
D. All of the above

*Myocarditis results from infections, drug hypersensitivity, radiation, chemicals or physical agents.*

**1051. In HIV myocarditis, the most common finding is?**
*Harrison's 20th Ed. Chapter 254 Page 1785*

A. Pericarditis
B. Left ventricular dysfunction
C. Right ventricular dysfunction
D. Conduction abnormalities

*In HIV patients, the most common finding is left ventricular dysfunction that in some cases appears to be due to infiltration of myocardium by virus.*

**1052. Chagas disease is caused by?**
*Harrison's 20th Ed. Chapter 254 Page 1786*

A. Toxoplasma gondii
B. Trypanosoma cruzi
C. Schistosoma haematobium
D. Dermatobia hominis

*Chagas disease caused by protozoan Trypanosoma cruzi is transmitted by the bite of insect vector reduvid bug.*

**1053. Protozoan Trypanosoma cruzi can be transmitted by?**
*Harrison's 20th Ed. Chapter 254 Page 1786*

A. Blood transfusion
B. Organ donation
C. Mother to fetus
D. All of the above

*Transmission of protozoan T. cruzi can also occur through blood transfusion, organ donation, from mother to fetus, and occasionally orally.*

**1054. Which of the following is a typical feature of Chagas' disease in ECG?**
*Harrison's 20th Ed. Chapter 254 Page 1786*

A. Atrial fibrillation
B. Ventricular tachyarrhythmias
C. Conduction system abnormalities
D. Nonspecific ST-T abnormalities

*Features typical of Chagas' disease are conduction system abnormalities, particularly sinus node and atrioventricular (AV) node dysfunction and right bundle branch block. Atrial fibrillation and ventricular tachyarrhythmias also occur.*

**1055. Multiple left ventricular aneurysm formation is a feature of which of the following?**
*Harrison's 20th Ed. Chapter 254 Page 1786*

A. Diphtheritic myocarditis
B. Myocarditis in patients with HIV
C. Chagas disease
D. Lyme carditis

*Cardiac involvement in Chagas heart disease is characterized by dilatation of cardiac chambers, fibrosis & thinning of ventricular wall, aneurysm formation in left ventricular apex and mural thrombi that may embolize to pulmonary and systemic circulations.*

**1056. Which of the following drug is used in the treatment of Chagas' disease?**
*Harrison's 20th Ed. Chapter 254 Page 1786*

A. Pentamidine
B. Benznidazole
C. Suramin
D. Melarsoprol

*Antiparasitic therapy for Chagas' disease include benznidazole and nifurtimox.*

**1057. West African trypanosomiasis is caused by?**
*Harrison's 20th Ed. Chapter 254 Page 1786*

A. Trypanosoma brucei gambiense
B. Trypanosoma brucei rhodesiense
C. Trypanosoma cruzi
D. All of the above

*African trypanosomiasis infection results from the tsetse fly bite. The West African form is caused by Trypanosoma brucei gambiense while the East African form is caused by Trypanosoma brucei rhodesiense.*

**1058. Toxoplasmosis can cause which of the following?**
*Harrison's 20th Ed. Chapter 254 Page 1786*

A. Myocarditis
B. Pericardial effusion
C. Constrictive pericarditis
D. All of the above

*Toxoplasmosis may present with encephalitis or chorioretinitis and, in the heart, can cause myocarditis, pericardial effusion, constrictive pericarditis and heart failure.*

**1059. Multidrug antituberculous regimens are effective in the treatment of?**
*Harrison's 20th Ed. Chapter 254 Page 1787*

A. Brucellosis
B. Whipple's disease
C. Clostridial infections
D. Psittacosis

*Multidrug antituberculous regimens are effective in the treatment of Whipple's disease caused by Tropheryma whipplei.*

**1060. Most common cardiac abnormality in Lyme disease is?**
*Harrison's 20th Ed. Chapter 254 Page 1787*

A. Myopericarditis
B. Left ventricular dysfunction
C. Right ventricular dysfunction
D. Conduction abnormalities

*In Lyme disease, conduction abnormalities are the most common manifestations of cardiac involvement.*

**1061. Giant cell myocarditis may occur in association with?**
*Harrison's 20th Ed. Chapter 254 Page 1787*

A. Thymoma
B. Thyroiditis
C. Pernicious anemia
D. All of the above

*Associated conditions of giant cell myocarditis are thymomas, thyroiditis, pernicious anemia, other autoimmune diseases.*

**1062. Myocarditis may result from hypersensitivity to which of the following drugs?**
*Harrison's 20th Ed. Chapter 254 Page 1788*

A. Thiazides
B. Antibiotics
C. Methyldopa
D. All of the above

*Myocarditis may result from hypersensitivity to antibiotics, thiazides, anticonvulsants, indomethacin, and methyldopa.*

**1063. Peripartum cardiomyopathy (PPCM) usually develops in which trimester of pregnancy?**
*Harrison's 20th Ed. Chapter 254 Page 1788*

A. First
B. Second
C. Third
D. All of the above

*Cardiac dilatation & CHF of unexplained cause may develop during last trimester of pregnancy or within 6 months after delivery.*

**1064. Likelihood of peripartum cardiomyopathy (PPCM) is more in?**
*Harrison's 20th Ed. Chapter 254 Page 1788*

A. Malnutrition
B. Increased maternal age & parity
C. Use of tocolytic therapy for premature labor
D. All of the above

**1065. Risk factor for peripartum cardiomyopathy (PPCM) is?**
*Harrison's 20th Ed. Chapter 254 Page 1788*

A. Blood group AB
B. Recurrent UTI
C. Preeclampsia or toxemia of pregnancy
D. All of the above

*Risk factors are increased maternal age, increased parity, twin pregnancy, malnutrition, use of tocolytic therapy for premature labor and preeclampsia or toxemia of pregnancy.*

**1066. Pregnancy-associated cardiomyopathy (PACM) refers to?**
*Harrison's 20th Ed. Chapter 254 Page 1788*

A. Heart failure occuring in successive pregnancies
B. Heart failure presenting earlier in pregnancy
C. Heart failure occuring after miscarriage
D. Any of the above

Heart failure presenting earlier in pregnancy has been termed pregnancy-associated cardiomyopathy (PACM).

**1067. Which of the following statements is false?**
*Harrison's 20th Ed. Chapter 254 Page 1788*

A. Chagas' disease is the most common infective cause of cardiomyopathy
B. Granulomatous myocarditis is the most common cause of noninfective inflammation
C. Alcohol is the most common toxin implicated in chronic DCM
D. None of the above

**1068. Polymorphisms of which of the following genes increases the likelihood of alcoholic cardiomyopathy?**
*Harrison's 20th Ed. Chapter 254 Page 1788*

A. Angiotensin-converting enzyme
B. $\beta_1$- adrenergic receptor
C. $\beta_2$- adrenergic receptor
D. All of the above

Polymorphisms of the genes encoding alcohol dehydrogenase and the angiotensin-converting enzyme increase the likelihood of alcoholic cardiomyopathy.

**1069. Alcohol consumption necessary to produce cardiomyopathy is?**
*Harrison's 20th Ed. Chapter 254 Page 1788*

A. 1 ounce of pure ethanol daily for 5 - 10 years
B. 2 ounces of pure ethanol daily for 5 - 10 years
C. 3 ounces of pure ethanol daily for 5 - 10 years
D. 4 ounces of pure ethanol daily for 5 - 10 years

Alcohol consumption necessary to produce cardiomyopathy in an otherwise normal heart is about 4 ounces of pure ethanol (five to six drinks) daily for 5 - 10 years.

**1070. "Holiday heart syndrome" is the term used for cardiotoxicity produced by?**
*Harrison's 20th Ed. Chapter 254 Page 1788*

A. Alcohol
B. Tobacco
C. Cocaine
D. Amphetamine

Holiday heart syndrome is a state of alcoholic cardiotoxicity presenting as recurrent supraventricular or ventricular tachyarrhythmias without overt heart failure due to alcoholic binge drinking.

**1071. Which of the following arrhythmias is most frequent in "Holiday heart syndrome"?**
*Harrison's 20th Ed. Chapter 254 Page 1788*

A. Atrial flutter
B. Atrial fibrillation
C. Ventricular premature depolarizations
D. Ventricular tachycardia

In holiday heart syndrome, atrial fibrillation is the most common arrhythmia, followed by atrial flutter and ventricular premature depolarizations.

**1072. What quantity of alcohol consumption has been shown to be cardio-protective?**
*Genes Nutr. 2010;5:111-120*

A. 10 - 20 grams / day
B. 20 - 30 grams / day
C. 30 - 40 grams / day
D. 40 - 50 grams / day

Alcohol consumption in moderate quantity (20 - 30 grams/day) appears to be cardio-protective.

**1073. Pathologic findings in CMP due to cocaine resemble those of?**
*Harrison's 20th Ed. Chapter 254 Page 1788*

A. Beri-beri heart disease
B. Diabetes
C. Pheochromocytoma
D. Hyperthyroidism

Cocaine & amphetamine related cardiomyopathy reveals microinfarcts due to small vessel ischemia, similar to those seen with pheochromocytoma.

**1074. Which of the following about cocaine is false?**
*Harrison's 20th Ed. Chapter 447 Page 3287*

A. Vasospastic
B. Enhances sympathetic activity
C. Psychostimulant
D. None of the above

**1075. Which of the following can lead to adrenergic crisis due to catecholamine excess?**
*Harrison's 20th Ed. Chapter 271 Page 1906*

A. Amphetamine overdose
B. Clonidine withdrawal
C. Interaction of tyramine-containing food with MAO inhibitors
D. All of the above

Adrenergic crisis due to catecholamine excess may be related to pheochromocytoma, cocaine or amphetamine overdose, clonidine withdrawal, acute spinal cord injuries, and an interaction of tyramine-containing compounds with monoamine oxidase inhibitors.

**1076. Which of the following drugs should be avoided while treating cocaine-induced cardiotoxicity?**
*Harrison's 20th Ed. Chapter 447 Page 3287*

A. Nitrates
B. Calcium channel blockers
C. Beta-adrenergic blockers
D. Benzodiazepines

Nitrates, calcium channel blockers (to reduce coronary spasm) & benzodiazepines are used to treat cocaine-induced cardiotoxicities. Beta-adrenergic blockers should be avoided.

**1077. Which of the following is the explanation for myocyte injury & fibrosis with use of doxorubicin?**
*Harrison's 20th Ed. Chapter 254 Page 1788*

A. Generation of ROS involving 5-lipoxygenase
B. Generation of ROS involving heme compounds
C. Generation of ROS involving vascular endothelial growth factor
D. Generation of ROS involving matrix metalloproteinase

Generation of reactive oxygen species (ROS) involving heme compounds is currently the favored explanation for myocyte injury and fibrosis with the use of anthracyclines like doxorubicin. Antineoplastic activity of anthracyclines is almost exclusively due to the ability to bind to DNA and act as a poison to topoisomerase II by inducing lethal double-strand DNA breaks.

**1078.** Which of the following is a cardioprotective agent when doxorubicin (Adriamycin) is given to a patient?
*Cancer Management and Research 2014:6 357–363*

A. Erythropoietin
B. Dexrazoxone
C. Amiodarone
D. Cyclophosphamide

*Iron chelator dexrazoxone is cardioprotective and reduces risk of doxorubicin (Adriamycin) cardiotoxicity. Recovery of cardiac function occurs with aggressive use of ACE inhibitors.*

**1079.** Dexrazoxane best relates to which of the following?
*Cancer Management and Research 2014:6 357–363*

A. British anti-Lewisite (BAL)
B. Ethylene diamine tetraacetic acid (EDTA)
C. Dimercaptosuccinic acid (DMSA)
D. Penicillamine

*Dexrazoxane is a water-soluble ring-closed analog of iron chelator ethylenediaminetetraacetic acid (EDTA). Unlike EDTA, dexrazoxane easily passes into cells. Upon hydrolysis, dexrazoxane opens into its EDTA-like form, ADR-925, which is a strong iron chelator that has the ability to displace iron from the anthracycline.*

**1080.** Which of the following drug is an anthracycline?
*Cancer Management and Research 2014:6 357–363*

A. Doxorubicin
B. Epirubicin
C. Daunorubicin
D. All of the above

**1081.** Which of the following drug is an anthracenedione?
*Cancer Management and Research 2014:6 357–363*

A. Etoposide
B. Teniposide
C. Mitoxantrone
D. All of the above

*Etoposide and teniposide are podophyllotoxins.*

**1082.** Dexrazoxane is a catalytic inhibitor of?
*Cancer Management and Research 2014:6 357–363*

A. DNA Topoisomerase I
B. DNA topoisomerase II
C. DNA topoisomerase IV
D. All of the above

*Dexrazoxane is a catalytic inhibitor of DNA topoisomerase II that is the same target as the DNA topoisomerase II poisonous anticancer agents like anthracyclines, anthracenediones and podophyllotoxins. Dexrazoxane does not induce lethal DNA double-strand breaks as do the topoisomerase poisons.*

**1083.** Trastuzumab interferes with?
*Harrison's 20th Ed. Chapter 254 Page 1788*

A. Human epidermal growth receptor 2
B. Vascular endothelial growth receptor
C. Peptide receptor radionuclides
D. All of the above

*Trastuzumab (Herceptin) is a monoclonal antibody that interferes with human epidermal growth receptor 2 (HER2) crucial for some tumor growth and for cardiac adaptation.*

**1084.** Which of the following drug causes dilated cardiomyopathy?
*Harrison's 20th Ed. Chapter 254 Page 1789*

A. Trastuzumab
B. Ifosfamide
C. Cyclophosphamide
D. All of the above

**1085.** Which of the following chemotherapeutic agents can cause recurrent coronary spasm?
*Harrison's 20th Ed. Chapter 254 Page 1789*

A. Cyclophosphamide
B. Ifosfamide
C. Cisplatin
D. All of the above

*5-Fluorouracil, cisplatin, and some other alkylating agents can cause recurrent coronary spasm.*

**1086.** Which of the following drugs can cause cardiotoxicity with chronic use?
*Harrison's 20th Ed. Chapter 254 Page 1789*

A. Hydroxychloroquine
B. Chloroquine
C. Emetine
D. All of the above

**1087.** Which of the following about a patient of pheochromocytoma is false?
*Harrison's 20th Ed. Chapter 254 Page 1789*

A. Very labile blood pressure & heart rate
B. Episodic palpitations
C. Postural hypotension
D. None of the above

**1088.** Heart failure with "preserved" ejection fraction best applies to?
*Harrison's 20th Ed. Chapter 254 Page 1789*

A. Hyperthyroidism
B. Hypothyroidism
C. Obesity
D. Diabetes

*Diabetes is a typical factor, along with hypertension, advanced age, and female gender, in heart failure with "preserved" ejection fraction.*

**1089.** Which of the following conditions is associated with a high risk of death in patients with viral myocarditis?
*Harrison's 20th Ed. Chapter 254 Page 1789*

A. Pulmonary hypertension
B. Pericarditis
C. Arrhythmias
D. Heart failure

*Patients with viral myocarditis & pulmonary hypertension are at a particularly high risk of death.*

**1090.** Deficiency of which of the following plays a pathogenetic role in peripartum cardiomyopathy?
*Harrison's 20th Ed. Chapter 254 Page 1789*

A. Gold
B. Zinc
C. Copper
D. Selenium

*Pathogenetic factors in peripartum cardiomyopathy include low socioeconomic status, high parity, prolonged lactation, excessive dietary salt intake & selenium deficiency.*

## 1091. "Wet beri-beri heart disease" is characterized by all except?
*Harrison's 20th Ed. Chapter 254 Page 1789*

A. Third heart sound
B. Cold extremities
C. Reduced ECG voltage
D. Prolongation of QT interval

"Wet beri-beri heart disease" is characterized by high cardiac output failure state & is associated with tachycardia, wide pulse pressure, S3, & warm extremities. ECG shows reduced voltage, diffuse T-wave abnormalities & prolongation of QT interval.

## 1092. While treating "wet beri-beri heart disease" with thiamine, which of the following drugs should be given?
*Harrison's 20th Ed. Chapter 254 Page 1789*

A. Digoxin
B. Theophylline
C. Quinidine
D. Diuretics

Response to thiamine in "wet beri-beri heart disease" is dramatic & must be accompanied by diuretics.

## 1093. Which of the following diseases is associated with selenium deficiency?
*Harrison's 20th Ed. Chapter 254 Page 1789*

A. Keshan Disease
B. Kallmann syndrome
C. Liddle's syndrome
D. Tay–Sachs disease

Specific diseases associated with selenium deficiency are Keshan Disease, Kashin-Beck Disease (Big Bone disease) and Myxedematous Endemic Cretinism. Keshan disease is an endemic cardiomyopathy found in children and young women residing in regions of China where dietary intake of selenium is low.

## 1094. Which of the following is best absorbed & utilized form of selenium?
*J Am College of Nutr. 2001;20:1-4*

A. Selenothiamine
B. Selenoarginine
C. Selenoleucine
D. Selenomethionine

Selenomethionine is considered to be the best absorbed and utilized form of selenium.

## 1095. Recommended Dietary Allowances (RDA) for selenium for adults is?
*J Am College of Nutr. 2001;20:1-4*

A. 50 µg/day
B. 500 µg/day
C. 5000 µg/day
D. 50000 µg/day

Recommended Dietary Allowances (RDA) for selenium for adults is 50-200 µg/day.

## 1096. Clinical syndrome of Hemochromatosis includes?
*Harrison's 20th Ed. Chapter 254 Page 1789*

A. Cirrhosis
B. Diabetes
C. Hypogonadism
D. All of the above

The clinical syndrome of Hemochromatosis includes cirrhosis, diabetes & hypogonadism.

## 1097. Which of the following is false about Hemochromatosis?
*Harrison's 20th Ed. Chapter 254 Page 1789*

A. May be due to iron overload as in hemolytic anemia
B. Iron deposited in perinuclear area of cardiomyocytes
C. Transferrin saturation > 60% for men
D. None of the above

## 1098. In right ventricular dysplasia, there is progressive replacement of right ventricular wall with?
*Harrison's 20th Ed. Chapter 254 Page 1790*

A. Elastic tissue
B. Collagen tissue
C. Adipose tissue
D. Mucopolysaccharides

RV dysplasia is a familial cardiomyopathy marked by progressive replacement of right ventricular wall with adipose tissue. Ventricular arrhythmias are common & sudden death is a constant threat.

## 1099. Which of the following is false about arrhythmogenic ventricular dysplasia?
*Harrison's 20th Ed. Chapter 254 Page 1790*

A. Can affect right ventricle
B. Can affect left ventricle
C. Can affect both ventricles
D. None of the above

Arrhythmogenic ventricular dysplasia can affect either or both ventricles.

## 1100. Which of the following is mostly affected in Arrhythmogenic Right Ventricular Dysplasia (ARVD)
*Harrison's 20th Ed. Chapter 254 Page 1790*

A. Nuclear membrane
B. Endoplasmic reticulum
C. Mitochondria
D. Desmosomes

ARVC/D is an autosomal dominant disorder caused by multiple mutations of several genes encoding proteins that constitute desmosomes, structures that maintain normal contacts between cells leading to detachment of myocytes with consequent myocyte apoptosis and fibrofatty replacement.

## 1101. Which of the following best relates to genetic defect in the desmosomal protein?
*Harrison's 20th Ed. Chapter 254 Page 1790*

A. Strabismus
B. Gait disturbance
C. Woolly hair
D. Cyanosis

Genetic defects in proteins of the desmosomal complex disrupt myocyte junctions & adhesions, leading to replacement of myocardium by deposits of fat. This same protein also affects hair & skin, leading to a distinct syndrome of "woolly hair" and thickened palms and soles.

## 1102. Drooping eyelids is a feature of?
*Neurol Genet 2018;4:e230, Harrison's 19th Ed. 207*

A. Hemochromatosis
B. Duchenne's and Becker's dystrophy
C. Mitochondrial myopathies
D. Hypothyroidism

Mitochondrial myopathies show the characteristic "ragged red fiber" appearance. Some patients with mitochondrial myopathy have characteristic drooping eyelids.

### 1103. Cardinal clinical feature of left ventricular noncompaction is?
*Harrison's 20th Ed. Chapter 254 Page 1790*

- A. Ventricular arrhythmias
- B. Embolic events
- C. Heart failure
- D. All of the above

The three cardinal clinical features of left ventricular noncompaction are ventricular arrhythmias, embolic events, and heart failure.

### 1104. Which of the following is false about Left Ventricular Noncompaction (LVNC)?
*Harrison's 20th Ed. Chapter 254 Page 1790*

- A. Congenital cardiomyopathy
- B. Abnormal embryogenesis
- C. Multiple deep trabeculations into myocardium
- D. None of the above

Left ventricular noncompaction (LVNC) is a congenital cardiomyopathy that may present at any age with symptoms of CHF, thromboembolism or ventricular arrhythmias due to arrest of normal embryogenesis, with persistence of multiple deep trabeculations into myocardium communicating with ventricular cavity, 2 layered structure of endomyocardium leading to LV contractile dysfunction. It is diagnosed echocardiographically.

### 1105. Left ventricular noncompaction is best related to?
*Harrison's 20th Ed. Chapter 254 Page 1790*

- A. Restanin
- B. Tafazzin
- C. Gibazin
- D. Frufin

Diagnostic criteria of left ventricular noncompaction includes presence of multiple trabeculations in left ventricle distal to papillary muscles, creating a "spongy" appearance of apex. It is associated with multiple genetic variants in sarcomeric and other proteins such as tafazzin.

### 1106. What does "tako tsubo" in Japanese language mean?
*Harrison's 20th Ed. Chapter 254 Page 1790, Q J Med 2003; 96:563–573*

- A. Japanese balloon
- B. Japanese parachute
- C. Japanese pot for fishing octopus
- D. Japanese fishing net

"Tako-tsubo" in Japanese language refers to a Japanese pot for fishing for octopus.

### 1107. Which of the following is false about Tako-Tsubo cardiomyopathy?
*Harrison's 20th Ed. Chapter 254 Page 1790*

- A. Also known as apical ballooning syndrome
- B. Severe chest discomfort preceded by stressful emotional or physical event
- C. Occurs mostly in women >50 years
- D. None of the above

Also known as apical ballooning syndrome, Tako-Tsubo (stress) cardiomyopathy is characterized by abrupt & severe chest discomfort preceded by a stressful emotional or physical event. It occurs mostly in women >50 years.

### 1108. Which of the following is false about Tako-Tsubo cardiomyopathy?
*Harrison's 20th Ed. Chapter 254 Page 1790*

- A. ST elevations &/or T-wave inversions in chest leads
- B. Normal coronary angiography
- C. ECG & Echo CG changes revert in 3-7 days
- D. None of the above

ECG in Tako-Tsubo (stress) cardiomyopathy shows ST-segment elevations and/or deep T-wave inversions in chest leads. Coronary angiography shows no obstruction in epicardial arteries. Severe akinesia of distal portion of left ventricle with EF reduction occurs. Troponins are mildly elevated. Changes are reversible in 3 - 7 days without consequences.

### 1109. Which of the following can present as dilated or restrictive disease?
*Harrison's 20th Ed. Chapter 254 Page 1791*

- A. Sarcoidosis
- B. Fabry's disease
- C. Carcinoid syndrome
- D. Amyloidosis

Sarcoidosis and hemochromatosis can present as dilated or restrictive disease.

### 1110. Overlapping types of cardiomyopathy are more common with?
*Harrison's 20th Ed. Chapter 254 Page 1791*

- A. Inflammatory myocarditis
- B. Toxic myocarditis
- C. Nutritional deficiencies
- D. Inherited metabolic disorders

Overlaps are particularly common with the inherited metabolic disorders, which can present as any of the three major phenotypes.

### 1111. Fabry's disease results from a deficiency of?
*Harrison's 20th Ed. Chapter 254 Page 1791*

- A. Alpha-galactosidase A
- B. Beta-galactosidase
- C. Sphingomyelinase
- D. Neuraminidase

Fabry's disease results from a deficiency of the lysosomal enzyme alpha galactosidase A.

### 1112. Which of the following about Fabry's disease is false?
*Harrison's 20th Ed. Chapter 254 Page 1791*

- A. Autosomal dominant disorder
- B. Disorder of glycosphingolipid metabolism
- C. Leg lymphedema without hypoproteinemia
- D. Enzyme therapy useful

Fabry's disease is an X-linked recessive disorder that may also cause clinical disease in female carriers. Clinically, it manifests with angiokeratomas (telangiectatic skin lesions), hypohidrosis, corneal & lenticular opacities, acroparesthesia; & small-vessel disease of kidney, heart & brain.

### 1113. Which of the following about angiokeratomas in Fabry's disease is false?
*Harrison's 20th Ed. Chapter 411 Page 3007*

- A. Do not blanch with pressure
- B. Mostly between umbilicus & knees "bathing suit area"
- C. Punctate, dark red to blue-black
- D. Asymmetric

Angiokeratomas are punctate, dark red to blue-black, flat or slightly raised, and usually symmetric; they do not blanch with pressure. They range from barely visible to several millimeters in diameter and have a tendency to increase in size and number with age. They are most dense between umbilicus & knees - the "bathing suit area". Angiokeratomas also occur in Fordyce scrotal angiokeratoma and several other very rare lysosomal storage diseases.

**1114. Cardiac Danon's Disease is due to mutations in?**
*Harrison's 20th Ed. Chapter 254 Page 1791*

A. LAMP1
B. LAMP2
C. LAMP3
D. LAMP4

Cardiac Danon Disease is caused by mutations in an X-linked lysosome-associated membrane protein (LAMP2).

**1115. Extreme left ventricular hypertrophy is seen in?**
*Harrison's 20th Ed. Chapter 254 Page 1791*

A. Fabry's disease
B. Gaucher's disease
C. Glycogen storage disease type III
D. Danon's disease

Danon's disease consists of skeletal myopathy, mental retardation and hepatic dysfunction. Extreme left ventricular hypertrophy appears early, often in childhood, and can progress rapidly to end-stage heart failure with low ejection fraction.

**1116. ECG of which of the following inherited metabolic cardiomyopathies with LVH shows ventricular preexcitation?**
*Harrison's 20th Ed. Chapter 254 Page 1791*

A. Fabry Disease
B. Friedreich's Ataxia
C. Cardiac Danon Disease
D. Glycogen Storage Cardiomyopathy

ECG in Cardiac Danon Disease shows severe LV hypertrophy & ventricular preexcitation. Deficiencies of LAMP2 and protein kinase, adenosine monophosphate (AMP)-activated gamma 2 noncatalytic subunit (PRKAG2) result in the accumulation of glycogen in heart and skeletal muscle. Their electrophysiologic abnormalities, particularly ventricular preexcitation and conduction defects distinguish them from patients with hypertrophic cardiomyopathy resulting from defects in sarcomere-protein genes.

# Restrictive Cardiomyopathy

**1117. The hallmark of the late secondary restrictive cardiomyopathies is an abnormal?**
*Harrison's 20th Ed. Chapter 254 Page 1791*

A. Systolic dysfunction
B. Diastolic dysfunction
C. Systolic + diastolic dysfunction
D. Any of the above

Hallmark of restrictive cardiomyopathies is abnormal diastolic function. Ventricular walls are excessively rigid & impede ventricular filling due to myocardial fibrosis, hypertrophy or infiltration. Infiltrative diseases leading to secondary RCM may show impairment of systolic function.

**1118. Which of the following is a feature of restrictive cardiomyopathy?**
*Harrison's 20th Ed. Chapter 254 Page 1791*

A. Both atria are enlarged
B. End-diastolic pressures are elevated in both ventricles
C. Preserved cardiac output
D. All of the above

**1119. Restrictive cardiomyopathy more commonly presents with clinical features related to?**
*Harrison's 20th Ed. Chapter 254 Page 1791*

A. Right heart
B. Left heart
C. Both ventricles
D. Any of the above

Restrictive cardiomyopathy presents with relatively more right-sided symptoms, such as edema, abdominal discomfort, and ascites, although filling pressures are elevated in both ventricles.

**1120. Which of the following is a clinical feature of restrictive cardiomyopathy?**
*Harrison's 20th Ed. Chapter 254 Page 1791*

A. S4 more common than S3
B. Rapid Y descent in jugular venous examination
C. Positive Kussmaul's sign
D. All of the above

**1121. Restrictive cardiomyopathies are due to?**
*Harrison's 20th Ed. Chapter 254 Page 1792*

A. Infiltration of abnormal substances between myocytes
B. Storage of abnormal metabolic products within myocytes
C. Fibrotic endomyocardial injury
D. Any of the above

Most restrictive cardiomyopathies are due to infiltration of abnormal substances between myocytes, storage of abnormal metabolic products within myocytes, or fibrotic injury.

**1122. Which of the following is the more common cause of secondary restrictive cardiomyopathy?**
*Harrison's 20th Ed. Chapter 254 Page 1792*

A. Amyloidosis
B. Sarcoidosis
C. Scleroderma
D. Hemochromatosis

Myocardial involvement with amyloid is a common cause of secondary RCM, although restriction is also seen in the transplanted heart, in hemochromatosis, glycogen deposition, endomyocardial fibrosis, sarcoidosis, hypereosinophilic disease, and scleroderma, following mediastinal irradiation, and in neoplastic infiltration.

**1123. Familial amyloidosis results from an autosomal dominant mutation in?**
*Harrison's 20th Ed. Chapter 254 Page 1792*

A. Calcitonin
B. Gelsolin
C. Transthyretin
D. Amyloid β protein

Familial amyloidosis results from an autosomal dominant mutation in transthyretin, a carrier protein for thyroxine and retinol.

**1124. Amyloidosis is best related to which of the following?**
*Harrison's 20th Ed. Chapter 254 Page 1793 Figure 254-14*

A. Glycosphingolipid
B. Congo red stain
C. Mucopolysaccharidoses
D. Hypereosinophilic syndrome

Congo red stain can be used to highlight amyloid.

### 1125. Amyloid fibrils infiltrate the myocardium, especially around?
*Harrison's 20th Ed. Chapter 254 Page 1793*

A. Cardiomyocyte
B. Coronary vessels
C. Lymphatics
D. Entry of SVC, IVC

*Amyloid fibrils infiltrate myocardium, especially around conduction system & coronary vessels.*

### 1126. Typical feature of amyloidosis is?
*Harrison's 20th Ed. Chapter 254 Page 1793*

A. Conduction block
B. Autonomic neuropathy
C. Renal involvement
D. All of the above

*Typical clinical features are conduction block, autonomic neuropathy, renal involvement, and occasionally thickened skin lesions.*

### 1127. 2D echocardiogram that shows refractile brightness in the septum is suggestive of?
*Harrison's 20th Ed. Chapter 254 Page 1793*

A. Endomyocardial fibrosis
B. Eosinophilic endomyocardial disease
C. Primary cardiac amyloidosis
D. All of the above

*2D echocardiogram that shows a characteristic refractile brightness in the septum suggestive of cardiac amyloidosis.*

### 1128. Which of the following go in favour of amyloidosis?
*Harrison's 20th Ed. Chapter 254 Page 1792*

A. Low voltage ECG
B. Hyperrefractile "glittering" of myocardium on 2D Echo
C. Both atria are dilated
D. All of the above

### 1129. Best overall prognosis is in which of the following?
*Harrison's 20th Ed. Chapter 254 Page 1793*

A. Primary amyloid
B. Immunoglobulin-associated amyloid
C. Abnormal transthyretin-associated cardiac amyloid
D. Senile cardiac amyloid

*The prognosis is worst for primary amyloid with a median survival of 6-12 months after symptoms of heart failure. Senile cardiac amyloid has the slowest progression and best overall prognosis.*

### 1130. Which of the following is beneficial in the treatment of AL amyloidosis?
*Blood 2011 118:827-828*

A. Rituximab
B. Bortezomib
C. Etoposide
D. Dasatinib

*Bortezomib has the highest activity that has ever been recorded for a single agent in AL amyloidosis.*

### 1131. Differentiation of constrictive pericarditis from restrictive cardiomyopathies is done by which of the following?
*N Engl J Med. 1997;336:273*

A. Apex impulse
B. Mitral regurgitation
C. Pericardial calcification
D. All of the above

*Apex impulse is easily palpable & mitral regurgitation is more common in RCM. Pericardial calcification on Chest X-ray/CT/MRI occurs commonly in constrictive pericarditis.*

### 1132. Löffler's endocarditis best relates to?
*Harrison's 20th Ed. Chapter 254 Page 1793*

A. Postcardiac injury syndrome
B. Hypoplastic left heart syndrome
C. Hypereosinophilic syndrome
D. Straight back syndrome

*Löffler's endocarditis is associated with a history of chronic hypereosinophilic syndrome, which is more common in men than women. Pericardial effusions are not common. Eosinophilic myocarditis or Löffler's endocarditis can lead to endomyocardial fibrosis.*

### 1133. In chronic hypereosinophilic syndrome, there is persistent hypereosinophilia of >1500 eos/μL for at least?
*Harrison's 20th Ed. Chapter 254 Page 1793*

A. 3 months
B. 6 months
C. 9 months
D. 12 months

*In chronic hypereosinophilic syndrome, there is persistent hypereosinophilia of >1500 eos/μL for at least 6 months.*

### 1134. Endomyocardial fibrosis most commonly affects which of the following age groups?
*Harrison's 20th Ed. Chapter 254 Page 1793*

A. Children and young adults
B. Middle aged
C. Elderly
D. Any of the above

*Endomyocardial fibrosis is a progressive disease of unknown cause that occurs mostly in children & young adults residing in tropical & subtropical Africa, particularly Uganda & Nigeria.*

### 1135. Fibrous endocardial lesions in endomyocardial fibrosis involve which of the following areas of heart?
*Harrison's 20th Ed. Chapter 254 Page 1793*

A. Inflow portion of right or left atria (or both)
B. Outflow portion of right or left atria (or both)
C. Inflow portion of right or left ventricle (or both)
D. Outflow portion of right or left ventricle (or both)

*Endomyocardial fibrosis is characterized by fibrous endocardial lesions of inflow portion of right or left ventricle (or both) & often involves atrioventricular valves, producing valvular regurgitation.*

### 1136. Endocardial fibrosis results from which of the following?
*Harrison's 20th Ed. Chapter 254 Page 1793*

A. Carcinoid syndrome
B. Fenfluramine
C. Phentermine
D. All of the above

*Carcinoid syndrome, use of anorexic agents like fenfluramine & phentermine result in endocardial fibrosis & stenosis and/or regurgitation of the tricuspid and/or pulmonary valve.*

# Hypertrophic Cardiomyopathy (HCM)

**1137. Hypertrophic cardiomyopathy is associated with?**
*Harrison's 20th Ed. Chapter 254 Page 1793*

A. Hypertension
B. Aortic valve disease
C. Systemic infiltrative or storage diseases
D. None of the above

*Hypertrophic cardiomyopathy is defined as left ventricular hypertrophy that develops in absence of causative hemodynamic factors like hypertension, aortic valve disease, or systemic infiltrative or storage diseases.*

**1138. Hypertrophic cardiomyopathy (HCM) is also called?**
*Harrison's 20th Ed. Chapter 254 Page 1793*

A. Hypertrophic obstructive cardiomyopathy (HOCM)
B. Asymmetric septal hypertrophy (ASH)
C. Idiopathic hypertrophic subaortic stenosis (IHSS)
D. All of the above

*The accepted terminology presently is hypertrophic cardiomyopathy with or without obstruction.*

**1139. Which of the following about HCM is false?**
*Harrison's 20th Ed. Chapter 254 Page 1794*

A. Autosomal dominant pattern of inheritance
B. Mutation in either MYH7 or MYBPC3
C. Age-dependent and incomplete penetrance
D. None of the above

*HCM is caused by mutations in β myosin heavy chain (MYH7) or myosin-binding protein C gene (MYBPC3).*

**1140. The defining phenotype of HCM is?**
*Harrison's 20th Ed. Chapter 254 Page 1794*

A. Asymmetric septal hypertrophy
B. Left ventricular outflow tract obstruction
C. Left ventricular hypertrophy
D. Endocardial fibrosis

*Defining phenotype of left ventricular hypertrophy is rarely present at birth & usually develops later in life.*

**1141. In MYBPC3 mutation carriers, the average age of HCM development is?**
*Harrison's 20th Ed. Chapter 254 Page 1794*

A. 20 years
B. 30 years
C. 40 years
D. 50 years

*In MYBPC3 mutation carriers, the average age of HCM disease development is 40 years.*

**1142. Hypertrophic cardiomyopathy mutations lead to?**
*Harrison's 20th Ed. Chapter 254 Page 1794*

A. Enhanced calcium sensitivity
B. Maximal force generation
C. ATPase activity
D. All of the above

*At the level of sarcomere, HCM mutations lead to enhanced calcium sensitivity, maximal force generation, and ATPase activity. All of these lead to abnormal energetics & impaired relaxation.*

**1143. Hypertrophic cardiomyopathy is characterized by?**
*Harrison's 20th Ed. Chapter 254 Page 1794*

A. Misaligned, disarrayed enlarged myofibrils & myocytes
B. Interstitial fibrosis
C. Microinfarction of hypertrophied myocardium
D. All of the above

*Hypertrophic cardiomyopathy is characterized by misalignment and disarray of the enlarged myofibrils and myocytes.*

**1144. Hypertrophic cardiomyopathy is characterized by?**
*Harrison's 20th Ed. Chapter 254 Page 1794*

A. Hypertrophy
B. Interstitial fibrosis
C. Microvascular disease
D. All of the above

*Interstitial fibrosis is detectable before overt hypertrophy develops in HCM.*

**1145. In HCM, maximal hypertrophy is seen in?**
*Harrison's 20th Ed. Chapter 254 Page 1795*

A. Interventricular septum
B. Midventricle
C. Ventricular apex
D. All of the above

*The interventricular septum is the typical location of maximal hypertrophy in HCM.*

**1146. Apical HCM (ApHCM) is also referred as?**
*Acta Cardiol Sin 2015;31:8386, Harrison's 19th Ed. 269e-10*

A. Ishimura syndrome
B. Yamaguchi's syndrome
C. Nishiyama syndrome
D. Takatsu syndrome

*Yamaguchi's syndrome is also called "Japanese heart disease".*

**1147. Which of the following is false about Yamaguchi's syndrome?**
*Acta Cardiol Sin. 2015;31:8386.*

A. Apical nonobstructive type of HCM
B. Giant T wave negativity in left precordial leads in ECG
C. "Ace of Spade" like configuration of LV cavity at end-diastole on left ventriculography
D. None of the above

*Typical features of apical nonobstructive type of HCM (Yamaguchi's syndrome, relatively common in Japan) include an audible fourth heart sound, giant T wave negativity in left precordial leads in ECG, a "Ace of spade" like configuration of left ventricular cavity at end-diastole on left ventriculography.*

**1148. Which of the following accompanies obstructive HCM?**
*Harrison's 20th Ed. Chapter 254 Page 1795*

A. AS
B. AR
C. MS
D. MR

*In HCM, mitral leaflet coaptation may lead to posteriorly directed mitral regurgitation.*

**1149. Which of the following is the most common monogenic cardiovascular disorder?**
*N Engl J Med. 2018;379:655-68*

A. Hypertrophic Cardiomyopathy
B. Marfan's syndrome
C. Sudden death associated with a prolonged QT syndrome
D. Monogenic hypertension

*About 65% of human monogenic disorders are autosomal dominant, 25% are autosomal recessive and 5% are X-linked. HCM is the most common monogenic cardiovascular disorder. Each child of a parent with HCM has a 50% chance of inheriting the condition. Spontaneous (de novo) mutations probably accounts for this disease burden. Sporadic (nonfamilial) HCM (i.e., sarcomere mutations in a patient without a family history of HCM) may be more common than currently thought. Genetic testing is the only reliable way to identify unaffected family members who may need to be screened for sudden death risk factors.*

**1150. Which of the following is false about HCM?**
*Cleveland Clinic J of Medicine 2018;85(5):399*

A. Dynamic obstruction of LV outflow tract is a key pathophysiologic mechanism
B. Transthoracic echocardiography is the first-line imaging test
C. β-blockers are the 1st line drugs for treating symptoms of HCM
D. None of the above

**1151. Which of the following diseases can mimic HCM?**
*N Engl J Med. 2018;379:655-68*

A. Lysosome-associated membrane protein 2 cardiomyopathy
B. Fabry's disease
C. Amyloidosis
D. All of the above

*Genetic testing can identify metabolic & storage phenocopies like lysosome-associated membrane protein 2 (LAMP2) cardiomyopathy, Fabry's disease, Pompe disease, PRKAG2, Danon disease and amyloidosis, that mimic HCM.*

**1152. Which of the following laboratory test will help differentiate HCM from Fabry disease?**
*Cleveland Clinic J of Medicine 2018;85(5):399*

A. Liver function tests
B. Renal function tests
C. Creatine kinase
D. Blood glucose levels

*Derangements in liver function & glucose levels will be evident in patients with glycogen storage disorders (Pompe disease). Renal dysfunction (serum creatinine) will be seen in patients with Fabry disease or amyloidosis. Creatine kinase may be elevated in patients with Danon disease.*

**1153. Which of the following is related to cellular metabolism?**
*Harrison's 20th Ed. Chapter 254 Page 1781 Table 254-3*

A. PRKAG2
B. MYH7
C. MYBPC3
D. All of the above

**1154. Gene defect in which of the following can cause HCM?**
*Harrison's 20th Ed. Chapter 254 Page 1781 Table 254-3*

A. Sarcomere
B. Z-disk and Cytoskeleton
C. Cellular Metabolism
D. All of the above

**1155. HCM⁺ refers to?**
*Harrison's 20th Ed. Chapter 254 Page 1781 Table 254-3*

A. HCM with preexcitation
B. HCM with dilated cardiomyopathy
C. HCM with restrictive cardiomyopathy
D. Any of the above

*HCM+ refers to HCM with preexcitation.*

**1156. Which of the following gene products is related to HCM⁺?**
*Harrison's 20th Ed. Chapter 254 Page 1781 Table 254-3*

A. PRKAG2 (γ-subunit of AMP kinase)
B. LAMP2 (lysosomal associated X-linked membrane protein)
C. GLA (α-galactosidase-A)
D. All of the above

**1157. HCMc refers to?**
*Harrison's 20th Ed. Chapter 254 Page 1781 Table 254-3*

A. HCM with cardiomyopathy
B. Congenital HCM
C. HCM with coronary artery disease
D. HCM with conduction disease

*HCMc refers to HCM with conduction disease.*

**1158. Clinical diagnosis of HCM is based on which of the following?**
*N Engl J Med. 2018;379:655-68*

A. Hypertrophied, nondilated left ventricle
B. Identified by echocardiography or MRI
C. Absence of another cardiac, systemic, metabolic, or syndromic disease
D. All of the above

*Clinical diagnosis of HCM is based on a hypertrophied, nondilated left ventricle, identified by means of echocardiography or magnetic resonance imaging (MRI) in the absence of another cardiac, systemic, metabolic, or syndromic disease. HCM is not characteristically a progressive disorder. Two or more major (but treatable) complications develop in only 10% of affected patients during their lifetime*

**1159. Which of the following is false about HCM?**
*Harrison's 20th Ed. Chapter 254 Page 1794*

A. Found in ~1 in 500 of general population
B. Systolic anterior motion of mitral valve is characteristic
C. Myocardial perfusion defects on thallium 201 radionuclide scintigraphy frequent
D. None of the above

*HCM is found in ~1 in 500 of the general population. Dynamic LV subaortic outflow tract pressure gradient due to midsystolic proximity of anterior mitral valve leaflet against hypertrophied septum is typical of obstructive HCM. Radionuclide scintigraphy with thallium 201 frequently shows myocardial perfusion defects even in asymptomatic patients.*

**1160. Which of the following is the most common cause of sudden death among young athletes?**
*Harrison's 20th Ed. Chapter 254 Page 1794, N Engl J Med. 2003;349:1064-75.*

A. Mitral valve prolapse syndrome
B. Hypertrophic cardiomyopathy
C. Thyrotoxicosis
D. Anxiety

*Hypertrophic cardiomyopathy is the most common cause of sudden death among young athletes.*

**1161. Which of the following is the most common cause of SCD in young competitive athletes?**
*Harrison's 20th Ed. Chapter 254 Page 1794*

A. MVP
B. Long QT syndrome
C. HCM
D. Tetralogy of Fallot

*HCM is the most common cause of SCD in young competitive athletes.*

**1162. Established risk marker for sudden death in cases of HCM is?**
*N Engl J Med. 2018;379:655-68*

A. Unexplained syncope
B. Extreme left ventricular wall thickness
C. HCM-related sudden death in a first-degree relative
D. All of the above

*Established risk markers for sudden death in cases of HCM are unexplained syncope, extreme left ventricular wall thickness, HCM-related sudden death in a first-degree relative, and multiple or prolonged episodes of nonsustained ventricular tachycardia.*

**1163. Differential diagnosis of large negative T-waves in ECG include?**
*The American Journal of Medicine 2014;127(1):31*

A. Acute coronary syndrome
B. Cocaine toxicity
C. Subarachnoid hemorrhage
D. All of the above

*Differential diagnosis of large negative T-waves in ECG include acute coronary syndrome, cocaine toxicity, neurological disorders (subarachnoid hemorrhage), and electrolyte abnormalities.*

**1164. In ECG, causes of giant T-wave inversion include?**
*Cleveland Clinic J of Medicine 2013;80(3):139*

A. Elevated intracranial pressure
B. Acute pancreatitis
C. Wolff-Parkinson-White syndrome
D. All of the above

*In ECG, causes of giant T-wave inversion include Apical hypertrophic obstructive cardiomyopathy, Subarachnoid hemorrhage, Cocaine abuse, Non-Q-wave myocardial infarction, Acute abdomen (acute pancreatitis), Complete heart block, Severe right ventricular hypertrophy, Elevated intracranial pressure, Post-pacemaker syndrome, Wolff-Parkinson-White syndrome.*

**1165. Systolic murmur in obstructive HCM is best heard at?**
*Cleveland Clinic J of Medicine 2018;85(5):399*

A. $A_1$ area
B. $A_2$ area
C. Pulmonary area
D. Lower left sternal border

*Hallmark of obstructive HCM is a systolic murmur which is typically harsh, diamond-shaped & begins after S1, since ejection is unimpeded early in systole. Murmur is best heard at lower left sternal border as well as at apex, where it is often more holosystolic & blowing in quality due to mitral regurgitation that usually accompanies obstructive HCM.*

**1166. In HCM, physical findings include?**
*Cleveland Clinic J of Medicine 2018;85(5):399*

A. Fourth heart sound
B. Systolic murmurs
C. Bifid carotid pulse
D. All of the above

*In HCM, physical findings are nonspecific and include systolic murmurs, bifid carotid pulse, a fourth heart sound, and a hyperdynamic precordium. Valsalva maneuver helps distinguish the murmur of left ventricular outflow tract obstruction in HCM from a murmur related to aortic stenosis by auscultation.*

**1167. Which of the following is the preferred method to provoke left ventricular outflow gradients?**
*N Engl J Med. 2018;379:655-68*

A. Amyl nitrite inhalation
B. Valsalva maneuver
C. Isoproterenol infusion
D. Exercise (stress) echocardiography

**1168. Maneuvers that increase the murmur of obstructive HCM include all except?**
*Harrison's 20th Ed. Chapter 254 Page 1795*

A. Valsalva maneuver
B. Tachycardia
C. Sudden standing
D. Passive leg raising

**1169. Maneuvers that decrease the murmur of obstructive HCM include all except?**
*Harrison's 20th Ed. Chapter 254 Page 1795*

A. Squatting
B. Sustained handgrip
C. Nitroglycerin
D. Passive leg raising

*Interventions that increase myocardial contractility like exercise, sympathomimetic amines & digitalis glycosides, and those that reduce ventricular volume like Valsalva maneuver, sudden standing, nitroglycerin, amyl nitrite or tachycardia, may all cause an increase in the gradient & the murmur. Conversely, elevation of arterial pressure by phenylephrine, squatting, sustained handgrip, augmentation of venous return by passive leg raising & expansion of the blood volume all increase ventricular volume & ameliorate the gradient & murmur.*

**1170. Left ventricular outflow tract obstruction is defined as a resting peak gradient of?**
*Cleveland Clinic J of Medicine 2018;85(5):399*

A. 10 mm Hg
B. 20 mm Hg
C. 30 mm Hg
D. 40 mm Hg

*Left ventricular outflow tract obstruction is defined as a resting peak gradient of 30 mm Hg or higher.*

**1171. In HCM, ubiquitous pathophysiologic abnormality is?**
*Harrison's 20th Ed. Chapter 254 Page 1795*

A. Systolic dysfunction
B. Diastolic dysfunction
C. Systolic + diastolic dysfunction
D. None of the above

*Ubiquitous pathophysiologic abnormality in HCM is diastolic dysfunction, characterized by increased stiffness of hypertrophied muscle. This results in elevated diastolic filling pressures & is present despite of a hyperdynamic left ventricle.*

**1172. In HCM, most common mutations occur in which of the following genes?**
*The American Journal of Medicine 2016;129:148-152*

A. Cardiac alpha-myosin heavy chain gene
B. Cardiac beta-myosin heavy chain gene
C. Cardiac myosin light chain gene
D. Cardiac troponins C, I, and T gene

In HCM, most common are mutations of the cardiac beta-myosin heavy chain gene and cardiac myosin-binding protein C gene. Others involve alpha-myosin heavy chains, cardiac troponins C, I, and T, actin, myosin light chains & titin.

**1173. In HCM, most common mutations of cardiac beta-myosin heavy chain gene is on?**
*The American Journal of Medicine 2016;129:148-152*

A. Chromosome 10
B. Chromosome 12
C. Chromosome 14
D. Chromosome 16

In HCM, most common mutations of cardiac beta-myosin heavy chain gene is on chromosome 14.

**1174. At what age, full genetic expression occurs in first-degree relatives of patients with familial HCM?**
*The American Journal of Medicine 2016;129:148-152*

A. 5 years
B. 10 years
C. 20 years
D. 30 years

Echocardiographic studies have confirmed that by age 20 years, full genetic expression occurs in about half of the first-degree relatives of patients with familial HCM.

**1175. What proportion of first-degree relatives of patients with familial HCM have evidence of the disease?**
*The American Journal of Medicine 2016;129:148-152*

A. One-fourth
B. One-third
C. One-half
D. Three-fourth

Echocardiographic studies have confirmed that about one-third of the first-degree relatives of patients with familial HCM have evidence of disease.

**1176. Hypertrophic cardiomyopathy commonly "masquerades" as?**
*The American Journal of Medicine 2016;129:148-152*

A. Asthma
B. Mitral prolapse
C. Coronary artery disease
D. All of the above

Hypertrophic cardiomyopathy is cardiology's "great masquerader."

**1177. In symptomatic HCM, the most common complaint is?**
*The American Journal of Medicine 2016;129:148-152*

A. Dyspnea
B. Palpitation
C. Angina pectoris
D. Syncope

In symptomatic HCM patients, most common complaint is dyspnea, due to diastolic ventricular dysfunction which impairs ventricular filling & leads to elevated LV diastolic, left atrial & pulmonary capillary pressures. Other symptoms include syncope, angina pectoris & fatigue. Symptoms are not closely related to the presence or severity of an outflow pressure gradient.

**1178. Mendelian transmission of single-gene defects may occur in?**
*Harrison's 20th Ed. Chapter 231 Page 1650*

A. Hypertrophic cardiomyopathy
B. Marfan syndrome
C. Long QT syndrome
D. All of the above

Familial clustering due to Mendelian transmission of single-gene defects may occur in hypertrophic cardiomyopathy, Marfan syndrome & sudden death associated with a prolonged QT syndrome. Essential hypertension or coronary atherosclerosis are often polygenic disorders.

**1179. Risk of sudden death in HCM correlates with all except?**
*Harrison's 20th Ed. Chapter 254 Page 1794*

A. Ventricular tachycardia on ambulatory monitoring
B. Marked ventricular septal hypertrophy (>30 mm)
C. Abnormal blood pressure response to exercise
D. Severity of symptoms

HCM patients at higher risk of sudden death are those with a history of resuscitation from sudden cardiac death, ventricular tachycardia on ambulatory monitoring or at electrophysiologic testing, marked ventricular hypertrophy (ventricular septal thickness >30 mm), syncope (in children), genetic mutations associated with an increased risk, abnormal blood pressure response to exercise & a family history of sudden death. There is no correlation between the risk of sudden death and the severity of symptoms, but there is an increased risk of death in patients with outflow gradients.

**1180. Left ventricular cavity in HCM is typically?**
*Harrison's 20th Ed. Chapter 254 Page 1794*

A. Small
B. Normal
C. Large
D. Any of the above

Left ventricular cavity typically is small in HCM, with vigorous posterior wall motion but reduced septal excursion.

**1181. In a hypertrophic cardiomyopathy phenotype, which of the following pathologic feature is possible?**
*The American Journal of Medicine 2016;129:148-152*

A. Abnormal anterior papillary muscle position in LV cavity
B. Mitral valve leaflets elongated and redundant
C. Narrowing of intramural small coronary arteries
D. All of the above

Systolic anterior motion (SAM) of the mitral valve results not from a Venturi effect, as previously believed, but rather from an early systolic flow interaction with the abnormally elongated anterior mitral valve leaflet pushing it into the left ventricular outflow tract.

**1182. Differential diagnosis of hypertrophic cardiomyopathy include?**
*Cleveland Clinic J of Medicine 2018;85(5):399*

A. Noncompaction cardiomyopathy
B. Hemochromatosis
C. 'Athlete's heart'
D. All of the above

Differential diagnosis of hypertrophic cardiomyopathy include hypertensive cardiomyopathy, Aortic valvulopathy (Aortic stenosis, Supra-aortic or subaortic membranes), Infiltrative cardiomyopathy like Amyloidosis, Fabry disease, Lysosomal diseases (Danon disease), Glycogen storage disorders (Pompe disease), Hemochromatosis, 'Athlete's heart' and Noncompaction cardiomyopathy.

**1183. In echocardiography of HCM, interventricular septum is how many times thicker than high posterior left ventricular free wall?**
*Cleveland Clinic J of Medicine 2018;85(5):399*

A. 0.5 times
B. 0.8 times
C. 1.1 times
D. 1.3 times

HCM echocardiogram, demonstrates LVH, with septum 1.3 or more times the thickness of high posterior left ventricular free wall.

**1184. Which of the following investigation is best for accurate measurements of regional hypertrophy and in identifying sites of regional fibrosis?**
*Harrison's 20th Ed. Chapter 254 Page 1794*

A. ECG
B. Echocardiography
C. CMRI
D. LV Angiography

Cardiac MRI is superior to echocardiography in providing accurate measurements of regional hypertrophy and in identifying sites of regional fibrosis.

**1185. Which of the following electrocardiographic findings can be seen in patients of HCM?**
*Cleveland Clinic J of Medicine 2018;85(5):399*

A. Left ventricular hypertrophy
B. Pseudoinfarct pattern with Q waves in anterolateral leads
C. Repolarization abnormalities
D. All of the above

More than 90% of HCM patients have ECG abnormalities. Common findings include Left ventricular hypertrophy, pseudoinfarct pattern with Q waves in anterolateral leads, repolarization changes like T-wave inversions & horizontal or down-sloping ST segments. Apical HCM presents with giant T-wave inversion (> 10 mm) in anterolateral leads, most prominent in V4, V5, and V6.

**1186. In HCM patients with circulatory shock requiring vasopressor support, which of the following should be used?**
*Cleveland Clinic J of Medicine 2018;85(5):399*

A. Digoxin
B. Phenylephrine
C. Norepinephrine
D. Dobutamine and Dopamine

Positive inotropic effect of vasopressors increases contractility & increases left ventricular outflow tract gradient. Therefore, Digoxin, Norepinephrine, dobutamine and dopamine should be avoided. In patients with circulatory shock requiring vasopressor support, pure alpha-agonists like phenylephrine is preferred, as they increase peripheral resistance without an inotropic effect.

**1187. Complications of HCM include?**
*N Engl M Med. 2004;350:1320-7*

A. Atrial fibrillation
B. Infective endocarditis
C. Sudden death
D. All of the above

Propensity for sudden death in HCM is genetic. Other complications include atrial fibrillation, infective endocarditis & end-stage heart failure.

**1188. Which of the following calcium channel blockers should be avoided in cases of obstructive HCM?**
*Harrison's 20th Ed. Chapter 254 Page 1796*

A. Verapamil
B. Diltiazem
C. Nifedipine
D. All of the above

Verapamil & diltiazem reduces stiffness of ventricle, reduces elevated diastolic pressures, increase exercise tolerance & reduces severity of outflow tract pressure gradients. Nifedipine should be avoided. Dihydropyridine calcium channel blockers should be avoided altogether, as they produce even more peripheral vasodilation and afterload reduction than nondihydropyridine calcium channel blockers.

**1189. Which of the following drugs should be avoided in cases of obstructive HCM?**
*Harrison's 20th Ed. Chapter 254 Page 1796*

A. Digitalis
B. Diuretics
C. Nitrates
D. All of the above

Digitalis, diuretics, nitrates, vasodilators are best avoided, particularly in patients with known left ventricular outflow tract pressure gradients. Any medication that causes afterload reduction, peripheral vasodilation, intravascular volume depletion, or positive inotropy can worsen the dynamic left ventricular outflow tract obstruction in a patient with HCM and should be avoided.

**1190. Which out of the following drugs should not be used in a case of obstrutive HCM?**
*Harrison's 20th Ed. Chapter 254 Page 1796*

A. Beta-blockers
B. Digitalis
C. Nondihydropyridine calcium blockers
D. Disopyramide

Beta blockers block the effects of catecholamines that exacerbate outflow tract obstruction & to slow the heart rate so that diastolic filling is enhanced. Disopyramide exerts negative inotropic effects that decreases the outflow gradient and thereby improve symptoms. Digitalis increases left ventricular outflow tract pressure gradients by increasing myocardial contractility.

**1191. Which of the following drug is protective against SCD in HCM?**
*N Engl J Med. 2018;379:655-68*

A. Amiodarone
B. Beta-adrenergic blockers
C. Disopyramide
D. Diltiazem

Amiodarone is effective in reducing the frequency of supraventricular as well as life-threatening ventricular arrhythmias and anecdotal data suggest that it may reduce the risk of SCD.

**1192. Which of the following is the treatment for nonobstructive HCM with heart failure?**
*N Engl J Med. 2018;379:655-68*

A. Heart transplantation
B. Implantable cardioverter – defibrillator (ICD) placement
C. Surgical septal myectomy
D. Alcohol septal ablation

1193. **Which of the following surgery can be considered for obstructive HCM?**

*Cleveland Clinic J of Medicine 2018;85(5):399*

- A. Ventricular septal myectomy
- B. Alcohol septal ablation
- C. Papillary muscle reorientation surgery
- D. All of the above

1194. **What is meant by "burned out HCM"?**

*Harrison's 20th Ed. Chapter 254 Page 1796*

- A. HCM not manifesting in offsprings
- B. HCM disappearing with advancing age
- C. HCM progressing to DCM with disappearance of preexisting outflow pressure gradient
- D. HCM with AR

Progression of HCM to left ventricular dilatation & dysfunction (DCM) with wall thinning & disappearance of a preexisting outflow pressure gradient is called burned out HCM. It occurs in 5 - 10% of patients & may be associated with nonresponsive CHF requiring cardiac transplantation.

## Aortic Valve Disease

**1195. The accelerated natural history of rheumatic valvular disease in Indian subcontinent is due to?**
*Harrison's 20th Ed. Chapter 256 Page 1802*

- A. Genetic predisposition
- B. Nutritional deficiencies
- C. Repeated infections with rheumatogenic streptococci
- D. All of the above

*Repeated infections with more virulent strains of rheumatogenic streptococci is perhaps the cause of accelerated natural history of rheumatic valvular disease in Indian subcontinent and in Southeast Asia.*

**1196. Severe aortic stenosis (AS) affects what percentage of the population above 75 years of age?**
*Harrison's 20th Ed. Chapter 256 Page 1802*

- A. 1.5%
- B. 2.5%
- C. 3.5%
- D. 4.5%

*Severe aortic stenosis (AS) is estimated to affect 3.5% of the population aged >75 years.*

**1197. Which of the following studies estimated the prevalence of moderate or severe mitral & aortic valve disease in US?**
*Harrison's 20th Ed. Chapter 256 Page 1802 Figure 256-2*

- A. Coronary Artery Risk Development in Young Adults (CARDIA)
- B. The Atherosclerosis Risk in Communities (ARIC)
- C. The Cardiovascular Health Study (CHS)
- D. All of the above

**1198. Aortic stenosis (AS) occurs in what percentage of all patients with chronic valvular heart disease?**
*Harrison's 20th Ed. Chapter 256 Page 1803*

- A. 10%
- B. 15%
- C. 25%
- D. 33%

*Aortic stenosis (AS) occurs in ~ one-fourth of all patients with chronic valvular heart disease.*

**1199. What percentage of adult patients with symptomatic valvular AS are male?**
*Harrison's 20th Ed. Chapter 256 Page 1803*

- A. 30%
- B. 50%
- C. 60%
- D. 80%

*80% of adult patients with symptomatic valvular AS are male.*

**1200. Degenerative calcification in AS occurs most commonly over and above which of the following?**
*Harrison's 20th Ed. Chapter 256 Page 1803*

- A. Bicuspid aortic valve (BAV)
- B. Chronic trileaflet aortic valve deterioration
- C. Previous rheumatic inflammation of aortic valve
- D. All of the above

*AS in adults is due to degenerative calcification of the aortic cusps and occurs most commonly on an existing disease like bicuspid aortic valve, chronic trileaflet deterioration, or previous rheumatic inflammation. Out of these, most cases have bicuspid aortic valve (BAV) disease.*

**1201. Process of aortic valve deterioration and calcification shares many features with?**
*Harrison's 20th Ed. Chapter 256 Page 1803*

- A. Atherosclerosis
- B. Apoptosis
- C. Mitochondrial diseases
- D. Neoplasia

*The process of aortic valve deterioration & calcification shares many features with vascular atherosclerosis, including endothelial dysfunction, lipid accumulation, inflammatory cell activation, cytokine release, and upregulation of several signaling pathways.*

**1202. Which of the following is central in the pathogenesis of aortic valve deterioration & calcification?**
*Harrison's 20th Ed. Chapter 256 Page 1803*

- A. Foam cell
- B. Myofibroblast
- C. Endothelial cell
- D. Macrophage

*In aortic valve deterioration & calcification, valvular myofibroblasts differentiate phenotypically into osteoblasts and actively produce bone matrix proteins that allow for the deposition of calcium hydroxyapatite crystals.*

**1203. Genetic polymorphisms involving which of the following is linked to the development of calcific AS?**
*Harrison's 20th Ed. Chapter 256 Page 1803*

- A. Vitamin D receptor
- B. Estrogen receptor
- C. Apolipoprotein E4
- D. All of the above

*Genetic polymorphisms involving the vitamin D receptor, the estrogen receptor in postmenopausal women, interleukin 10 and apolipoprotein E4 have been linked to the development of calcific AS and a strong familial clustering of cases.*

**1204. Polymorphism & elevated levels of which of the following is associated with aortic-valve calcification and incident aortic stenosis?**
*N Engl J Med. 2014;371:744-56*

- A. HDLc
- B. Triglycerides
- C. Lipoprotein(a)
- D. All of the above

*In a genome wide linkage meta-analysis of three large population-based studies, a specific lipoprotein(a) polymorphism was shown to be associated with elevated serum levels of lipoprotein(a), aortic-valve calcification, and incident aortic stenosis.*

**1205. Population-based studies have shown associations between calcific valve disease and?**
*N Engl J Med. 2014;371:744-56*

A. Male sex
B. Elevated levels of serum low-density lipoprotein cholesterol
C. Elevated levels of serum lipoprotein(a)
D. All of the above

Population-based studies have shown associations between calcific valve disease and older age, male sex, elevated serum levels of low-density lipoprotein (LDL) cholesterol & lipoprotein(a), hypertension, smoking, diabetes, and metabolic syndrome.

**1206. Specific populations at increased risk for aortic stenosis include?**
*N Engl J Med. 2014;371:744-56*

A. Mediastinal irradiation
B. Renal failure
C. Disorders of calcium metabolism
D. All of the above

Specific populations at increased risk for aortic stenosis include patients with a history of mediastinal irradiation, renal failure, familial hypercholesterolemia, or disorders of calcium & phosphate metabolism.

**1207. Which of the following is false about aortic valve sclerosis?**
*Harrison's 20th Ed. Chapter 256 Page 1803*

A. Focal thickening of the leaflets
B. Focal calcification of the leaflets
C. No obstruction
D. None of the above

Aortic valve sclerosis means focal thickening and calcification of the leaflets not severe enough to cause obstruction.

**1208. What percentage of persons over 65 years exhibit aortic valve sclerosis?**
*Harrison's 20th Ed. Chapter 256 Page 1803*

A. 30%
B. 50%
C. 60%
D. 80%

**1209. What percentage of persons over 65 years exhibit frank aortic stenosis?**
*Harrison's 20th Ed. Chapter 256 Page 1803*

A. 2%
B. 4%
C. 8%
D. 10%

About 30% of persons older than 65 years exhibit aortic valve sclerosis, whereas 2% exhibit frank stenosis.

**1210. Among persons older than age 65, presence of aortic valve sclerosis is associated with an excess risk of?**
*Harrison's 20th Ed. Chapter 256 Page 1803*

A. Hypertension
B. Myocardial infarction
C. Left ventricular hypertrophy
D. Cardiomyopathy

Presence of aortic valve sclerosis is associated with an excess risk of cardiovascular death and myocardial infarction (MI) among persons older than age 65.

**1211. What is the prevalence of aortic stenosis among adults between the ages of 50 and 59 years?**
*N Engl J Med. 2014;371:744-56*

A. About 0.1%
B. About 0.2%
C. About 0.3%
D. About 0.4%

The prevalence of aortic stenosis is only about 0.2% among adults between the ages of 50 and 59 years.

**1212. What is the prevalence of AS among octogenarians?**
*N Engl J Med. 2014;371:744-56*

A. About 10%
B. About 20%
C. About 30%
D. About 40%

The prevalence of aortic stenosis is about 9.8% in octogenarians. Overall prevalence is 2.8% in adults older than 75 years of age.

**1213. What is the rate of death at 2 years in patients with symptomatic aortic-valve disease?**
*N Engl J Med. 2014;371:744-56*

A. Over 30%
B. Over 40%
C. Over 50%
D. Over 60%

Although mortality is not increased when aortic stenosis is asymptomatic, the rate of death is >50% at 2 years in patients with symptomatic aortic-valve disease unless aortic-valve replacement is performed promptly.

**1214. A rheumatic etiology of aortic stenosis is favored by?**
*Harrison's 20th Ed. Chapter 256 Page 1803*

A. History of rheumatic fever
B. Rheumatic involvement of mitral valve
C. Associated AR
D. All of the above

Rheumatic AS is almost always associated with involvement of the mitral valve and with AR.

**1215. Autotaxin is involved in which of the following in the pathogenesis of calcific aortic stenosis?**
*Harrison's 20th Ed. Chapter 256 Page 1804 Figure 256-3*

A. Lipid infiltration
B. Inflammation
C. Fibro-calcific response
D. All of the above

Valvular interstitial cells (VIC) are critical participants in the formation of disorganized collagen (fibrosis) and calcium hydroxyapatite (bone) deposition in the pathogenesis of calcific aortic stenosis.

**1216. Which of the following is the most common congenital heart valve defect?**
*Harrison's 20th Ed. Chapter 256 Page 1803*

A. Congenital pulmonic stenosis
B. Bicuspid aortic valve (BAV)
C. Congenital mitral stenosis
D. Congenital tricuspid stenosis

A bicuspid aortic valve (BAV) is the most common congenital heart valve defect and occurs in 0.5–1.4% of the population with a 2—4:1 male to female predominance.

**1217. Inheritance pattern of bicuspid aortic valve disease is?**
*Harrison's 20th Ed. Chapter 256 Page 1803*

A. Autosomal recessive with incomplete penetrance
B. Autosomal recessive with complete penetrance
C. Autosomal dominant with incomplete penetrance
D. Autosomal dominant with complete penetrance

*Inheritance pattern of bicuspid aortic valve disease is autosomal dominant with incomplete penetrance.*

**1218. Bicuspid aortic valve disease may be associated with?**
*Harrison's 20th Ed. Chapter 256 Page 1803*

A. Ellis-van Creveld syndrome
B. Noonan syndrome
C. Holt-Oram syndrome
D. Turner's syndrome

*X-linked inheritance is suggested by prevalence of BAV disease in patients with Turner's syndrome.*

**1219. Prevalence of BAV disease among first-degree relatives of an affected individual is?**
*Harrison's 20th Ed. Chapter 256 Page 1803*

A. ~ 5%
B. ~ 10%
C. ~ 15%
D. ~ 20%

*Prevalence of BAV disease among 1° relatives of an affected individual is ~10%.*

**1220. Mutation in which of the following gene may be associated with BAV disease?**
*Harrison's 20th Ed. Chapter 256 Page 1803*

A. NOTCH1
B. NOTCH2
C. NOTCH3
D. NOTCH4

*Mutation in NOTCH1 gene on chromosome 9q34-35 has been described in some families suffering from BAV disease. Abnormalities in endothelial nitric oxide synthase and NKX2.5 have been implicated as well.*

**1221. Which of the following occur commonly among patients with BAV disease?**
*Harrison's 20th Ed. Chapter 256 Page 1803*

A. Aortic coarctation
B. Ascending aortic aneurysm
C. Aortic dissection
D. All of the above

**1222. In BAV disease, which of the following is the most common bicuspid variant?**
*Harrison's 20th Ed. Chapter 256 Page 1803*

A. Left-right cusp fusion
B. Right-left cusp fusion
C. Lateral-medial cusp fusion
D. Medial-lateral cusp fusion

*Right-left cusp fusion is the most common bicuspid variant.*

**1223. Shone's complex consists of all except?**
*Harrison's 20th Ed. Chapter 256 Page 1803*

A. Parachute like mitral valve
B. Supravalvular mitral ring
C. Asymmetric septal hypertrophy
D. Coarctation of aorta

*Shone's complex is a rare congenital heart disease (Shone, 1963) typically consisting of four obstructive left heart lesions namely parachute like mitral valve, supravalvular mitral ring, subaortic stenosis, and coarctation of aorta. BAV can be a component of Shone's complex. The severity of mitral obstruction is the most significant indicator of survival and long-term prognosis.*

**1224. Shone's complex or Shone's anomaly is found in what percentage of all congenital heart diseases?**
*Heart Views. 2016;17(1):23-26*

A. 0.1%
B. 0.3%
C. 0.6%
D. 0.9%

*Shone's complex or Shone's anomaly is 0.6% of all congenital heart diseases.*

**1225. Heyde's syndrome best relates to?**
*N Engl J Med. 2014;371:744-56*

A. Thromboxane A2
B. Prostacyclin I2
C. von Willebrand factor
D. Angiotensin II

*In some patients with aortic stenosis, angiodysplastic gastrointestinal bleeding is seen in association with an acquired deficiency of von Willebrand factor multimers, a condition known as Heyde's syndrome. Unfolding of the von Willebrand multimers owing to abnormal shear stress as blood passes through the narrow valve results in cleavage by a specific plasma metalloproteinase. Low levels of von Willebrand factor also affect platelet function and may confer a predisposition to angiogenesis. These abnormalities typically normalize after valve replacement.*

**1226. Lp(a) is best related to?**
*Harrison's 20th Ed. Chapter 400 Page 2890 Table 400-1*

A. ApoB-48
B. ApoC- III
C. ApoB-100
D. ApoE

*Lp(a) is a cholesterol-rich particle lipoprotein similar to LDL consisting of a covalently linked molecule of apolipoprotein B100 with a molecule of apolipoprotein(a). Apo(a) is synthesized in the liver and attached to apoB- 100 by a disulfide linkage. The major site of clearance of Lp(a) is liver.*

**1227. Which of the following produce obstruction to LV outflow?**
*Harrison's 20th Ed. Chapter 256 Page 1803*

A. Hypertrophic obstructive cardiomyopathy
B. Fibromuscular / membranous subaortic stenosis
C. Supravalvular aortic stenosis
D. All of the above

*Hypertrophic obstructive cardiomyopathy, discrete fibromuscular / membranous subaortic stenosis and supravalvular AS produce obstruction to LV outflow.*

**1228. Laplace relation is?**
*Harrison's 20th Ed. Chapter 256 Page 1803*

A. Systolic wall stress = (Pressure x Radius) / Wall thickness
B. Systolic wall stress = (Pressure x Wall thickness) / Radius
C. Systolic wall stress = (Wall thickness x Radius) / Pressure
D. Systolic wall stress = (Pressure + Radius) / Wall thickness

*Systolic stress developed by myocardium is predicted by Laplace relation (S = Pr/h, where S = systolic wall stress, P = pressure, r = radius, and h = wall thickness).*

**1229. In normal sized adults, severe obstruction to LV outflow is considered when effective aortic orifice area is?**
*Harrison's 20th Ed. Chapter 256 Page 1803*

A. 0.6 cm$^2$/m$^2$ body surface area
B. 0.8 cm$^2$/m$^2$ body surface area
C. 1.0 cm$^2$/m$^2$ body surface area
D. 1.2 cm$^2$/m$^2$ body surface area

*A mean systolic pressure gradient >40 mm Hg with a normal CO or an effective aortic orifice area < ~1.0 cm$^2$ (or ~<0.6 cm$^2$/m$^2$ body surface area in a normal-sized adult) i.e., < ~ one-third of the normal orifice is considered to represent severe obstruction to LV outflow.*

**1230. In AS, hypertrophied LV compresses coronary arteries causing ischemia of?**
*Harrison's 20th Ed. Chapter 256 Page 1804*

A. Subendocardium
B. Myocardium
C. Epicardium
D. All of the above

*Hypertrophied LV in AS causes an increase in myocardial oxygen requirements. Capillary density is reduced relative to wall thickness, compressive forces are increased, and the elevated LV end-diastolic pressure reduces the coronary driving pressure. Subendocardium is especially vulnerable to ischemia by this mechanism.*

**1231. Which of the following is not a cardinal symptom of aortic stenosis?**
*Harrison's 20th Ed. Chapter 256 Page 1804*

A. Exertional dyspnea
B. Angina pectoris
C. Syncope
D. Palpitation

*Exertional dyspnea, angina pectoris and syncope are the three cardinal symptoms in patients with pure or predominant AS.*

**1232. Which of the following excludes the possibility of pure or predominant severe aortic stenosis?**
*Harrison's 20th Ed. Chapter 256 Page 1804*

A. Atrial fibrillation
B. Absence of systolic thrill
C. Bisferiens pulse
D. All of the above

*AF in AS suggests the possibility of associated mitral valve disease.*

**1233. In aortic stenosis, systolic thrill is generally present at?**
*Harrison's 20th Ed. Chapter 256 Page 1805*

A. Base of heart
B. In suprasternal notch
C. Along carotid arteries
D. All of the above

*Systolic thrill is present at the base of heart, in suprasternal notch & along carotid arteries (commonly left).*

**1234. Which of the following is false about aortic stenosis murmur?**
*Harrison's 20th Ed. Chapter 256 Page 1805*

A. High pitched
B. Rough & rasping in character
C. Ejection systolic
D. Loudest in second right intercostal space

*Murmur of AS is ejection (mid) systolic murmur commencing shortly after S1, increasing in intensity to reach a peak toward middle of ejection & ending just before aortic valve closure. It is characteristically low-pitched, rough & rasping in character & loudest at the base of heart in 2nd right intercostal space. It is transmitted along carotid arteries.*

**1235. In Gallavardin effect, murmur of AS radiates to which of the following?**
*Harrison's 20th Ed. Chapter 256 Page 1805*

A. Apex
B. Carotids
C. Back
D. None of the above

*Occasionally, murmur of AS may be transmitted downward to the apex, where it is loudest with musical quality (Gallavardin effect) and may be confused with systolic murmur of MR. In almost all patients with severe obstruction & preserved CO, the murmur of AS is at least grade III/VI.*

**1236. Intensity of a cardiac murmur is graded (1-6) according to?**
*Am J Cardiol. 2008;102(8):1107-10*

A. Morrison scale
B. Mogagni scale
C. Levine scale
D. Osler scale

*Murmurs were described first by Laennec in 1819. The intensity of a cardiac murmur is graded according to the Levine scale of 1 to 6 grades of intensity.*

**1237. Echocardiographically, which of the following is characteristic of congenitally bicuspid valves?**
*Harrison's 20th Ed. Chapter 256 Page 1805*

A. Leaflet calcification and restriction
B. Eccentric closure of the aortic valve cusps
C. Distortion of the subvalvular apparatus
D. All of the above

*The key findings on TTE in AS are thickening, calcification, and reduced systolic opening of the valve leaflets and LV hypertrophy. Eccentric closure of the aortic valve cusps is characteristic of congenitally bicuspid valves.*

**1238. Aortic stenosis is called "mild", when the aortic valve area is?**
*Harrison's 20th Ed. Chapter 256 Page 1805*

A. 1.0–1.5 cm$^2$
B. 1.5–2.0 cm$^2$
C. 2.0–2.5 cm$^2$
D. 2.5–3.0 cm$^2$

**1239. Aortic stenosis is called "moderate", when the aortic valve area is?**
*Harrison's 20th Ed. Chapter 256 Page 1805*

A. 1.0 – 1.5 cm$^2$
B. 1.5 – 2.0 cm$^2$
C. 2.0 – 2.5 cm$^2$
D. 2.5 – 3.0 cm$^2$

*Mitral stenosis is called "moderate", when the mitral valve orifice is 1.0 cm$^2$–1.5 cm$^2$.*

**1240. Aortic stenosis is called "severe", when aortic valve area is?**
*Harrison's 20th Ed. Chapter 256 Page 1805*

A. < 1.5 cm²
B. < 1.0 cm²
C. < 0.5 cm²
D. < 0.2 cm²

**1241. Aortic sclerosis is defined echocardiographically as focal thickening or calcification of valve cusps with a peak Doppler transaortic velocity of?**

*Harrison's 20th Ed. Chapter 256 Page 1805*

A. ≤ 2.5 meters/second
B. ≤ 3.5 meters/second
C. ≤ 4.5 meters/second
D. ≤ 5.5 meters/second

*Aortic sclerosis is defined echocardiographically as focal thickening or calcification of the valve cusps with a peak Doppler transaortic velocity of ≤2.5 meters/second at a peak gradient <25 mm Hg.*

**1242. Which of the following chest X-ray findings indicate that valvular AS is not severe?**

*Harrison's 20th Ed. Chapter 256 Page 1805*

A. Little overall cardiac enlargement
B. Proximal ascending aorta not dilated
C. Absence of valvular calcification
D. Absence of pulmonary congestion

*In chest X-ray, absence of valvular calcification in adults suggests that severe valvular AS is not present.*

**1243. Following onset of symptoms in AS, which of the following leads to early death?**

*Harrison's 20th Ed. Chapter 256 Page 1806*

A. Angina pectoris
B. Syncope
C. Congestive heart failure
D. None of the above

*After onset of symptoms in AS, life expectancy in angina pectoris & syncope is 3 years, dyspnea - 2 years and congestive heart failure - 1.5 to 2 years.*

**1244. Endocarditis prophylaxis is advised to AS patients with?**

*Harrison's 20th Ed. Chapter 256 Page 1807*

A. Significant LV hypertrophy
B. Associated aortic regurgitation
C. Prior history of endocarditis
D. All of the above

*The need for endocarditis prophylaxis is restricted to AS patients with a prior history of endocarditis.*

**1245. Operation is indicated in patients with severe AS who are?**

*Harrison's 20th Ed. Chapter 256 Page 1807*

A. Symptomatic severe AS
B. LV systolic dysfunction (EF <50%)
C. BAV disease
D. All of the above

**1246. Very severe AS is defined by?**

*Harrison's 20th Ed. Chapter 256 Page 1807*

A. Mean gradient > 30 mm Hg
B. Mean gradient > 40 mm Hg
C. Mean gradient > 50 mm Hg
D. Mean gradient > 60 mm Hg

*Very severe AS is defined by an aortic valve jet velocity >5 m/s or mean gradient >60 mm Hg.*

**1247. Long-term postoperative survival correlates with?**

*Harrison's 20th Ed. Chapter 256 Page 1807*

A. Aortic valve area
B. Duration of symptoms
C. Preoperative LV function
D. All of the above

*Long-term postoperative survival correlates with preoperative LV function.*

**1248. Dobutamine stress echocardiography is considered positive if after dobutamine challenge, there is?**

*Harrison's 20th Ed. Chapter 256 Page 1807*

A. ≥ 5% increase in stroke volume
B. ≥ 10% increase in stroke volume
C. ≥ 20% increase in stroke volume
D. ≥ 30% increase in stroke volume

*Dobutamine stress echocardiography is considered positive by an ≥20% increase in stroke volume after dobutamine challenge.*

**1249. Homograft AVR is usually reserved for patients with?**

*Harrison's 20th Ed. Chapter 256 Page 1807*

A. Rheumatic valvulitis
B. Aortic valve endocarditis
C. Traumatic aortic valve
D. All of the above

*Homograft AVR is usually reserved for patients with aortic valve endocarditis.*

**1250. Transcatheter aortic valve replacement (TAVR) is associated with postprocedural?**

*Harrison's 20th Ed. Chapter 256 Page 1807*

A. Stroke
B. Paravalvular AR
C. Heart block
D. All of the above

**1251. Paradoxical, low-flow, low-gradient severe aortic stenosis is staged as?**

*Harrison's 20th Ed. Chapter 256 Page 1806 Figure 256-4*

A. D1
B. D2
C. D3
D. D4

*With aortic stenosis, stage D1 refers to symptomatic patients with severe AS and a high valve gradient (>40 mm Hg mean gradient). Stage D2 refers to patients with symptomatic, severe, low flow, low-gradient aortic stenosis and low LVEF. Stage D3 characterizes patients with symptomatic, severe, low-flow, low gradient AS and preserved LVEF (paradoxical, low-flow, low-gradient severe aortic stenosis).*

**1252. Which of the following trials relate to aortic valve replacement?**

*Harrison's 20th Ed. Chapter 256 Page 1808 Figure 256-6*

A. CORP-2 trial
B. PARTNER I trial
C. SYNTAX trial
D. FREEDOM trial

# Aortic Regurgitation

**1253. Severe LV hypertrophy is present when a wall thickness is?**
*Harrison's 19th Ed. 1532*

- A. > 5 mm
- B. > 10 mm
- C. > 15 mm
- D. > 20 mm

*Severe LV hypertrophy is present when a wall thickness is > 15 mm.*

**1254. Aortic regurgitation can occur due to?**
*Harrison's 20th Ed. Chapter 257 Page 1809*

- A. Membranous subaortic stenosis
- B. Ventricular septal defect
- C. Myxomatous degeneration
- D. All of the above

**1255. Which of the following is the cause of aortic regurgitation due to primary valve disease?**
*Harrison's 20th Ed. Chapter 257 Page 1809, Table 257-1*

- A. Aortic dissection
- B. Hypertension
- C. Ankylosing spondylitis
- D. Marfan's syndrome

**1256. Which of the following is the cause of aortic regurgitation due to both primary valve disease & primary aortic root disease?**
*Harrison's 20th Ed. Chapter 257 Page 1809, Table 257-1*

- A. Aortitis
- B. Bicuspid aortic valve
- C. Marfan's syndrome
- D. Rheumatic fever

*Causes of AR due to primary valve disease include congenital (bicuspid), endocarditis, rheumatic fever, myxomatous (prolapse), traumatic, syphilis and ankylosing spondylitis. Causes of AR due to primary aortic root disease include aortic dissection, cystic medial degeneration (Marfan's syndrome, bicuspid aortic valve, nonsyndromic familial aneurysm), aortitis and hypertension.*

**1257. Coexistence of hemodynamically significant AS with AR occurs in which of the following?**
*Harrison's 20th Ed. Chapter 257 Page 1810*

- A. Congenital AR
- B. Syphilis
- C. Marfan's syndrome
- D. All of the above

*Coexistence of hemodynamically significant AS with AR occurs almost exclusively in patients with rheumatic or congenital AR.*

**1258. Which of the following is the cause of aortic regurgitation due to both primary valve disease & primary aortic root disease?**
*Harrison's 20th Ed. Chapter 257 Page 1810*

- A. Syphilis
- B. Bicuspid aortic valve
- C. Ankylosing spondylitis
- D. All of the above

*Both syphilis & ankylosing spondylitis affect aortic valves. They may also be associated with cellular infiltration & scarring of media of thoracic aorta, leading to aortic dilation, aneurysm formation, & severe aortic regurgitation.*

**1259. Which of the following condition predisposes to AR?**
*Harrison's 20th Ed. Chapter 257 Page 1810*

- A. Marfan syndrome
- B. Ankylosing spondylitis
- C. Bicuspid aortic valve
- D. All of the above

*Conditions that predispose to AR are bicuspid aortic valve, IE, Marfan syndrome, or ankylosing spondylitis.*

**1260. At autopsy, heart of which of the following lesions is heaviest?**
*Harrison's 20th Ed. Chapter 257 Page 1810*

- A. Chronic AS
- B. Chronic AR
- C. HOCM
- D. Dilated cardiomyopathy

*At autopsy, hearts of patients with chronic AR may be among the largest encountered sometimes weighing >1000 grams.*

**1261. Early sign of LV dysfunction in chronic AR is?**
*Harrison's 20th Ed. Chapter 257 Page 1810*

- A. Elevation of LA pressure
- B. Reduction in LVEF
- C. Elevation of PA wedge pressure
- D. Elevation of LV end-diastolic pressure

*In chronic AR, both LV preload & afterload increase. When adaptive measures fail, LV function deteriorates, end-diastolic volume rises further and the forward stroke volume and EF decline. An early sign of LV dysfunction is a reduction in the EF. Deterioration of LV function often precedes the development of symptoms.*

**1262. A large fraction of coronary blood flow occurs during?**
*Harrison's 20th Ed. Chapter 257 Page 1810*

- A. Systole
- B. Diastole
- C. Systole + diastole
- D. Any of the above

*A large fraction of coronary blood flow occurs during diastole.*

**1263. Myocardial ischemia occurs in AR because of?**
*Harrison's 20th Ed. Chapter 257 Page 1810*

- A. LV dilation
- B. Elevated LV systolic tension
- C. Low arterial pressure
- D. All of the above

*Myocardial ischemia, particularly of the subendocardium, occurs in AR because of myocardial oxygen requirements are elevated by LV dilation, hypertrophy, and elevated LV systolic tension, and coronary blood flow may be compromised due to low arterial pressure.*

**1264. Which of the following is a cause of acute severe AR?**
*Harrison's 20th Ed. Chapter 257 Page 1810*

A. Infective endocarditis
B. Aortic dissection
C. Nonpenetrating cardiac injury
D. All of the above

Acute severe AR results from infective endocarditis, aortic dissection, or trauma (Nonpenetrating cardiac injury leading to rupture or avulsion of the aortic valve).

**1265. Which of the following about AR is false?**
*Harrison's 20th Ed. Chapter 257 Page 1810*

A. 3/4th of patients with predominant valvular AR are men
B. Primary valvular AR with rheumatic mitral valve disease more common in women
C. Exertional dyspnea is the first symptom of diminished cardiac reserve
D. None of the above

**1266. Which of the following is a symptom of chronic severe AR?**
*Harrison's 20th Ed. Chapter 257 Page 1810*

A. Vomiting
B. Gait disturbance
C. Vertigo
D. Diaphoresis

Exertional dyspnea is followed by orthopnea, paroxysmal nocturnal dyspnea, and excessive diaphoresis. Nocturnal angina that does not respond satisfactorily to sublingual nitroglycerin may be accompanied by marked diaphoresis.

**1267. Diaphoresis is a predominant symptom of which of the following valvular heart disease?**
*Harrison's 20th Ed. Chapter 257 Page 1810*

A. AS
B. AR
C. MS
D. MR

**1268. In free AR, booming "pistol-shot" sound heard over femoral arteries is called?**
*Harrison's 20th Ed. Chapter 257 Page 1810*

A. Corrigan's pulse
B. Quincke's pulse
C. Traube's sign
D. Duroziez's sign

In free AR, booming "pistol-shot" sound heard over femoral arteries is termed as Traube's sign.

**1269. Large-volume 'collapsing' water hammer peripheral pulse seen in AR is named after?**
*J Postgrad Med. 2008;54:163-5*

A. Corrigan
B. Watson
C. de Musset
D. Duroziez

Large-volume 'collapsing' water hammer peripheral pulse seen in AR is named after Watson. Other peripheral signs of AR include Corrigan's pulse (rapid upstroke & collapse of carotid artery pulse), de Musset's sign (head nodding in time with heart beat), Quincke's sign (pulsation of capillary bed in nails), Traube's sign (systolic & diastolic murmurs described as 'pistol shots' heard over femoral artery when it is gradually compressed), Duroziez's sign (a double sound heard over femoral artery when it is compressed distally), Lighthouse sign (blanching & flushing of forehead), Landolfi's sign (alternating constriction & dilatation of pupil), Becker's sign (pulsations of retinal vessels), Müller's sign (pulsations of uvula), Mayen's sign (diastolic drop of BP >15 mm Hg with arm raised), Rosenbach's sign (pulsatile liver), Gerhardt's sign (enlarged spleen), Hill's sign - a >20 mm Hg difference in popliteal & brachial systolic cuff pressures in chronic severe AR, Lincoln sign (pulsatile popliteal artery), Sherman sign (dorsalis pedis pulse is quickly located & unexpectedly prominent in age >75 years).

**1270. Which of the following is a feature of murmur of chronic AR?**
*Harrison's 20th Ed. Chapter 257 Page 1811*

A. High-pitched, blowing
B. Decrescendo diastolic murmur
C. Heard best in III intercostal space along left sternal border
D. All of the above

As the severity of AR increases, decrescendo brief diastolic murmur becomes louder and longer and becomes holodiastolic.

**1271. Decrescendo diastolic murmur of AR is best heard with?**
*Harrison's 20th Ed. Chapter 257 Page 1811*

A. Patient sitting up
B. Patient leaning forward
C. Breath held in forced expiration
D. All of the above

When the murmur of AR is soft, it can be heard best with the diaphragm of the stethoscope and with the patient sitting up, leaning forward, and with the breath held in forced expiration.

**1272. The murmur of AR is typically heard best in?**
*Harrison's 20th Ed. Chapter 257 Page 1811*

A. II left ICS parasternally
B. III left ICS parasternally
C. IV left ICS parasternally
D. V left ICS parasternally

Murmur of chronic AR is typically high-pitched, blowing, decrescendo diastolic murmur, heard best in 3rd intercostal space along left sternal border. It seldom causes thrill.

**1273. When murmur of AR is heard best along right sternal border, it suggests that AR is?**
*Harrison's 20th Ed. Chapter 257 Page 1811*

A. Accompanied by significant MS
B. Accompanied by Infective endocarditis
C. Due to aneurysmal dilatation of aortic root
D. Due to severe hypertension

When murmur of AR is heard best along right sternal border, it suggests that AR is caused by aneurysmal dilatation of aortic root.

**1274. "Cooing" or musical diastolic murmurs of AR suggests?**
*Harrison's 20th Ed. Chapter 257 Page 1811*

A. Vegetations of the aortic leaflet
B. Fenestrations in the aortic leaflet
C. Eversion of an aortic cusp
D. Any of the above

"Cooing" or musical diastolic murmur of AR suggest eversion of aortic cusp vibrating in regurgitant stream.

**1275. Austin Flint (1812-86) was a physician of which country?**
*N Engl J Med. 2010;363:2164*

A. American
B. United Kingdom
C. Australia
D. Canada

Austin Flint, an American physician (1812-1886) was a pioneer in the use of the stethoscope. His "A Treatise on the Principles and Practice of Medicine" (1866) was a leading textbook of medicine.

**1276. Which of the following murmur is heard in chronic AR?**
*Harrison's 20th Ed. Chapter 257 Page 1811*

A. Decrescendo diastolic murmur
B. Mid-systolic ejection murmur
C. Mid-to-late diastolic murmur
D. All of the above

**1277. The auscultatory features of AR are intensified by?**
*Harrison's 20th Ed. Chapter 257 Page 1811*

A. Inhalation of amyl nitrite
B. Strenuous and sustained handgrip
C. Valsalva maneuver
D. All of the above

The auscultatory features of AR are intensified by strenuous and sustained handgrip, which augments systemic vascular resistance.

**1278. Which of the following is a hemodynamic effect of amly nitrite?**
*N Engl J Med. 1966;275:1007*

A. Decrease in systemic arterial pressure
B. Decrease in duration of contraction of left ventricle
C. Increase in heart rate
D. All of the above

Major hemodynamic effects of amly nitrite include a decrease in systemic arterial pressure, vascular resistance, stroke work, circulation time and duration of contraction of the left ventricle, ejection and diastolic filling period; an increase in heart rate, cardiac index and ejection velocity; and no change in stroke volume or minute work.

**1279. Which of the following is a feature of acute severe AR?**
*Harrison's 20th Ed. Chapter 257 Page 1811*

A. Soft $S_1$
B. Pulse pressure not wide
C. Soft, short, early diastolic murmur of AR
D. All of the above

**1280. Most common pathologic condition associated with aortic aneurysm is?**
*N Engl J Med. 2004;351:1539-46*

A. Syphilis
B. Atherosclerosis
C. Tuberculosis
D. Marfan's syndrome

**1281. In ECG of patient with AR, which of the following findings usually signify a poor prognosis?**
*Harrison's 20th Ed. Chapter 257 Page 1811*

A. No electrocardiographic abnormalities
B. ST depression & T-wave inversion in I, aVL
C. ST depression & T-wave inversion in $V_5$ & $V_6$
D. QRS prolongation

Left axis deviation and/or QRS prolongation denote diffuse myocardial disease and signify a poor prognosis.

**1282. On echocardiogram, which of the following can be found in a patient of AR?**
*Harrison's 20th Ed. Chapter 257 Page 1811*

A. Increased systolic excursion of posterior LV wall
B. High-frequency diastolic fluttering of anterior mitral leaflet
C. Dilatation of aortic annulus
D. All of the above

A rapid, high-frequency fluttering of the anterior mitral leaflet produced by the impact of the regurgitant jet is a characteristic finding in 2D echocardiogram of AR patient.

**1283. Which of the following findings in color flow Doppler imaging suggest severe AR?**
*Harrison's 20th Ed. Chapter 257 Page 1811*

A. Central jet width > 65% of left ventricular outflow tract
B. Regurgitant volume > 60 mL/beat
C. Regurgitant fraction > 50%
D. All of the above

With severe AR, central jet width assessed by color flow Doppler imaging exceeds 65% of left ventricular outflow tract, regurgitant volume is ≥60 mL/beat, regurgitant fraction is >=50%, and diastolic flow reversal in the proximal descending thoracic aorta is seen.

**1284. In chronic severe AR, the apex is displaced?**
*Harrison's 20th Ed. Chapter 257 Page 1811*

A. Downward
B. Leftward
C. Posteriorly
D. All of the above

**1285. Which of the following is contraindicated in the treatment of acute aortic regurgitation?**
*Harrison's 20th Ed. Chapter 257 Page 1811*

A. Intravenous diuretics
B. Vasodilators (sodium nitroprusside)
C. Intra-aortic balloon counterpulsation
D. Surgery

Patients with acute severe AR may respond to IV diuretics and vasodilators like sodium nitroprusside. Surgery is the treatment of choice and is usually necessary within 24 hours of diagnosis. Intraaortic balloon counterpulsation is contraindicated. Beta blockers are also best avoided as they may reduce CO further.

**1286. In AR, which of the following drugs can delay the need for surgery?**
*Harrison's 20th Ed. Chapter 257 Page 1811*

A. Digitalis glycosides
B. Diuretics
C. Nondihydropyridine calcium channel blockers
D. Long-acting nifedipine

**1287. In AR, operation should be carried out in?**
*Harrison's 20th Ed. Chapter 257 Page 1811*

A. LVEF < 50%
B. LV end-systolic dimension > 50 mm
C. Acute, severe AR
D. All of the above

Surgery should be carried out in asymptomatic patients with severe AR and progressive LV dysfunction defined by an LVEF <50%, an LV end-systolic dimension >50 mm or end-systolic volume >55 mL/m², or an LV diastolic dimension >65 mm.

**1288. In "55 rule" for gauging the timing of surgery for AR, 55 refers to?**
*N Engl J Med. 1997;337:37*

A. Ejection fraction
B. Shortening fraction
C. Mean pressure gradient
D. Maximum velocity

"55 rule" has been useful in gauging the timing of surgery for AR. Aortic-valve surgery should be performed before the ejection fraction falls below 55 percent or the endsystolic dimension exceeds 55 mm.

## Mitral Stenosis

**1289. Which of the following condition affects the mitral valve?**
*Circulation. 2004;109:e38-e41*

A. Obstruction
B. Leakage
C. Bulging backward during valve closure
D. All of the above

There are 3 main conditions that affect the valve: Obstruction (stenosis), leakage (regurgitation), and bulging backward during valve closure (prolapse). Prolapse is the most common, occurring in up to 5% of the population, whereas stenosis is the least common, accounting for <1% of cardiac diagnoses in the US, although it is more frequently seen in developing nations.

**1290. Which of the following is not a cause of obstruction to left atrial outflow?**
*Harrison's 20th Ed. Chapter 258 Page 1813*

A. Systemic lupus erythematosus
B. Rheumatoid arthritis
C. Wegener's granulomatosis
D. Cor triatriatum

Rheumatic fever is the leading cause of mitral stenosis (MS). Other less common etiologies of obstruction to left atrial outflow include congenital mitral valve stenosis, cor triatriatum, mitral annular calcification with extension onto the leaflets, systemic lupus erythematosus, rheumatoid arthritis, left atrial myxoma, and infective endocarditis with large vegetations.

**1291. What proportion of all patients with rheumatic heart disease & a history of rheumatic fever have pure or predominant MS?**
*Harrison's 20th Ed. Chapter 258 Page 1814*

A. 10%
B. 20%
C. 30%
D. 40%

Pure or predominant MS occurs in ~40% of all patients with rheumatic heart disease and a history of rheumatic fever.

**1292. Which of the following is a component of Shone's Syndrome?**
*Am J Cardiol. 1963; 11:714-25*

A. Parachute mitral valve
B. Subaortic stenosis
C. Coarctation of aorta
D. All of the above

Shone syndrome is a collection of eight left-sided obstructive heart lesions. These affect blood flow to and from the left ventricle. The lesions are Cor Triatriatum, Supramitral Ring, Parachute mitral valve, Subaortic stenosis, Bicuspid Aortic Valve, Coarctation of the Aorta, Hypoplastic (stiff) left ventricle and Small Aortic Arch.

**1293. What proportion of all patients with mitral stenosis are female?**
*Circulation. 2004;109:e38-e41*

A. One-fourth
B. One-third
C. Two-third
D. Three-fourth

**1294. The mitral valve (MV) apparatus comprises of?**
*Arch Cardiovasc Dis. 2013;106:111-5*

A. Mitral valve annulus
B. Anterior and posterior MV leaflets
C. Chordae, and anteromedial & posterolateral papillary muscles
D. All of the above

The mitral valve (MV) apparatus is comprised of the mitral valve annulus, anterior and posterior MV leaflets, chordae, and anteromedial and posterolateral papillary muscles.

**1295. Which of the following statements is false?**
*Arch Cardiovasc Dis. 2013;106:111-5*

A. Anterior & posterior leaflets have roughly the same area
B. Annulus is a saddle-shaped structure
C. Posterior leaflet occupies two thirds of the annulus
D. None of the above

**1296. Which of the following statements about MS is false?**
*Arch Cardiovasc Dis. 2013;106:111-5*

A. Congenital MS is a disease of newborn and infancy
B. Rheumatic MS typically presents in III & IV decades of life
C. Degenerative MS presents in the VII & VIII decades of life
D. None of the above

**1297. Which of the following statements about MS is false?**
*Arch Cardiovasc Dis. 2013;106:111-5*

A. Degenerative MS has more annular & basal leaflet calcification
B. Calcification in rheumatic MS primarily affects leaflet tips
C. Calcification in congenital MS is minimal or absent
D. None of the above

The hallmark of degenerative MS is mitral annular calcification (MAC).

**1298. Which of the following statements about MS is false?**
*Arch Cardiovasc Dis. 2013;106:111-5*

A. In rheumatic MS, commissural fusion is the norm
B. In degenerative MS, the commissures are open
C. In congenital MS, commissures are absent
D. None of the above

**1299. In rheumatic MS, chronic inflammation leads to?**
*Harrison's 20th Ed. Chapter 258 Page 1814*

A. Fusion of mitral commissures
B. Fusion & shortening of chordae tendineae
C. Rigidity of valvular cusps
D. All of the above

**1300.** Which of the following term define the appearance of valve orifice in MS?

*Harrison's 20th Ed. Chapter 258 Page 1814*

- A. Pigeon chest
- B. Parrot peek
- C. Camel back
- D. Fish-mouth

In rheumatic MS, chronic inflammation leads to diffuse thickening of valve leaflets with fibrosis often with calcific deposits. Mitral commissures fuse, chordae tendineae fuse and shorten, valvular cusps become rigid, and the pathologic process eventually leads to narrowing at apex of the funnel-shaped ("fish-mouth") valve.

**1301.** In patients of MS without atrial fibrillation (AF), thrombi arise more frequently from?

*Harrison's 20th Ed. Chapter 258 Page 1814*

- A. Mitral valve leaflets
- B. Chordae tendineae
- C. Left atrial appendage
- D. Mitral commissures

**1302.** In patients of MS with atrial fibrillation (AF), thrombi arise more frequently from?

*Harrison's 20th Ed. Chapter 258 Page 1814*

- A. Mitral valve leaflets
- B. Chordae tendineae
- C. Left atrial appendage
- D. Mitral commissures

Thrombus formation & arterial embolization may arise from calcific valve itself, but in patients with atrial fibrillation (AF), thrombi arise more frequently from the dilated left atrium (LA), particularly from within the left atrial appendage.

**1303.** The mitral valve's annulus is shaped more like a?

*BJA Education. 2017; 17(1):1-9*

- A. M
- B. D
- C. O
- D. Any of the above

The mitral valve's annulus is a saddle-shaped structure which is shaped more like a 'D' than an 'O'.

**1304.** Which of the following coronary artery is closest to the annulus of the mitral valve?

*BJA Education. 2017;17(1):1-9*

- A. Right coronary artery
- B. Left circumflex artery
- C. Left anterior descending artery
- D. Posterior descending artery

The left circumflex artery follows the line of annulus as it passes anteriorly around base of the heart, a position that places it at risk during any mitral valve surgery.

**1305.** Which of the following regarding papillary muscles and chorda tendinae is false?

*BJA Education. 2017;17(1):1-9*

- A. Anterolateral muscle receives a dual blood supply from left anterior descending and circumflex artery
- B. Posteromedial muscle is supplied by right coronary artery
- C. Primary chordae are attached to free edge of valve leaflet, and secondary chordae are attached to ventricular surface of leaflet
- D. None of the above

**1306.** Number of discrete segments or scallops on posterior mitral leaflet is?

*BJA Education. 2017;17(1):1-9*

- A. 1
- B. 2
- C. 3
- D. 4

There are three discrete segments or scallops on anterior leaflet (A1, A2, and A3) and posterior leaflet (P1, P2, and P3).

**1307.** In normal adults, which of the following parameter of the mitral valve orifice is 4-6 cm²?

*Harrison's 20th Ed. Chapter 258 Page 1814*

- A. Diameter
- B. Circumference
- C. Area
- D. Radius

In normal adults, the area of the mitral valve orifice is 4-6 cm².

**1308.** Significant obstruction of mitral valve orifice is considered when the orifice is less than approximately?

*Harrison's 20th Ed. Chapter 258 Page 1814*

- A. 1 cm²
- B. 2 cm²
- C. 3 cm²
- D. 4 cm²

Mitral valve orifice area of < ~2 cm² is considered "significant obstruction" because blood can flow from LA to LV only if propelled by an abnormally elevated left atrioventricular pressure gradient.

**1309.** Mitral stenosis is called "severe", when the mitral valve opening is reduced to?

*Harrison's 20th Ed. Chapter 258 Page 1814*

- A. < 1.5 cm²
- B. < 1 cm²
- C. < 0.5 cm²
- D. < 0.2 cm²

When the mitral valve opening is reduced to < 1.5 cm² it is referred to as "severe" MS. When the mitral valve opening is reduced to < 1 cm² it is referred to as "very severe" MS.

**1310.** In severe MS, LA pressure required to maintain a normal cardiac output is?

*Harrison's 20th Ed. Chapter 258 Page 1814*

- A. ~ 10 mm Hg
- B. ~ 15 mm Hg
- C. ~ 20 mm Hg
- D. ~ 25 mm Hg

In severe MS, LA pressure of ~25 mm Hg is required to maintain a normal cardiac output.

**1311. Hemodynamic variable of importance in mitral stenosis is?**
*Harrison's 20th Ed. Chapter 258 Page 1814*

A. Transvalvular pressure gradient
B. Cardiac output
C. Heart rate
D. All of the above

*Hemodynamic severity of MS depends on transvalvular pressure gradient and the flow rate which depends on the cardiac output and heart rate.*

**1312. Clinical and hemodynamic features of MS are influenced importantly by?**
*Harrison's 20th Ed. Chapter 258 Page 1814*

A. Cardiac output
B. Heart rate
C. Transvalvular pressure gradient
D. Pulmonary arterial pressure (PAP)

*The clinical and hemodynamic features of MS are influenced importantly by the level of the PAP.*

**1313. "Second stenosis" refers to which of the following?**
*Harrison's 20th Ed. Chapter 258 Page 1814*

A. Passive backward transmission of elevated LA pressure
B. Pulmonary arteriolar constriction
C. Interstitial edema in walls of small pulmonary vessels
D. Organic obliterative changes in pulmonary vascular bed

*Pulmonary hypertension results from passive backward transmission of elevated LA pressure; pulmonary arteriolar constriction ("second stenosis"), interstitial edema in walls of small pulmonary vessels and organic obliterative changes in pulmonary vascular bed.*

**1314. Severe pulmonary hypertension results in?**
*Harrison's 20th Ed. Chapter 258 Page 1814*

A. RV enlargement
B. Secondary tricuspid regurgitation (TR)
C. Pulmonic regurgitation (PR)
D. All of the above

*Severe pulmonary hypertension results in RV enlargement, secondary tricuspid regurgitation (TR) and pulmonic regurgitation (PR), as well as right-sided heart failure.*

**1315. Which of the following about mitral stenosis is false?**
*Harrison's 20th Ed. Chapter 258 Page 1814*

A. Latent period between initial attack of rheumatic carditis & development of symptoms due to MS is ~ 2 decades
B. Infective endocarditis is rare in isolated MS
C. Hemoptysis is rarely fatal
D. None of the above

**1316. Most patients of MS begin to experience disability in?**
*Harrison's 20th Ed. Chapter 258 Page 1814*

A. II decade of life
B. III decade of life
C. IV decade of life
D. V decade of life

**1317. Once MS patient becomes seriously symptomatic, MS progresses inexorably to death within?**
*Harrison's 20th Ed. Chapter 258 Page 1814*

A. 6 months to 1 year
B. 1–2 years
C. 2–5 years
D. 5–7 years

*Once MS patient becomes seriously symptomatic, MS progresses inexorably to death within 2–5 years.*

**1318. LA pressure gets markedly elevated by sudden changes in?**
*Harrison's 20th Ed. Chapter 258 Page 1814*

A. Heart rate
B. Volume status
C. Cardiac output
D. All of the above

**1319. Which of the following marks a turning point in the disease course of MS?**
*Harrison's 20th Ed. Chapter 258 Page 1814*

A. Development of orthopnea
B. Development of paroxysmal nocturnal dyspnea
C. Development of paroxysmal AF
D. Development of persistent AF

*Development of persistent AF marks a turning point in the course of an MS patient. It is associated with acceleration of the rate at which symptoms progress.*

**1320. In MS, hemoptysis results from rupture of?**
*Harrison's 20th Ed. Chapter 258 Page 1814*

A. Alveolar capillaries
B. Pulmonary arterioles
C. Bronchial arterioles
D. Pulmonary-bronchial venous connections

*Hemoptysis results from rupture of pulmonary-bronchial venous connections secondary to pulmonary venous hypertension in patients who have elevated LA pressures without markedly elevated pulmonary vascular resistances and is rarely fatal.*

**1321. In MS, hemoptysis results from?**
*Harrison's 20th Ed. Chapter 258 Page 1814*

A. Pulmonary-bronchial venous connections
B. Recurrent pulmonary emboli
C. Pulmonary infections
D. All of the above

**1322. Which of the following occurs in the pulmonary vascular bed MS?**
*Harrison's 20th Ed. Chapter 258 Page 1814*

A. Fibrous thickening of the walls of alveoli
B. Fibrous thickening of the walls of pulmonary capillaries
C. Interstitial edema in walls of small pulmonary vessels
D. All of the above

**1323. Which of the following PFT variable is reduced in MS?**
*Harrison's 20th Ed. Chapter 258 Page 1814*

A. Vital capacity
B. Total lung capacity
C. Maximal breathing capacity
D. All of the above

*In addition to interstitial edema in walls of small pulmonary vessels and organic obliterative changes in pulmonary vascular bed, fibrous thickening of walls of alveoli & pulmonary capillaries occurs commonly in MS. Vital capacity, total lung capacity, maximal breathing capacity, and oxygen uptake per unit of ventilation are reduced.*

**1324. The incidence of systemic embolization in MS is?**
*Harrison's 20th Ed. Chapter 258 Page 1814*

A. 1–2%
B. 2–5%
C. 5–10%
D. 10–20%

*The incidence of systemic embolization is 10–20% in MS.*

**1325. In MS, systemic embolization occurs more frequently in?**
*Harrison's 20th Ed. Chapter 258 Page 1814*

A. Patients with AF
B. In older patients
C. In those with a reduced cardiac output
D. All of the above

*Thrombi form in left atria, particularly in enlarged atrial appendages of patients with MS. Systemic embolization, incidence of which is 10–20%, occurs more frequently in patients with AF, in older patients (>65 years), and in those with a reduced CO.*

**1326. Which of the following may rarely be present in MS?**
*Harrison's 20th Ed. Chapter 258 Page 1815*

A. Malar flush with pinched and blue facies
B. Prominent a waves in jugular venous pulse
C. Diastolic thrill at cardiac apex
D. Parasternal heave

**1327. Which of the following is false about auscultation in MS?**
*Harrison's 20th Ed. Chapter 258 Page 1815*

A. $S_1$ is accentuated and delayed
B. OS follows $A_2$ by 0.05–0.12 seconds
C. $A_2$ - OS interval varies directly with severity of MS
D. None of the above

*A2 - OS time interval varies inversely with the severity of the MS.*

**1328. Which of the following correlates with the severity of mitral stenosis?**
*Harrison's 20th Ed. Chapter 258 Page 1815*

A. Loudness of opening snap
B. Duration of mid-diastolic murmur
C. Duration of presystolic accentuation
D. All of the above

*Duration of low-pitched, rumbling, diastolic murmur correlates with the severity of the stenosis in patients with preserved CO. The A2 - OS time interval varies inversely with the severity of MS.*

**1329. In patients with MS with RV failure, pleural effusion is on which side?**
*Harrison's 20th Ed. Chapter 258 Page 1815*

A. Right
B. Left
C. Bilateral
D. Any of the above

*Pleural effusion, particularly in right pleural cavity, may occur in patients with MS and RV failure.*

**1330. In MS, which of the following findings can be found along left sternal border?**
*Harrison's 20th Ed. Chapter 258 Page 1815*

A. Pansystolic murmur
B. High-pitched, diastolic, decrescendo blowing murmur
C. Soft, grade I or II/VI systolic murmurs
D. All of the above

*With severe pulmonary hypertension, a pansystolic murmur, louder during inspiration, produced by functional TR may be audible along the left sternal border. Graham Steell murmur of PR, a high-pitched, diastolic, decrescendo blowing murmur along the left sternal border, results from dilation of pulmonary valve ring due to severe pulmonary hypertension. Soft, grade I or II/VI systolic murmurs are commonly heard at the apex or along the left sternal border in patients with pure MS and do not necessarily signify the presence of MR.*

**1331. Carvallo's sign best relates to?**
*Harrison's 20th Ed. Chapter 258 Page 1815*

A. Right heart murmur
B. Phases of breathing
C. Elicited along the left sternal border
D. All of the above

**1332. Which of the following is found in the ECG of a patient of MS?**
*Harrison's 20th Ed. Chapter 258 Page 1815*

A. Tall and peaked P wave in lead II
B. Upright P wave in lead V1
C. Normal QRS complex
D. All of the above

**1333. Which of the following echocardiographic technique is most useful in evaluating a patient of MS?**
*Harrison's 20th Ed. Chapter 258 Page 1815*

A. M-mode Echocardiography
B. 2D Echocardiography with Color Doppler studies
C. Transthoracic echocardiography (TTE) with color flow and spectral Doppler imaging
D. All of the above

*Transthoracic echocardiography (TTE) with color flow and spectral Doppler imaging provides critical information in evaluation of a patient of MS.*

**1334. Transesophageal echocardiography (TEE) in MS is especially indicated to exclude?**
*Harrison's 20th Ed. Chapter 258 Page 1815*

A. Left atrial myxoma
B. Presence of LA thrombus
C. Presence of LV thrombus
D. All of the above

*TEE is especially indicated to exclude the presence of LA thrombus prior to percutaneous mitral balloon valvotomy (PMBV). TEE is utilised to perform precise 3D reconstruction of the MV and its apparatus. Cardiac computed tomography (CCT) has also emerged as a valuable tool for studying cardiac calcifications including calcific valvular lesions.*

**1335. Which of the following is a chest X-ray sign of pulmonary venous hypertension in MS?**
*Harrison's 20th Ed. Chapter 258 Page 1815*

A. Stag's antler sign
B. Hands-up sign
C. Inverted moustache sign
D. All of the above

*On CxR, in pulmonary venous hypertension, prominence of upper lobe pulmonary veins is seen and is called Stag's antler sign. It is the earliest sign of pulmonary venous hypertension. This sign is also known as hands-up sign or inverted moustache sign.*

**1336. In MS, Kerley B lines on X-ray chest are apparent when the resting mean LA pressure exceeds approximately?**
*Harrison's 20th Ed. Chapter 258 Page 1815*

A. 10 mm Hg
B. 15 mm Hg
C. 20 mm Hg
D. 25 mm Hg

Kerley B lines are fine, dense, opaque, horizontal lines most prominent in the lower and mid-lung fields resulting from distention of interlobular septae and lymphatics with edema when resting mean LA pressure > ~20 mm Hg.

**1337. Which of the following about Kerley's A lines is false?**
*Circulation. 1972;XLV:1323*

A. Linear opacities on CxR chest
B. Extend from periphery to hila
C. Caused by distention of anastomotic channels between peripheral & central lymphatics
D. None of the above

Kerley's A lines are linear opacities extending from periphery to hila caused by distention of anastomotic channels between peripheral & central lymphatics. They do not bifurcate and they do not follow the normal branching pattern of bronchi and vessels. These lines are most commonly seen in the upper lobes, are slightly curved rather than straight.

**1338. Which of the following about Kerley's B lines is false?**
*Circulation. 1972;XLV:1323*

A. Short horizontal lines on CxR chest
B. Situated perpendicularly to pleural surface at lung base
C. Represent edema of interlobular septa
D. None of the above

Kerley's B lines are short horizontal lines situated perpendicularly to pleural surface at lung base. They represent edema of the interlobular septa. B lines are "short, sharp lines seen only at the bases, usually less than an inch long and running transversely outward to touch the pleural margin. These are the most commonly recognized of the Kerley lines.

**1339. Which of the following about Kerley's C lines is false?**
*Circulation. 1972;XLV:1323*

A. Reticular opacities at lung base
B. Represent Kerley's B lines en face
C. Suggest cardiogenic pulmonary edema
D. None of the above

Kerley's C lines are reticular opacities at the lung base, representing Kerley's B lines en face suggesting cardiogenic pulmonary edema. C lines are "fine interlacing lines givinlg a network appearance.

**1340. Which of the following is false about Austin Flint murmur?**
*Harrison's 20th Ed. Chapter 258 Page 1815*

A. Apical
B. Mid-diastolic
C. Not intensified in presystole
D. None of the above

Apical mid-diastolic murmur associated with severe AR (Austin Flint murmur) is differentiated from MS because it is not intensified in presystole & becomes softer with administration of amyl nitrite.

**1341. Which of the following features differentiates atrial septal defect from MS?**
*Harrison's 20th Ed. Chapter 258 Page 1815*

A. Absence of LA enlargement
B. Absence of Kerley B lines
C. Fixed splitting of $S_2$
D. All of the above

Atrial septal defect may be mistaken for MS as in both conditions there is clinical, ECG, and chest X-ray evidence of RV enlargement and accentuation of pulmonary vascularity. Absence of LA enlargement and of Kerley B lines and the demonstration of fixed splitting of S2 with a grade 2 or 3 mid-systolic murmur at the mid to upper left sternal border all favor atrial septal defect over MS.

**1342. Auscultatory findings change markedly with body position in which of the following?**
*Harrison's 20th Ed. Chapter 258 Page 1815*

A. Mitral stenosis
B. Tricuspid stenosis
C. Left atrial myxoma
D. Atrial septal defect

The auscultatory findings in left atrial myxoma change markedly with body position.

**1343. Levels of which of the following is elevated in left atrial myxoma?**
*Harrison's 20th Ed. Chapter 258 Page 1815*

A. Interleukin 2 (IL-2)
B. Interleukin 4 (IL-4)
C. Interleukin 6 (IL-6)
D. Interleukin 8 (IL-8)

In LA myxoma, elevated levels of serum IgG and interleukin 6 (IL-6) are found.

**1344. Which of the following is a feature of left atrial myxoma?**
*Harrison's 20th Ed. Chapter 258 Page 1815*

A. Systemic manifestations
B. Elevated serum IgG
C. Echo-producing mass in the LA with TTE
D. All of the above

**1345. Anticoagulants are administered for how long to MS patients who have suffered systemic and/or pulmonary embolization?**
*Harrison's 20th Ed. Chapter 258 Page 1816*

A. At least 3 months
B. At least 6 months
C. At least 1 year
D. Life long

**1346. Anticoagulants should be administered for how long to patients with MS who have atrial fibrillation?**
*Harrison's 20th Ed. Chapter 258 Page 1816*

A. At least 3 months
B. At least 6 months
C. At least 1 year
D. Life long

**1347. In MS with AF of relatively recent origin, cardioversion is undertaken after patient has had anticoagulant treatment for?**
*Harrison's 20th Ed. Chapter 258 Page 1816*

A. 1 week
B. 2 weeks
C. 3 weeks
D. 4 weeks

Cardioversion should be undertaken after the patient has had at least 3 consecutive weeks of anticoagulant treatment to a therapeutic INR.

**1348. In patients with MS and AF, conversion to sinus rhythm is rarely sustained when?**

*Harrison's 20th Ed. Chapter 258 Page 1816*

- A. LA is enlarged
- B. AF has been present for more than 1 year
- C. Severe MS
- D. All of the above

Conversion to sinus rhythm is rarely successful or sustained in patients with severe MS, particularly those in whom the LA is especially enlarged or in whom AF has been present for more than 1 year.

**1349. Mitral valvotomy is indicated in the symptomatic patient with isolated MS whose effective orifice is less than?**

*Harrison's 20th Ed. Chapter 258 Page 1816*

- A. 1.0 cm$^2$/m$^2$ body surface area
- B. 1.5 cm$^2$/m$^2$ body surface area
- C. 2.0 cm$^2$/m$^2$ body surface area
- D. 2.5 cm$^2$/m$^2$ body surface area

Mitral valvotomy is indicated in symptomatic patients with isolated MS whose effective orifice is < ~1.0 cm$^2$/m$^2$ body surface area or <1.5 cm$^2$ in normal-sized adults.

**1350. In pregnant patient with MS, percutaneous mitral balloon valvuloplasty (PMBV) is performed with?**

*Harrison's 20th Ed. Chapter 258 Page 1816*

- A. CT
- B. MRI
- C. TEE
- D. Any of the above

In the pregnant patient with MS not responding to intensive medical treatment, PMBV is the preferred strategy and is performed with TEE and no or minimal X-ray exposure.

**1351. Successful mitral valvotomy is defined as a reduction in the mean mitral valve gradient by?**

*Harrison's 20th Ed. Chapter 258 Page 1817*

- A. 10%
- B. 20%
- C. 30%
- D. 50%

Successful mitral valvotomy is defined by a 50% reduction in the mean mitral valve gradient and a doubling of the mitral valve area.

**1352. Operative mortality is maximum in which of the following?**

*Harrison's 20th Ed. Chapter 258 Page 1817 Table 258-2*

- A. Aortic valve replacement with coronary artery bypass
- B. Mitral valve replacement with coronary artery bypass
- C. Mitral valve replacement
- D. Aortic valve replacement

**1353. Operative mortality is maximum in which of the following?**

*Harrison's 20th Ed. Chapter 258 Page 1817 Table 258-2*

- A. Aortic valve repair
- B. Mitral valve repair
- C. Tricuspid valve surgery
- D. Pulmonic valve replacement

# Mitral Regurgitation

**1354. Which of the following is a component of mitral valve apparatus?**
*Harrison's 20th Ed. Chapter 259 Page 1818*

A. Chordae tendineae
B. Papillary muscles
C. Subjacent myocardium
D. All of the above

*Five functional components of the mitral valve apparatus are leaflets, annulus, chordae tendineae, papillary muscles, and subjacent myocardium. Dysfunction in any of these may cause MR.*

**1355. Which of the following is used to classify Mitral Regurgitation?**
*J Thorac Cardiovasc Surg. 1980;79:338-48*

A. Gorman
B. Miller
C. Carpentier
D. Lamas

**1356. Modified Carpentier classification of mitral regurgitation is based on?**
*J Thorac Cardiovasc Surg. 1980;79:338-48*

A. Regurgitant volume
B. Regurgitant fraction
C. Leaflet motion
D. All of the above

*Carpentier et al. introduced a pathophysiologic classification of MR. The basis of this classification is mitral leaflet motion. MR with normal motion is type I, with increased motion is type II and with restricted motion is type III.*

**1357. Acute MR can occur in which of the following?**
*Harrison's 20th Ed. Chapter 259 Page 1818*

A. Infective endocarditis
B. Acute myocardial infarction with papillary muscle rupture
C. Blunt chest wall trauma
D. All of the above

*Acute MR can occur in infective endocarditis, papillary muscle rupture (post Acute MI), following blunt chest wall trauma, and rupture of chordae tendineae in MVP & IE.*

**1358. Which of the following statements is false?**
*Harrison's 20th Ed. Chapter 259 Page 1818*

A. Posteromedial papillary muscle has singular blood supply
B. Transient, acute MR can occur during angina pectoris
C. In acute MI, anterolateral papillary muscle is involved much more frequently
D. None of the above

*With acute MI, posteromedial papillary muscle is involved much more frequently than anterolateral papillary muscle because of its singular blood supply.*

**1359. Which of the following is a cause of chronic primary MR?**
*Harrison's 20th Ed. Chapter 259 Page 1818 Table 259-1*

A. Ischemic cardiomyopathy
B. Dilated cardiomyopathy
C. Radiation
D. HOCM (with SAM)

*Causes of chronic primary MR i.e. those (affecting leaflets & chordae) include myxomatous, rheumatic fever, IE (healed), congenital and radiation. Causes of chronic secondary MR include ischemic cardiomyopathy, dilated cardiomyopathy, HOCM (with SAM) and chronic AF with LA enlargement and annular dilatation.*

**1360. In secondary (functional) MR, regurgitation is caused by?**
*Harrison's 20th Ed. Chapter 259 Page 1818*

A. Left ventricular remodeling with annular enlargement
B. Papillary muscle displacement
C. Leaflet tethering
D. All of the above

*In secondary (functional) MR, leaflets & chordae tendineae are usually normal but regurgitation is caused by LV remodeling with annular enlargement, papillary muscle displacement, leaflet tethering, or their combination.*

**1361. Chronic MR can result from all except?**
*Harrison's 20th Ed. Chapter 259 Page 1818*

A. Ankylosing spondylitis
B. Hypertrophic obstructive cardiomyopathy (HOCM)
C. Mitral valve prolapse (MVP)
D. Dilated cardiomyopathy

*Chronic MR can result from rheumatic disease, mitral valve prolapse (MVP), extensive mitral annular calcification, congenital valve defects, hypertrophic obstructive cardiomyopathy (HOCM), and dilated cardiomyopathy.*

**1362. Which of the following about functional (secondary) MR is false?**
*Harrison's 20th Ed. Chapter 259 Page 1818*

A. Leaflets are structurally normal
B. Chordae tendineae are structurally normal
C. Annular enlargement
D. None of the above

**1363. MR associated with which of the following is dynamic in nature?**
*Harrison's 20th Ed. Chapter 259 Page 1818*

A. HOCM
B. Acute myocardial infarction
C. Dilated cardiomyopathy
D. All of the above

*The MR associated with both MVP and HOCM is usually dynamic in nature.*

**1364. Chronic MR is frequently secondary to?**
*Harrison's 20th Ed. Chapter 259 Page 1818*

A. Ventricular remodeling
B. Leaflet tethering
C. Fibrosis of a papillary muscle
D. All of the above

*Chronic MR is frequently secondary to ischemia and may occur as a consequence of ventricular remodeling, papillary muscle displacement, and leaflet tethering or with fibrosis of a papillary muscle in patients with healed MI and ischemic cardiomyopathy.*

**1365.** MR occurs universally in patients with nonischemic forms of dilated cardiomyopathy when left ventricular end-diastolic dimension is?
*Harrison's 20th Ed. Chapter 259 Page 1818*

A. 3.0 cm
B. 4.0 cm
C. 5.0 cm
D. 6.0 cm

Annular dilatation and ventricular remodeling contribute to MR that occurs universally among patients with nonischemic forms of dilated cardiomyopathy once the left ventricular end-diastolic dimension reaches 6.0 cm.

**1366.** In severe chronic MR, enlargement of LA places tension on?
*Harrison's 20th Ed. Chapter 259 Page 1818*

A. Anterior mitral leaflet
B. Posterior mitral leaflet
C. Chordae tendineae
D. All of the above

Chronic severe MR is progressive since enlargement of LA places tension on posterior mitral leaflet, pulling it away from the mitral orifice & thereby aggravating valvular dysfunction.

**1367.** Significant pulmonary hypertension at rest is defined as?
*J Am Heart Assoc. 2014;3:e000748*

A. Pulmonary artery systolic pressure [PASP] >20 mm Hg
B. Pulmonary artery systolic pressure [PASP] >30 mm Hg
C. Pulmonary artery systolic pressure [PASP] >40 mm Hg
D. Pulmonary artery systolic pressure [PASP] >50 mm Hg

Significant pulmonary hypertension is defined as pulmonary artery systolic pressure (PASP) >50 mm Hg at rest or >60 mm Hg with exercise.

**1368.** Which of the following defines severe MR?
*Harrison's 20th Ed. Chapter 259 Page 1818*

A. Regurgitant volume ≥ 60 mL/beat
B. Regurgitant fraction (RF) ≥ 50%
C. Effective regurgitant orifice area ≥ 0.40 cm$^2$
D. All of the above

Severe nonischemic MR is defined by a regurgitant volume ≥60 mL/beat, regurgitant fraction (RF) ≥50%, and effective regurgitant orifice area ≥0.40 cm$^2$. Severe ischemic MR is usually associated with an effective regurgitant orifice area of >0.3 cm$^2$.

**1369.** Acute severe MR & chronic severe MR are differentiated by?
*Harrison's 20th Ed. Chapter 259 Page 1819*

A. V wave in the LA pressure pulse
B. Frequency of acute pulmonary edema
C. Decrescendo configuration of systolic murmur
D. All of the above

In acute severe MR, v wave in LA pressure pulse is prominent. Acute pulmonary edema is common. Murmur is early in timing and decrescendo in configuration. In chronic severe MR, LA v wave is relatively less prominent. Murmur is classically holosystolic in timing and plateau in configuration.

**1370.** In mitral regurgitation due to papillary muscle dysfunction, the systolic murmur commences in?
*Harrison's 20th Ed. Chapter 259 Page 1819*

A. Early systole
B. Midsystole
C. Late systole
D. All of the above

**1371.** Which of the following is not ordinarily heard with isolated MR?
*Harrison's 20th Ed. Chapter 259 Page 1819*

A. Holosystolic murmur
B. $S_3$
C. $S_4$
D. Presystolic murmur

In chronic MR, S1 is generally absent, soft, or buried in the holosystolic murmur. In severe MR, aortic valve may close prematurely, resulting in wide but physiologic splitting of S2. Low-pitched S3 occurring 0.12–0.17 seconds after A2 is caused by sudden tensing of papillary muscles, chordae tendineae and valve leaflets. Short, rumbling, mid-diastolic murmur, even in the absence of structural MS may follow. S4 is heard in acute severe MR in sinus rhythm. A presystolic murmur is not ordinarily heard with isolated MR.

**1372.** Systolic murmur of MR, transmitted to base of heart indicates primary involvement of?
*Harrison's 20th Ed. Chapter 259 Page 1819*

A. Anterior mitral leaflet
B. Posterior mitral leaflet
C. Both mitral leaflets
D. Mitral valve annulus

In patients with ruptured chordae tendineae or primary involvement of the posterior mitral leaflet with prolapse or flail, regurgitant jet is eccentric, directed anteriorly, & strikes LA wall adjacent to aortic root. In this situation, systolic murmur is transmitted to base of heart.

**1373.** In patients with which of the following, systolic murmur may have a cooing or "seagull" quality?
*Harrison's 20th Ed. Chapter 259 Page 1819*

A. Mitral valve prolapse (MVP)
B. Ruptured chordae tendineae
C. Acute rheumatic fever
D. HOCM

In patients with ruptured chordae tendineae, systolic murmur of MR may have a cooing or "sea gull" quality.

**1374.** In patients with which of the following, systolic murmur may have a musical quality?
*Harrison's 20th Ed. Chapter 259 Page 1819*

A. Mitral valve prolapse (MVP)
B. Ruptured chordae tendineae
C. Acute rheumatic fever
D. HOCM

In patients with a flail leaflet, murmur of MR may have a musical quality. Systolic murmur of chronic MR not due to MVP is intensified by isometric exercise (handgrip) but is reduced during the strain phase of the Valsalva maneuver.

**1375.** Rheumatic heart disease is the cause of chronic MR in what percentage of cases?
*Harrison's 17th Ed. 1469*

A. 25%
B. 33%
C. 50%
D. 66%

Rheumatic heart disease is the cause of chronic MR in only about one-third of cases and occurs more frequently in males.

**1376.** Which of the following best relates to Cabot - Locke murmur?
*N Engl J Med. 2010;363:22*

A. Hyperthyroidism
B. Anemia
C. Pericarditis
D. Endocarditis

Cabot - Locke murmur is a diastolic murmur heard best at the left sternal border. It sounds similar to aortic insufficiency but does not have a decrescendo. Murmur resolves with treatment of anemia. Richard Cabot was an American physician and Frank Locke was his colleague.

# Mitral Valve Prolapse

**1377. Barlow's syndrome refers to?**
*Harrison's 20th Ed. Chapter 260 Page 1821*

A. Bicuspid aortic stenosis
B. Atrial myxoma
C. Mitral valve prolapse
D. HOCM

*MVP is also termed systolic click-murmur syndrome, Barlow's syndrome, floppy-valve syndrome, and billowing mitral leaflet syndrome.*

**1378. John Barlow belonged to which country?**
*N Engl J Med. 2010;363:22*

A. South Africa
B. United Kingdom
C. Australia
D. Canada

*South African physician John Barlow first submitted his work on mitral-valve prolapse to the journal Circulation, but the manuscript was refused for its "overstated conclusion." After considerable abbreviation of the paper, it was finally accepted & published in 1968 by British Heart Journal.*

**1379. Which of the following statements about MVP is false?**
*Harrison's 20th Ed. Chapter 260 Page 1822*

A. Reduced production of type III collagen
B. Increased concentrations of acid mucopolysaccharide
C. Posterior leaflet is more affected than anterior
D. None of the above

**1380. Mitral valve prolapse has association with heritable disorder like?**
*Harrison's 20th Ed. Chapter 260 Page 1822*

A. Down syndrome
B. Osteogenesis imperfecta
C. Turner syndrome
D. Hemophilia

*MVP is a frequent finding in patients with heritable disorders of connective tissue, including Marfan syndrome, osteogenesis imperfecta & Ehler-Danlos syndrome.*

**1381. Mitral valve prolapse (MVP) may occur as a sequel to?**
*Harrison's 20th Ed. Chapter 260 Page 1822*

A. Acute rheumatic fever
B. Ischemic heart disease
C. Various cardiomyopathies
D. All of the above

*MVP may occur as a sequel to acute rheumatic fever, in ischemic heart disease, and in various cardiomyopathies.*

**1382. Mitral valve prolapse (MVP) is associated with which of the following?**
*Harrison's 20th Ed. Chapter 260 Page 1822*

A. Ostium primum atrial septal defect
B. Ostium secundum atrial septal defect
C. Ventricular septal defect
D. Patent ductus arteriosus

*Mitral valve prolapse (MVP) is associated with 20% of patients with ostium secundum ASD.*

**1383. Which of the following may be an associated feature of MVP?**
*Harrison's 20th Ed. Chapter 260 Page 1822*

A. Inguinal hernias
B. Joint dislocations
C. Meniscal tears
D. All of the above

**1384. Which of the following valve may be affected in MVP?**
*Harrison's 20th Ed. Chapter 260 Page 1822*

A. Mitral valve
B. Tricuspid valve
C. Aortic valve
D. All of the above

**1385. Ventricular arrhythmias in MVP result from stress placed on?**
*Harrison's 20th Ed. Chapter 260 Page 1822*

A. Mitral annulus
B. Posterior mitral leaflet
C. Chordae tendineae
D. Papillary muscles

*MVP causes ventricular arrhythmias due to excessive stress on papillary muscles which lead to dysfunction & ischemia of papillary muscles and subjacent ventricular myocardium.*

**1386. Which of the following valvular heart disease is more common in male?**
*Harrison's 20th Ed. Chapter 260 Page 1822*

A. Rheumatic MR
B. Mitral stenosis (MS)
C. MVP
D. AR with associated mitral valve disease

**1387. Which of the following valvular heart disease is more common in female?**
*Harrison's 20th Ed. Chapter 260 Page 1822*

A. Rheumatic MR
B. MVP
C. Adult patients with symptomatic valvular AS
D. Patients with pure or predominant valvular AR

**1388. Which of the following valvular heart disease is more common in female?**
*Harrison's 20th Ed. Chapter 260 Page 1822*

A. Rheumatic MR
B. Tricuspid Stenosis
C. Adult patients with symptomatic valvular AS
D. Patients with pure or predominant valvular AR

**1389. Sudden death occurs most often in MVP patients with?**
*Harrison's 20th Ed. Chapter 260 Page 1822*

A. Severe MR
B. Depressed left ventricle (LV) systolic function
C. Flail leaflet
D. All of the above

*Sudden death is a very rare complication of MVP and occurs most often in patients with severe MR & depressed left ventricle systolic function or among patients with a flail leaflet.*

### 1390. In MVP, nonejection systolic click occurs how many seconds after S1?
*Harrison's 20th Ed. Chapter 260 Page 1822*

A. 0.11 seconds
B. 0.12 seconds
C. 0.13 seconds
D. 0.14 seconds

*In MVP, the mid- or late (nonejection) systolic click occurs 0.14 seconds or more after S1 and is due to sudden tensing of slack, elongated chordae tendineae or due to prolapsing mitral leaflet when it reaches its maximum excursion.*

### 1391. Which of the following about MVP is false?
*Harrison's 20th Ed. Chapter 260 Page 1822*

A. Systolic clicks may be multiple
B. High-pitched, late systolic crescendo-decrescendo murmur
C. Late systolic murmur heard best at apex
D. None of the above

*In MVP, the late systolic murmur is high-pitched, crescendo-decrescendo configuration ("whooping" or "honking") and is heard best at the apex.*

### 1392. Systolic click & murmur of MVP occur earlier in all of the following except?
*Harrison's 20th Ed. Chapter 260 Page 1822*

A. Standing
B. Squatting
C. During the strain phase of Valsalva maneuver
D. All of the above

*In MVP, systolic click & murmur occur earlier with standing, during strain phase of Valsalva maneuver, and with any intervention that decreases LV volume. Conversely, squatting & isometric exercises, which increase LV volume, diminish click-murmur complex of MVP thus moving it away from S1.*

### 1393. Most frequent serious sequelae of mitral valve prolapse is?
*Harrison's 20th Ed. Chapter 260 Page 1822*

A. Infective endocarditis
B. Sudden cardiac death
C. Severe mitral regurgitation
D. None of the above

*Sudden death is a rare complication & occurs in patients with severe MR & depressed LV systolic function. MVP is the commonest cause of isolated severe MR requiring surgical treatment.*

### 1394. Which view in echocardiography is best to diagnose mitral valve prolapse?
*Harrison's 20th Ed. Chapter 260 Page 1822*

A. Parasternal long-axis view
B. Parasternal short-axis view
C. Four-chamber view
D. All of the above

### 1395. "Classic" mitral valve prolapse is defined as?
*Harrison's 20th Ed. Chapter 260 Page 1823*

A. Prolapse of mitral valve
B. Prolapse > 2 mm beyond long-axis annular plane
C. Thickening of the valve leaflets
D. All of the above

*Echocardiographic definition of MVP is systolic displacement (in the parasternal long axis view) of mitral valve leaflets by at least 2 mm into LA superior to the plane of the mitral annulus.*

### 1396. Which of the following is true in mitral valve prolapse syndrome?
*Lancet. 2005;365:507*

A. Expansion of spongiosa layer by proteoglycans
B. Structural alterations of collagen in all components of leaflet
C. Structurally abnormal chordae tendinae
D. All of the above

### 1397. Non-prolapse related systolic clicks are documented in?
*Lancet. 2005;365:507*

A. Bicuspid aortic stenosis
B. Atrial myxoma
C. Pericarditis
D. All of the above

### 1398. Which of the following echocardiographic parameters is useful to risk stratify patients with mitral valve prolapse?
*Lancet. 2005;365:507*

A. Leaflet thickness
B. Redundancy
C. Increased left-ventricular diameter
D. All of the above

### 1399. Transthoracic echocardiography (TTE) does not exclude?
*Lancet. 2005;365:507*

A. Medial scallop prolapse
B. Middle scallop prolapse
C. Lateral scallop prolapse
D. None of the above

### 1400. Patients with mitral valve prolapse at increased risk of complications are?
*Lancet. 2005;365:507*

A. Depressed left ventricular systolic function
B. Moderate-severe mitral regurgitation
C. Mitral leaflet thickness greater than 5 mm
D. All of the above

### 1401. In MVP, which of the following echocardiographic finding predicts a greater risk of severe MR?
*Lancet. 2005;365:507*

A. Presence of thickened leaflets
B. Posterior leaflet prolapse
C. Increased left ventricular dimensions
D. All of the above

# Tricuspid Valve Disease

**1402. Which of the following about tricuspid stenosis is false?**
*Harrison's 20th Ed. Chapter 261 Page 1823*

- A. Generally congenital in origin
- B. More common in women than men
- C. Does not occur as an isolated lesion
- D. Rheumatic TS commonly associated with TR

*Tricuspid stenosis (TS) is generally rheumatic in origin and more common in women than men. It does not occur as an isolated lesion and is usually associated with MS. Rheumatic TS is commonly associated with some degree of TR. Nonrheumatic causes of TS are rare.*

**1403. Systemic venous congestion sets in when mean RA - RV diastolic pressure gradient is?**
*Harrison's 20th Ed. Chapter 261 Page 1823*

- A. 1 mm Hg
- B. 2 mm Hg
- C. 3 mm Hg
- D. 4 mm Hg

*A diastolic pressure gradient between the RA and RV defines TS. A mean diastolic pressure gradient of 4 mm Hg is usually sufficient to elevate the mean RA pressure to levels that result in systemic venous congestion (hepatomegaly, ascites, edema).*

**1404. In Tricuspid stenosis (TS), jugular veins may show?**
*Harrison's 20th Ed. Chapter 261 Page 1824*

- A. Giant 'a' wave
- B. Less conspicuous 'v' wave
- C. Slow 'y' descent
- D. All of the above

*In TS with sinus rhythm, jugular veins are distended with giant "a" waves. "v" waves are less conspicuous with a slow "y" descent.*

**1405. Which of the following statements is false?**
*Harrison's 20th Ed. Chapter 261 Page 1824*

- A. Development of MS precedes that of TS
- B. Presence of TS can mask clinical features of MS
- C. TS is almost always accompanied by significant TR
- D. None of the above

*Presence of TS can mask hemodynamic & clinical features of MS. Development of MS generally precedes that of TS. TS is almost always accompanied by significant TR.*

**1406. Murmur of which of the following valvular heart disease is heard best over the xiphoid process?**
*Harrison's 20th Ed. Chapter 261 Page 1824*

- A. TS
- B. TR
- C. VSD
- D. All of the above

*Murmur of TS is best heard along left sternal margin and over xiphoid process.*

**1407. In sinus rhythm, murmur of TS is most prominent during?**
*Harrison's 20th Ed. Chapter 261 Page 1824*

- A. Early diastole
- B. Mid systole
- C. Presystole
- D. All of the above

*Murmur of TS is most prominent during presystole in patients with sinus rhythm. It is augmented during inspiration, reduced during expiration and during the strain phase of Valsalva maneuver.*

**1408. Which of the following is false about combined MS & TS?**
*Harrison's 20th Ed. Chapter 261 Page 1824*

- A. Absence of ECG evidence of RVH
- B. Prominence of RA & SVC without enlarged PA on CxR
- C. Less evidence of pulmonary vascular congestion
- D. None of the above

*In combined MS & TS there is absence of ECG evidence of right ventricular hypertrophy (RVH) in a patient with right-sided heart failure. Chest X-ray shows prominence of RA & superior vena cava without much enlargement of PA with less evidence of pulmonary vascular congestion.*

**1409. Severe TS is characterized by a valve area of?**
*Harrison's 20th Ed. Chapter 261 Page 1824*

- A. ≤ 2 cm$^2$
- B. ≤ 1.5 cm$^2$
- C. ≤ 1 cm$^2$
- D. ≤ 0.5 cm$^2$

*Severe TS is characterized by a valve area ≤1 cm$^2$ or pressure half-time of ≥190 ms.*

**1410. Thromboembolic complications are most when mechanical valves are used for which valve replacement?**
*Harrison's 20th Ed. Chapter 261 Page 1824*

- A. Mitral
- B. Tricuspid
- C. Aortic
- D. Pulmonary

*Mechanical valves in the tricuspid position are more prone to thromboembolic complications than in other positions.*

**1411. Functional tricuspid regurgitation (TR) may be observed in?**
*Harrison's 20th Ed. Chapter 261 Page 1824*

- A. Inferior MI
- B. Ischemic cardiomyopathy
- C. Idiopathic dilated cardiomyopathy
- D. All of the above

**1412. Severe pulmonary artery hypertension is defined when pulmonary artery systolic pressure is?**
*Harrison's 20th Ed. Chapter 261 Page 1824*

- A. > 25 mm Hg
- B. > 35 mm Hg
- C. > 45 mm Hg
- D. > 55 mm Hg

*Severe pulmonary artery hypertension is defined when pulmonary artery systolic pressure is > 55 mm Hg.*

**1413. Carcinoid heart disease predominantly affects which of the following heart valves?**
*Harrison's 20th Ed. Chapter 261 Page 1824*

A. Mitral
B. Tricuspid
C. Aortic
D. Pulmonary

Infarction of RV papillary muscles, tricuspid valve prolapse, carcinoid heart disease, endomyocardial fibrosis, radiation, infective endocarditis, and trauma may produce TR.

**1414. Carcinoid syndrome may cause?**
*Harrison's 20th Ed. Chapter 261 Page 1824*

A. Tricuspid regurgitation
B. Pulmonic stenosis
C. Pulmonic regurgitation
D. All of the above

Carcinoid syndrome may cause TR, pulmonic stenosis and/or regurgitation.

**1415. Which of the following is seen in jugular venous pulsations in tricuspid regurgitation?**
*Harrison's 20th Ed. Chapter 261 Page 1824*

A. No x descent
B. Prominent c-v wave
C. Rapid y descent
D. All of the above

In severe TR, RA pressure pulse shows no x descent during early systole but a prominent c-v wave with a rapid y descent.

**1416. In RA pressure pulse, prominent c-v wave with rapid y descent is typical of?**
*Harrison's 20th Ed. Chapter 261 Page 1824*

A. Ebstein's anomaly
B. Tricuspid regurgitation
C. Constrictive pericarditis
D. All of the above

In severe TR, RA pressure pulse may exhibit no x descent during early systole but a prominent c-v wave with a rapid y descent.

**1417. Carvallo's sign is related to which of the following?**
*Harrison's 20th Ed. Chapter 261 Page 1825*

A. Aortic regurgitation
B. Mitral regurgitation
C. Tricuspid regurgitation
D. Pericarditis

A prominent RV pulsation along the left parasternal region and a blowing holosystolic murmur along the lower left sternal margin, which may be intensified during inspiration & reduced during expiration or the strain of the Valsalva maneuver (Carvallo's sign), are characteristic findings of TR.

**1418. A positive hepatojugular reflex is seen in?**
*Harrison's 20th Ed. Chapter 261 Page 1825*

A. TS
B. TR
C. PS
D. All of the above

In TR, systemic venous congestion causes right-sided heart failure manifesting as marked hepatomegaly, ascites, pleural effusions, edema, systolic pulsations of liver, and a positive hepatojugular reflex.

**1419. Hepatic vein systolic flow reversal on Doppler echocardiography is a feature of?**
*Harrison's 20th Ed. Chapter 261 Page 1825*

A. TS
B. TR
C. PS
D. All of the above

**1420. On Doppler examination, "hepatic vein systolic flow reversal" is a feature of?**
*Harrison's 20th Ed. Chapter 261 Page 1825*

A. Constrictive pericarditis
B. Tricuspid regurgitation
C. SVC obstruction
D. All of the above

On Doppler examination, severe TR is accompanied by hepatic vein systolic flow reversal.

# Pulmonic Valve Disease

**1421.** Which of the following about pulmonic valve stenosis (PS) is false?
*Harrison's 20th Ed. Chapter 262 Page 1826*

- A. Essentially a congenital disorder
- B. Pulmonic valve is typically domed
- C. Very rarely affected by the rheumatic process
- D. None of the above

**1422.** Dysplastic pulmonic valves are seen as part of which of the following syndrome?
*Harrison's 20th Ed. Chapter 262 Page 1826*

- A. Down syndrome
- B. Parkes-Weber syndrome
- C. Noonan syndrome
- D. Williams syndrome

*Dysplastic pulmonic valves are seen as part of the Noonan syndrome.*

**1423.** Severe PS is defined by a peak systolic gradient across the pulmonic valve of?
*Harrison's 20th Ed. Chapter 262 Page 1826*

- A. > 30 mm Hg
- B. > 40 mm Hg
- C. > 50 mm Hg
- D. > 60 mm Hg

**1424.** PS rarely progresses in patients with peak gradients of?
*Harrison's 20th Ed. Chapter 262 Page 1826*

- A. < 30 mm Hg
- B. < 40 mm Hg
- C. < 50 mm Hg
- D. < 60 mm Hg

*Severe PS is defined by a peak systolic gradient across the pulmonic valve of > 50 mm Hg. PS rarely progresses in patients with peak gradients <30 mm Hg.*

**1425.** Which of the following is a right-sided acoustic event that decreases in intensity with inspiration?
*Harrison's 20th Ed. Chapter 262 Page 1826*

- A. Third heart sound
- B. Fourth heart sound
- C. Systolic murmur
- D. Ejection sound (click)

*The ejection sound is the only right-sided acoustic event that decreases in intensity with inspiration.*

**1426.** Which of the following heart valves is least affected by infective endocarditis?
*Harrison's 20th Ed. Chapter 262 Page 1826*

- A. Mitral
- B. Tricuspid
- C. Aortic
- D. Pulmonary

*Pulmonic valve is affected by rheumatic fever far less frequently than the other valves, and it is uncommonly a nidus for infective endocarditis.*

**1427.** Which of the following is false about 'Graham Steell murmur'?
*Harrison's 20th Ed. Chapter 262 Page 1827*

- A. High-pitched
- B. Decrescendo, diastolic
- C. Along left sternal border
- D. None of the above

*Graham Steell murmur due to severe pulmonary hypertension is a high-pitched, decrescendo, diastolic blowing murmur along the left sternal border.*

**1428.** Pulmonic regurgitation occurs universally among patients who have undergone which of the following?
*Harrison's 20th Ed. Chapter 262 Page 1827*

- A. Mustard operation
- B. Repair of tetralogy of Fallot
- C. Senning operation
- D. Ross procedure

*Pulmonic regurgitation occurs universally among patients who have undergone childhood repair of tetralogy of Fallot with reconstruction of the RV outflow tract.*

## Multiple and Mixed Valvular Heart Disease

**1429. Which of the following drug can cause aortic insufficiency?**
*Harrison's 20th Ed. Chapter 262 Page 1827*

A. Methysergide
B. Fenfluramine
C. Penicillin
D. Cisplatin

*Aortic insufficiency can be caused by serotonin reuptake inhibitors, specifically medications containing fenfluramine or dexfenfluramine isotopes, and dopamine agonists.*

**1430. Which of the following can produce mixed valve lesions?**
*Harrison's 20th Ed. Chapter 262 Page 1827*

A. Mediastinal radiation
B. Carcinoid heart disease
C. Marfan's syndrome
D. All of the above

**1431. An enlarged azygos vein in the frontal projection indicates?**
*Harrison's 20th Ed. Chapter 262 Page 1829*

A. RA hypertension
B. LA hypertension
C. Increased pulmonary vascular resistance (PVR)
D. All of the above

*An enlarged azygos vein in the frontal projection indicates RA hypertension.*

**1432. Bioprosthetic valves are indicated in?**
*Harrison's 20th Ed. Chapter 262 Page 1829*

A. Elderly (> 65 years)
B. Women who expect to become pregnant
C. In whom anticoagulation is contraindicated
D. All of the above

*Bioprostheses are preferred for patients >65 years, for women who expect to become pregnant & for those who refuse to take anticoagulation or for whom anticoagulation is contraindicated.*

## Congenital Heart Disease in the Adult

**1433. Pregnant women with certain CHD, may not tolerate?**
*Harrison's 20th Ed. Chapter 264 Page 1831*
- A. Elevated pulmonary artery (PA) pressures
- B. Decreased ventricular function
- C. Symptomatic left-sided obstructive lesions
- D. All of the above

**1434. Which of the following agents are teratogenic and contraindicated during pregnancy?**
*Harrison's 20th Ed. Chapter 264 Page 1831*
- A. Angiotensin converting enzyme (ACE) inhibitors
- B. Angiotensin receptor blockers
- C. Endothelin-receptor blockers
- D. All of the above

**1435. Which of the following occurs in pregnancy?**
*British Medical Bulletin. 2008;85:151-180*
- A. 50% expansion in blood volume & cardiac output
- B. Increase in heart rate from 6th week, peaking at III trimester
- C. Decrease in systemic vascular resistance (SVR)
- D. All of the above

**1436. Which of the following can occur during pregnancy in woman with CHD?**
*British Medical Bulletin. 2008;85:151-180*
- A. Endocarditis
- B. Arrhythmias
- C. Aortic dissection
- D. All of the above

**1437. Which of the following condition can lead to aortic dissection during pregnancy in woman with CHD?**
*British Medical Bulletin. 2008;85:151-180*
- A. Coarctation of aorta
- B. Bicuspid aortic valve
- C. Marfan syndrome
- D. All of the above

*Potential risk of adverse cardiovascular events during pregnancy in woman with CHD include arrhythmias, thromboembolic events, heart failure or pulmonary oedema, aortic dissection (for patients with coarctation of aorta, bicuspid aortic valve and Marfan syndrome), endocarditis and even death.*

**1438. A fetal echocardiogram is advised for parents with CHD between?**
*Harrison's 20th Ed. Chapter 264 Page 1831, British Medical Bulletin. 2008;85:151-180*
- A. 12 and 14 weeks of gestation
- B. 14 and 18 weeks of gestation
- C. 18 and 22 weeks of gestation
- D. 22 and 25 weeks of gestation

*A fetal echocardiogram between 18 and 22 weeks of gestation is advised for parents with CHD.*

**1439. The heart starts to form in which week of gestation?**
*Harrison's 20th Ed. Chapter 264 Page 1831*
- A. II
- B. III
- C. IV
- D. V

**1440. The heart is nearly fully formed by which week of gestation?**
*Harrison's 20th Ed. Chapter 264 Page 1831*
- A. VII
- B. VIII
- C. IX
- D. X

*The heart starts to form in the third week of gestation, and is nearly fully formed by 8 weeks' gestation.*

**1441. Cells of the second heart field contribute to the formation of?**
*Harrison's 20th Ed. Chapter 264 Page 1831*
- A. Atria
- B. RV
- C. Outflow tract
- D. All of the above

**1442. Which of the following is essential for septation of the outflow tracts and formation of the semilunar valves?**
*Harrison's 20th Ed. Chapter 264 Page 1831*
- A. Mesodermal precardiac cells
- B. Cells of the second heart field
- C. Cardiac neural crest cells
- D. All of the above

**1443. The most common birth defects have origin in?**
*Harrison's 20th Ed. Chapter 264 Page 1831*
- A. Cardiovascular system
- B. Central nervous system
- C. Gastrointestinal system
- D. Urogenital system

*The most common birth defects are cardiovascular in origin.*

**1444. Which of the following is the most commonly occurring birth defect?**
*Harrison's 20th Ed. Chapter 264 Page 1831*
- A. Cleft palate
- B. Flat foot
- C. Congenital heart disease
- D. Strabismus

*CHD is the most commonly occurring birth defect.*

**1445. What percentage of children born with Trisomy 21 have a CHD?**
*Harrison's 20th Ed. Chapter 264 Page 1832*

A. 10%
B. 25%
C. 50%
D. 75%

Children born with Trisomy 21 have a 50% chance of having CHD, most commonly defects in the atrioventricular canal.

**1446. DiGeorge syndrome is characterized by?**
*Harrison's 20th Ed. Chapter 264 Page 1832*

A. Conotruncal defects
B. Psychiatric disorders
C. Disabilities in cognitive function
D. All of the above

**1447. Noonan syndrome is characterized by?**
*Harrison's 20th Ed. Chapter 264 Page 1832*

A. Dysplastic pulmonary valve
B. Facial abnormalities
C. Lymphatic abnormalities
D. All of the above

**1448. Hypercalcemia is a feature of?**
*Harrison's 20th Ed. Chapter 264 Page 1832*

A. Down syndrome
B. DiGeorge syndrome
C. Noonan syndrome
D. Williams syndrome

**1449. Mutation in PTPN11 gene causes which of the following?**
*Harrison's 20th Ed. Chapter 264 Page 1832*

A. Williams syndrome
B. Down syndrome
C. Noonan syndrome
D. DiGeorge/velocardiofacial syndrome

**1450. Which of the following is a congenital etiology for right heart dilation?**
*Harrison's 20th Ed. Chapter 264 Page 1832 Table 264-3*

A. Ebstein anomaly
B. Arrhythmogenic RV cardiomyopathy
C. Uhl's anomaly
D. All of the above

**1451. Which of the following is a feature of Uhl's anomaly?**
*Ann Pediatr Card. 2015;8:71-3*

A. Absence of myocardium in parietal wall of right ventricle
B. Apposition of endocardium & epicardium, no adipose tissue
C. Papillary muscles of tricuspid valve are normally muscularized
D. All of the above

Uhl's Anomaly is a rare cardiac condition in which there is total absence of right ventricular myocardium resulting in apposition of the endocardium and epicardium. The septal wall, septomarginal trabeculation and the papillary muscles of the tricuspid valve are normally muscularized.

**1452. Which of the following shunt lesions cause right heart dilation?**
*Harrison's 20th Ed. Chapter 264 Page 1832 Table 264-3*

A. Gerbode defect
B. Coronary sinus septal defect
C. Partial anomalous pulmonary venous return
D. All of the above

**1453. In Gerbode defect, abnormal shunting occurs between?**
*Harrison's 20th Ed. Chapter 264 Page 1832 Table 264-3*

A. RV - LA
B. LV - RA
C. LV - RV
D. LA - RA

Gerbode defect is defined as abnormal shunting between the left ventricle and right atrium resulting from either a congenital defect or prior cardiac insults. Surgeon Frank Gerbode at Stanford University described it as "the lesion consists of a high ventricular septal defect associated with a defect of the septal leaflet of the tricuspid valve which allows left ventricular blood to enter the right atrium".

**1454. In Gerbode defect, physical examination finding include?**
*J Clin Diagn Res. 2015;9(9):OD06–OD08*

A. Pansystolic murmur similar to that of a VSD
B. Unvarying with respiration
C. Thrill along the left sternal border
D. All of the above

**1455. Congenital heart disease complicates what percentage of all live births?**
*British Medical Bulletin. 2008;85:151-180*

A. ~ 1%
B. ~ 2%
C. ~ 3%
D. ~ 4%

CHD complicates ~1% of all live births in general population, but occurs in 4% of offspring of women with CHD.

**1456. Which of the following arches develop as the internal carotid arteries?**
*Circulation. 2006;114:1873-1882*

A. 1
B. 2
C. 3
D. 4

Truncus arteriosus & aortic sac initially develop six paired symmetric arches. Development of arch 3 results in internal carotid arteries, left arch 4 as the aortic arch and right subclavian artery, and part of arch 6 as the patent ductus arteriosus.

**1457. Sinus venosus receives which of the following veins?**
*Circulation. 2006;114:1873-1882*

A. Umbilical vein
B. Vitelline vein
C. Common cardinal vein
D. All of the above

Sinus venosus receives the umbilical, vitelline, and common cardinal veins.

### 1458. Which of the following congenital heart disease is more common in females?
*N Engl J Med. 2000;342:256-263*

A. ASD
B. Congenital valvular AS
C. Coarctation of aorta
D. Complete transposition of great vessels

*ASD occurs more frequently in females. Congenital valvular AS, Coarctation of aorta and Complete transposition of great vessels is more frequent in males.*

### 1459. Which of the following ASD type is false?
*N Engl J Med. 2000;342:256-263*

A. Ostium secundum is in the region of the fossa ovalis
B. Ostium primum is in the lower part of the atrial septum
C. Sinus venosus is in the upper atrial septum
D. None of the above

*Ostium secundum defects make up 75 percent of all atrial septal defects, ostium primum defects make up 15 percent, and sinus venosus defects make up 10 percent.*

### 1460. Which of the following ASD type is associated with anomalous pulmonary venous connection?
*N Engl J Med. 2000;342:256-263*

A. Sinus venosus ASD
B. Ostium primum ASD
C. Ostium secundum ASD
D. Patent foramen ovale

*ASD in sinus venosus type is high up in the atrial septum near the entry of superior vena cava into right atrium. It is associated frequently with anomalous pulmonary venous connection from the right lung to the superior vena cava or right atrium.*

### 1461. ASD occurs in the basal portion of the interventricular septum in which of the following?
*N Engl J Med. 2000;342:256-263*

A. Sinus venosus ASD
B. Ostium primum ASD
C. Ostium secundum ASD
D. Patent foramen ovale

### 1462. Mitral-valve prolapse occurs with?
*N Engl J Med. 2000;342:256-263*

A. Sinus venosus ASD
B. Ostium primum ASD
C. Ostium secundum ASD
D. Patent foramen ovale

*Additional cardiac abnormalities may occur with each type of defect; these include mitral-valve prolapse (with ostium secundum defects), mitral regurgitation (due to a cleft in the anterior mitral-valve leaflet, which occurs with ostium primum defects), and partial anomalous drainage of the pulmonary veins into the right atrium or venae cavae (with sinus venosus defects).*

### 1463. Which of the following ASD is more common in Down syndrome?
*Harrison's 19th Ed. 1520*

A. Sinus venosus ASD
B. Ostium primum ASD
C. Ostium secundum ASD
D. Patent foramen ovale

### 1464. Which out of the following ASD is most common?
*Harrison's 20th Ed. Chapter 264 Page 1832*

A. Sinus venosus ASD
B. Ostium primum ASD
C. Ostium secundum ASD
D. Patent foramen ovale

### 1465. Which out of the following ASD is in the region of fossa ovalis?
*Harrison's 20th Ed. Chapter 264 Page 1832*

A. Sinus venosus ASD
B. Ostium primum ASD
C. Ostium secundum ASD
D. Patent foramen ovale

### 1466. Patent foramen ovale (PFO) persists in what proportion of adults?
*Harrison's 20th Ed. Chapter 264 Page 1832*

A. 5%
B. 15%
C. 25%
D. 35%

*Patent foramen ovale (PFO) is the persistence of patency of the flap valve of fossa ovalis. It is not associated with right-sided cardiac dilation. PFO persists in ~25% of adults.*

### 1467. ASD is considered a large shunt, with substantial hemodynamic consequences, when its diameter is more than?
*N Engl J Med. 2000;342:256-263*

A. 0.5 cm
B. 1.0 cm
C. 1.5 cm
D. 2.0 cm

*A small ASD (<0.5 cm in diameter) is associated with a small shunt and no hemodynamic sequelae. A sizable defect (>2 cm in diameter) may be associated with a large shunt, with substantial hemodynamic consequences.*

### 1468. A small ASD is characterized by a ratio of pulmonary to systemic flow of less than?
*N Engl J Med. 2000;342:256-263*

A. 0.5
B. 1.0
C. 1.5
D. 2.0

*A small defect with minimal left-to-right shunting (characterized by a ratio of pulmonary to systemic flow of <1.5) usually causes no symptoms or hemodynamic abnormalities and therefore does not require closure.*

### 1469. Flow across the atrial septal defect itself produces which of the following murmur?
*N Engl J Med. 2000;342:256-263*

A. Systolic
B. Diastolic
C. Continuous
D. No murmur

*Flow across the atrial septal defect itself does not produce a murmur.*

**1470. Mid-diastolic rumbling murmur in ASD is loudest at?**
*N Engl J Med. 2000;342:256-263*

A. 3rd intercostal space, along left sternal border
B. 3rd intercostal space, along right sternal border
C. 4th intercostal space, along left sternal border
D. 4th intercostal space, along right sternal border

**1471. Which of the following cardiac murmurs can be heard in various types of compensated ASD?**
*N Engl J Med. 2000;342:256-263*

A. Midsystolic pulmonary outflow murmur
B. Mid-diastolic left parasternal murmur
C. Apical holosystolic murmur
D. All of the above

*Increased flow across the pulmonic valve is responsible for a midsystolic pulmonary outflow murmur. Mid-diastolic murmur at fourth intercostal space and along left sternal border indicates increased flow across tricuspid valve. In ostium primum ASD, apical holosystolic murmur indicates associated mitral or tricuspid regurgitation or a ventricular septal defect (VSD).*

**1472. In ASD, second heart sound is widely split and is relatively fixed in relation to?**
*Harrison's 20th Ed. Chapter 264 Page 1832*

A. Respiration
B. Posture
C. Heart rate
D. All of the above

*In ASD, second heart sound is widely split and is relatively fixed in relation to respiration.*

**1473. Which of the following is key to wide and fixed splitting of the second heart sound in ASD?**
*N Engl J Med. 2000;342:256-263*

A. No respiratory changes in right & left atrial stroke volumes
B. No respiratory changes in right & left ventricular stroke volumes
C. No respiratory changes in pulmonary artery
D. No respiratory changes in pulmonary vasculature

*Wide & fixed splitting of S2 in ASD is due to prolonged RV ejection and increased PA capacitance which delays pulmonary valve closure. Splitting of S2 is fixed because phasic changes in systemic venous return to right atrium during respiration are accompanied by reciprocal changes in volume of shunted blood from left atrium to the right atrium, thereby minimizing the respiratory changes in right & left ventricular stroke volumes that are normally responsible for physiologic splitting.*

**1474. In adults with an ASD and atrial fibrillation, the physical findings may be confused with?**
*Harrison's 19th Ed. 1521*

A. Mitral stenosis
B. Tricuspid stenosis
C. Pulmonary stenosis
D. Mitral regurgitation

*In adults with an ASD and atrial fibrillation, physical findings may be confused with mitral stenosis with pulmonary hypertension because the tricuspid diastolic flow murmur and widely split second heart sound may be mistakenly thought to represent the diastolic murmur of mitral stenosis and the mitral "opening snap," respectively.*

**1475. Which of the following statements about ostium secundum type of ASD is false?**
*Harrison's 20th Ed. Chapter 264 Page 1832*

A. ECG shows left axis deviation
B. $S_2$ widely split and relatively fixed
C. Middiastolic rumbling murmur
D. Midsystolic pulmonary ejection murmur

*In ostium secundum ASD, ECG shows right-axis deviation and an rSr' pattern in right precordial leads representing enlargement of the RV outflow tract.*

**1476. In ECG of cases of ostium primum ASD, which of the following is true?**
*N Engl J Med. 2000;342:256-263*

A. Right-axis deviation
B. Left superior axis deviation
C. Left inferior axis deviation
D. Left-axis deviation

**1477. In ECG of cases of ostium primum ASD, which of the following is true?**
*N Engl J Med. 2000;342:256-263*

A. Clockwise rotation of frontal plane QRS loop
B. Counterclockwise rotation of frontal plane QRS loop
C. Clockwise rotation of sagittal plane QRS loop
D. Counterclockwise rotation of sagittal plane QRS loop

*In ostium primum ASD, the RV conduction defect is accompanied by left superior axis deviation and counterclockwise rotation of the frontal plane QRS loop.*

**1478. Which of them is a finding in echocardiogram of a patient of ASD?**
*N Engl J Med. 2000;342:256-263*

A. Pulmonary arterial dilatation
B. RV and RA dilatation
C. Abnormal (paradoxical) ventricular septal motion
D. All of the above

*In ASD, echocardiography reveals pulmonary arterial and RV and RA dilatation with abnormal (paradoxical) ventricular septal motion in the presence of a significant right heart volume overload. ASD may be visualized directly by two-dimensional imaging, color-flow imaging, or echocontrast.*

**1479. Which of the following about atrial septal defect is false?**
*N Engl J Med. 2000;342:256-263*

A. Sinus venosus ASD cases rarely die before 5th decade
B. Ostium secundum ASD cases rarely die before 5th decade
C. Risk of infective endocarditis in ASD is low
D. None of the above

*Closure by an appropriate method should be advised in uncomplicated secundum ASD with significant left-to-right shunting, i.e., pulmonary-to-systemic flow ratios 2:1. Patients with sinus venosus or ostium secundum ASDs rarely die before the fifth decade. Risk of infective endocarditis is quite low unless ASD is complicated by valvular regurgitation or has recently been repaired with a patch or device.*

**1480. Ebstein's anomaly is a disease of?**
*Harrison's 20th Ed. Chapter 264 Page 1832*

A. Right atrium
B. Right ventricle
C. Right ventricular outflow tract
D. All of the above

*Ebstein's anomaly is a disease of the entire right ventricle.*

### 1481. Ebstein anomaly is the result of?
*Harrison's 20th Ed. Chapter 264 Page 1832*

A. Failure of delamination of TV leaflets from ventricular myocardium
B. Failure of delamination of TV leaflets from atrial myocardium
C. Failure of septation of ventricular myocardium
D. Failure of septation of atrial myocardium

Ebstein anomaly is due to embryologic failure of delamination or "peeling away" of tricuspid valve leaflets from the ventricular myocardium, resulting in adherence of the valve leaflets to the underlying myocardium.

### 1482. Which of the following about Ebstein anomaly is false?
*Harrison's 20th Ed. Chapter 264 Page 1832*

A. Apical & posterior displacement of dilated TV annulus
B. Dilation of the "atrialized" portion of the RV
C. Fenestrations, redundancy & tethering of anterior leaflet of TV
D. None of the above

Ebstein anomaly consists of apical & posterior displacement of dilated tricuspid valve annulus, dilation of "atrialized" portion of RV, and fenestrations, redundancy & tethering of anterior leaflet of tricuspid valve.

### 1483. Most common finding in Ebstein's anomaly is?
*Harrison's 20th Ed. Chapter 264 Page 1832*

A. MS
B. MR
C. TS
D. TR

Ebstein's Anomaly is characterized by a downward displacement of tricuspid valve into right ventricle, due to anomalous attachment of dysplastic tricuspid leaflets. This results in tricuspid regurgitation.

### 1484. Which of the following signs is related to Ebstein anomaly?
*Harrison's 20th Ed. Chapter 264 Page 1832*

A. McConnell's sign
B. Broadbent's sign
C. Sail sign
D. Ewart's sign

In Ebstein anomaly, there are few hemodynamic correlates for the observed auscultatory events. Multiple components of the first sound and "ejection" sounds are frequently described. 'Sail sound' in patients with Ebstein's anomaly is not simply a closing sound of tricuspid valve, but a complex closing sound which includes a sudden stopping sound after the redundant anterior and/or other tricuspid leaflets balloon out at systole.

### 1485. An interatrial communication is present in what percentage of patients with Ebstein's anomaly?
*Circulation. 2007;115:277-285*

A. 50% – 60%
B. 60% – 70%
C. 70% – 80%
D. 80% – 90%

An interatrial communication is present in 80% to 94% of patients with Ebstein's anomaly.

### 1486. Which of the following is false about Ebstein anomaly?
*Circulation. 2007;115:277-285*

A. Jugular venous pulse rarely shows a large V wave
B. Widely split S2 and several added sounds
C. Marked enlargement of the right atrium
D. None of the above

On examination, the jugular venous pulse rarely shows a large V wave despite severe regurgitation of the tricuspid valve because the large right atrium engulfs the increased volume. S1 & S2 heart sounds are widely split, and a S3 or S4 heart sound is often present, resulting in a "triple" or "quadruple" rhythm.

### 1487. Patients with Ebstein's anomaly and an interatrial communication are at risk for?
*N Engl J Med. 2000;342(5):334-342*

A. Paradoxical embolization
B. Brain abscess
C. Sudden death
D. All of the above

### 1488. Which of the following is false about ECG in Ebstein anomaly?
*Circulation. 2007;115:277-285*

A. Tall and broad P waves
B. Complete or incomplete right bundle-branch block
C. Complete heart block is rare
D. None of the above

### 1489. On CxR, cardiac silhouette of typical Ebstein's anomaly is similar to that of?
*Circulation. 2007;115:277-285*

A. Mitral stenosis
B. Pericardial effusion
C. Partially anomalous pulmonary venous drainage
D. Tetralogy of Fallot

The cardiac silhouette may vary from almost normal to the typical Ebstein's anomaly configuration consisting of a globe-shaped heart (due to right atrial enlargement) with a narrow waist similar to that seen with pericardial effusion. Vascularity of pulmonary fields is either normal or decreased. Cardiothoracic ratio 0.65 carries a poor prognosis.

### 1490. Wolff–Parkinson–White syndrome occurs frequently in which of the following CHD?
*Harrison's 20th Ed. Chapter 264 Page 1832, British Medical Bulletin. 2008;85:151-180*

A. Tetralogy of Fallot
B. Ebstein's anomaly
C. ASD
D. All of the above

Wolff–Parkinson–White syndrome occurs in ~20% of patients with Ebstein's anomaly.

### 1491. Most common congenital cardiac anomaly recognized at birth is?
*Harrison's 20th Ed. Chapter 264 Page 1833*

A. ASD
B. VSD
C. PDA
D. Coarctation of the Aorta

VSD are the most common congenital anomaly recognized at birth. However, they account for only ~10% of CHD in the adult, due to the high rate of spontaneous closure of small VSDs during the early years of life.

### 1492. Which of the following about ventricular septal defect is false?
*N Engl J Med. 2000;342:256-263*

A. Occur with similar frequency in boys and girls
B. 25%–40% close spontaneously by the age of 2 years
C. 90% close by the age of 10 years
D. None of the above

### 1493. Which of the following about ventricular septal defect is false?
*N Engl J Med. 2000;342:256-263*

A. 70% are located in membranous portion of IVS
B. 20% are located in muscular portion of IVS
C. 5% are located just below the aortic valve
D. None of the above

*VSD located just below the aortic valve undermine the valve annulus and cause aortic regurgitation. 5% of VSD are located near the junction of mitral & tricuspid valves (atrioventricular canal defects).*

### 1494. The risk associated with surgery for VSD is prohibitive once the ratio of pulmonary to systemic vascular resistance exceeds?
*N Engl J Med. 2000;342:256-263*

A. 0.6
B. 0.7
C. 0.8
D. 0.9

*Once the ratio of pulmonary to systemic vascular resistance exceeds 0.7, the risk associated with surgery is prohibitive.*

### 1495. Which of the following gene can cause septal defects?
*Circulation. 2006;114:2190-2197*

A. TBX5
B. GATA4
C. NKX2.5
D. All of the above

### 1496. Which of the following is false about VSD?
*Circulation. 2006;114:2190-2197*

A. Smaller defects are loudest and may have a thrill
B. Murmurs are typically holosystolic or pansystolic
C. Large defects with no shunt do not have a VSD murmur
D. None of the above

### 1497. Which of the following is false about VSD?
*Circulation. 2006;114:2190-2197*

A. Endocarditis is a lifelong risk in unoperated patients
B. Chamber enlargement is a measure of the degree of shunting
C. Small VSD have no apparent ECG & radiographic abnormality
D. None of the above

### 1498. Which of the following about ductus arteriosus is false?
*Harrison's 20th Ed. Chapter 264 Page 1834*

A. Originates from bifurcation of pulmonary artery
B. Ends at aorta just distal to left subclavian artery
C. Continuous murmur best heard at upper left sternal edge
D. None of the above

*Patent ductus arteriosus (PDA) is a vascular structure that connects the proximal descending aorta to the roof of the main pulmonary artery near the origin of the left branch pulmonary artery.*

### 1499. Incidence of PDA is higher than average in?
*N Engl J Med. 2000;342:256-263*

A. Pregnancies complicated by persistent perinatal hypoxemia
B. Maternal rubella infection
C. Infants born at high altitude or prematurely
D. All of the above

*Rubella infection during the first trimester of pregnancy, particularly in the first 4 weeks, is associated with a high incidence of PDA. It has been reported to be associated with fetal valproate syndrome.*

### 1500. PDA occurs with increased frequency in which of the following genetic syndromes?
*Circulation. 2006;114:1873-1882*

A. Trisomy 21
B. Carpenter's syndrome
C. Holt-Oram syndrome
D. All of the above

*PDA occurs with increased frequency in trisomy 21, 4p- syndrome, Carpenter's syndrome, Holt-Oram syndrome, and incontinentia pigmenti.*

### 1501. Which of the following about moderate or large patent ductus arteriosus is false?
*N Engl J Med. 2000;342:256-263*

A. Bounding peripheral arterial pulses
B. Widened pulse pressure
C. Hyperdynamic left ventricular impulse
D. None of the above

### 1502. Which of the following about continuous "machinery" or Gibson's murmur of PDA is false?
*N Engl J Med. 2000;342:256-263*

A. Heard in second left anterior intercostal space
B. Begins shortly after S1
C. Peaks in intensity at or immediately after S2
D. None of the above

*In PDA, S1 heart sound is normal. A continuous "machinery" murmur, audible in II left anterior intercostal space, begins shortly after S1, peaks in intensity at or immediately after S2 (thereby obscuring it), and declines in intensity during diastole. As pulmonary vascular obstruction and hypertension develop, the continuous murmur decreases in duration and intensity and eventually disappears and a pulmonary ejection click and a diastolic decrescendo murmur of pulmonary regurgitation may appear.*

### 1503. Differential cyanosis is best related to?
*Harrison's 20th Ed. Chapter 234 Page 1667*

A. ASD
B. VSD
C. Patent ductus arteriosus
D. Tetralogy of Fallot

*In PDA, severe pulmonary vascular disease results in reversal of flow through ductus therby unoxygenated blood is shunted to descending aorta leading to cyanosis and clubbing of the toes, but not fingers because the right-to-left ductal shunting is distal to the subclavian arteries. This is called differential cyanosis.*

### 1504. Which of the following about patent ductus arteriosus is false?
*N Engl J Med. 2000;342:256-263*

A. Rarely closes spontaneously after infancy
B. Elevated risk of infective endocarditis
C. May become aneurysmal & calcified leading to rupture
D. None of the above

### 1505. Infective endocarditis involves which of the following in a case of PDA?
*N Engl J Med. 2000;342:256-263*

A. Aortic side of ductus arteriosus
B. Pulmonary side of ductus arteriosus
C. Mid portion of ductus arteriosus
D. Any of the above

*Infective endocarditis involves the pulmonary side of the ductus arteriosus or the pulmonary artery opposite the duct orifice, from which septic pulmonary emboli may arise.*

### 1506. Leading cause of death in adults with PDA is?
*N Engl J Med. 2000;342:256-263*

A. Infective endarteritis
B. Cardiac arrhythmia
C. Brain abscess
D. Restrictive lung disease

Leading causes of death in adults with patent ductus are cardiac failure & infective endarteritis.

### 1507. Which of the following is the most common form of cyanotic CHD after infancy?
*Harrison's 20th Ed. Chapter 264 Page 1834*

A. Tetralogy of Fallot (TOF)
B. Ebstein's Anomaly
C. Transposition of the Great Arteries
D. Eisenmenger's syndrome

### 1508. Which of the following about Tetralogy of Fallot is false?
*Cleveland Clinic J of Medicine. 2010;77(11):822-828*

A. Occurs in ~1 in 3,600 live births
B. Occurs in 3.5% of infants born with congenital heart disease
C. Accounts for 10% of all cases
D. None of the above

Tetralogy of Fallot occurs in approximately 1 in 3,600 live births or 3.5% of infants born with congenital heart disease. It is the most common type of cyanotic congenital heart disease, accounting for 10% of all cases.

### 1509. Which of the following is a component of Tetralogy of Fallot?
*Harrison's 20th Ed. Chapter 264 Page 1835*

A. Right ventricular hypertrophy
B. Overriding aorta
C. Membranous ventricular septal defect
D. All of the above

The four components of Tetralogy of Fallot are right ventricular hypertrophy, overriding aorta, membranous ventricular septal defect, and right ventricular outflow tract obstruction.

### 1510. In Tetralogy of Fallot, severity of which of the following determines the clinical presentation?
*Harrison's 20th Ed. Chapter 264 Page 1835*

A. Size of VSD
B. Aortic override of the VSD
C. RV outflow obstruction
D. RV hypertrophy

The four components of the tetralogy of Fallot are malaligned VSD, obstruction to RV outflow, aortic override of the VSD, and RV hypertrophy due to the RV's response to aortic pressure via the large VSD. The severity of RV outflow obstruction determines the clinical presentation.

### 1511. "Pink tetralogy of Fallot" refers to?
*J Cardiovasc Comput Tomogr. 2010;4(1):58-61*

A. Noncyanotic TOF
B. Pulmonary stenosis is mild
C. Ventricular septal defect is in balance
D. All of the above

"Pink tetralogy of Fallot" refers to the the noncyanotic patient in whom pulmonary stenosis is mild and ventricular septal defect is in balance.

### 1512. Tetrology of Fallot may be seen in?
*International Journal of Current Advanced Research. 2018;07(5):12979-12981*

A. CATCH 22
B. DiGeorge syndrome
C. Shprintzen syndrome
D. All of the above

### 1513. Which of the following abnormalities may occur in association with tetralogy of Fallot?
*N Engl J Med. 2000;342(5):334-342*

A. Right aortic arch
B. Atrial septal defect
C. Coronary arterial anomalies
D. All of the above

Abnormalities that may occur in association with tetralogy of Fallot include right aortic arch (25%), atrial septal defect (10%) -so called pentalogy of Fallot, and coronary arterial anomalies (10%).

### 1514. Which of the following is not a part of Trilogy of Fallot?
*J Pract Cardiovasc Sci. 2016;2:114-9*

A. Atrial septal defect
B. Valvular pulmonary stenosis
C. Infundibular pulmonary stenosis
D. Right ventricular hypertrophy

### 1515. Which of the following coronary artery is anomalous in TOF?
*Harrison's 20th Ed. Chapter 264 Page 1835*

A. Right coronary artery
B. Left anterior descending coronary artery
C. Left circumflex coronary artery
D. Posterior descending coronary artery

~7% of patients with TOF have an anomalous coronary artery, most commonly, anomalous left anterior descending coronary artery from the right coronary cusp.

### 1516. Which of the following affect the magnitude of right-to-left shunting in TOF?
*N Engl J Med. 2000;342(5):334-342*

A. Changes in pulmonary vascular resistance
B. Changes in systemic vascular resistance
C. Size of VSD
D. All of the above

Since the resistance to flow across right ventricular outflow tract is relatively fixed, changes in systemic vascular resistance affect the magnitude of right-to-left shunting. A decrease in systemic vascular resistance increases right-to-left shunting, whereas an increase in systemic resistance decreases right-to-left shunting.

### 1517. Which of the following about TOF is false?
*N Engl J Med. 2000;342(5):334-342*

A. Most patients have cyanosis from birth or beginning in first year
B. Hypoxic "spells" do not occur in adolescents or adults
C. Without surgical intervention, most patients die in childhood
D. None of the above

**1518. In TOF, hypoxic "spells" are characterized by?**
*N Engl J Med. 2000;342(5):334-342*

A. Tachypnea
B. Hyperpnea
C. Worsening cyanosis
D. All of the above

**1519. Which of the following about TOF is false?**
*J Pract Cardiovasc Sci. 2016;2:114-9*

A. Normal JVP
B. Aortic ejection sound
C. Congestive heart failure rare
D. None of the above

**1520. Which of the following is a complication of chronic cyanosis?**
*N Engl J Med. 2000;342(5):334-342*

A. Abnormalities of hemostasis
B. Cerebral abscesses or stroke
C. Endocarditis
D. All of the above

*Complications of chronic cyanosis include erythrocytosis, hyperviscosity, abnormalities of hemostasis, cerebral abscesses or stroke, and endocarditis.*

**1521. Which of the following may also be present in TOF?**
*N Engl J Med. 2000;342(5):334-342*

A. Pulmonary valve stenosis
B. Unilateral absence of a pulmonary artery
C. Right-sided aortic arch & descending thoracic aorta
D. All of the above

*In tetralogy of Fallot, severity of hypoplasia of the RV outflow tract varies from mild to complete (pulmonary atresia). Pulmonary valve stenosis and supravalvular and peripheral pulmonary arterial obstruction may coexist. Rarely, there is unilateral absence of a pulmonary artery (usually left). A right-sided aortic arch and descending thoracic aorta occur in 25%.*

**1522. Which of the following is a clinical finding in TOF?**
*N Engl J Med. 2000;342(5):334-342*

A. Normal S1
B. Single S2
C. Systolic ejection murmur along the left sternal border
D. All of the above

*In TOF, second heart sound is single, since its pulmonary component is inaudible.*

**1523. Which of the following about ECG findings in Tetralogy of Fallot is false?**
*N Engl J Med. 2000;342(5):334-342*

A. Right-axis deviation
B. Right ventricular hypertrophy
C. T wave inversion very rare
D. None of the above

**1524. Which of the following about chest X-ray findings in Triology of Fallot is false?**
*J Pract Cardiovasc Sci. 2016;2:114-9*

A. Cardiomegaly
B. Dilated PA
C. Normal shape of the heart
D. None of the above

**1525. Which of the following about chest X-ray findings in Tetralogy of Fallot is false?**
*N Engl J Med. 2000;342(5):334-342*

A. Enlarged heart
B. Boot-shaped heart (coeur en sabot)
C. Oligemic lung fields
D. Concavity in the region of pulmonary conus

*In Tetralogy of Fallot, chest X-ray shows a normal-sized or small heart, boot-shaped (coeur en sabot) with a prominent right ventricle and a concavity in the region of pulmonary conus. Pulmonary vascular markings are typically diminished, and the aortic arch and knob may be on the right side.*

**1526. Which of the following is an operative procedure for Tetralogy of Fallot?**
*N Engl J Med. 2000;342(5):334-342*

A. Waterston operation
B. Potts operation
C. Blalock–Taussig operation
D. All of the above

*Procedures for correction of TOF involve anastomosis of a systemic artery to a pulmonary artery. Waterston operation (a side-to-side anastomosis of ascending aorta and right pulmonary artery), Potts operation (a side-to-side anastomosis of the descending aorta to the left pulmonary artery), and Blalock–Taussig operation (end-to-side anastomosis of the subclavian artery to the pulmonary artery).*

**1527. Which of the following about treatment in TOF is false?**
*Harrison's 20th Ed. Chapter 264 Page 1835*

A. Reoperation in adults is mostly for severe PR
B. Ventricular and atrial arrhythmias common
C. Aortic regurgitation common
D. Endocarditis risk eliminated after surgical repair

*Most adults with tetralogy of Fallot have had some form of previous surgical intervention. Reoperation in adults is most commonly for severe pulmonary regurgitation. Ventricular & atrial arrhythmias require treatment. Aortic root has a medial tissue defect & it is commonly enlarged & associated with aortic regurgitation. Endocarditis remains a risk despite surgical repair.*

**1528. On a resting ECG, QRS duration of what duration is associated with ↑ risk of VT & sudden death in patients with repaired TOF?**
*Harrison's 20th Ed. Chapter 264 Page 1835*

A. ≥ 100 ms
B. ≥ 120 ms
C. ≥ 160 ms
D. ≥ 180 ms

*On a resting ECG, QRS duration of ≥ 180 ms is associated with ↑ risk of VT & sudden death in patients with repaired TOF.*

**1529. On a resting ECG, what rate of change in QRS duration is associated with ↑ risk of VT & sudden death in patients with TOF?**
*Cleveland Clinic J of Medicine. 2010;77(11):822-828*

A. > 1.5 ms/year
B. > 2.5 ms/year
C. > 3.5 ms/year
D. > 4.5 ms/year

*In TOF, a relatively rapid increase (> 3.5 ms/year) in QRS duration is strongly associated with ventricular arrhythmias & sudden death, even if the QRS duration is not markedly prolonged. Reduced heart rate variability also is a marker of risk of sudden cardiac death in TOF.*

**1530. The most common re-intervention in a repaired TOF patient is?**
*Harrison's 20th Ed. Chapter 264 Page 1835*

A. Closure of residual VSDs
B. Dilation and/or stenting of the RVOT
C. Pulmonary valve replacement (PVR)
D. Catheter ablation for arrhythmias

*The most common re-intervention in a repaired TOF patient is pulmonary valve replacement (PVR).*

**1531. Which of the following is false about Transposition of the great arteries (TGA)?**
*Harrison's 20th Ed. Chapter 264 Page 1835*

A. Aorta arises from the RV and the PA arises from the LV
B. D-loop TGA is the more common form of TGA
C. VSD is the most common additional congenital defect in TGA
D. None of the above

**1532. Which communication in TGA provides compatibility with life?**
*Harrison's 20th Ed. Chapter 264 Page 1835*

A. Atrial septal defect (ASD)
B. Ventricular septal defect (VSD)
C. Patent ductus arteriosus (PDA)
D. All of the above

*Without interchamber or intravascular communications, this circulation is incompatible with life. Presence of ASD, VSD or PDA, allow for some interchamber or intravascular mixing, and provide partial relief of cyanosis and sustenance of life, at the expense of increased pulmonary blood flow.*

**1533. Which is the most common communication in complete transposition of the great arteries?**
*Harrison's 20th Ed. Chapter 264 Page 1835*

A. ASD
B. VSD
C. PDA
D. All of the above

*Most patients of complete transposition of the great arteries have an interatrial communication, two-thirds have a patent ductus arteriosus, and about one-third have an associated VSD.*

**1534. Which of the following procedure is used for correction of TGA?**
*Harrison's 20th Ed. Chapter 264 Page 1835*

A. Mustard procedure
B. Senning procedure
C. Rastelli procedure
D. All of the above

**1535. Which of the following about L-loop TGA is false?**
*Harrison's 20th Ed. Chapter 264 Page 1836*

A. Also called congenitally corrected TGA
B. Atrioventricular discordance
C. Ventriculoarterial discordance
D. None of the above

**1536. Associated congenital anomaly with L-loop TGA is?**
*Harrison's 20th Ed. Chapter 264 Page 1836*

A. Dextrocardia
B. ASDs
C. Pulmonary stenosis
D. All of the above

*Patients with L-loop TGA commonly have associated congenital anomalies, including dextrocardia, ASDs, a dysplastic tricuspid valve and pulmonary stenosis.*

**1537. Transposition of great arteries is associated with which of the following genetic syndromes?**
*Front Pediatr. 2013;1:11*

A. Turner
B. Noonan
C. Williams
D. None of the above

*Transposition of great arteries is very rarely associated with the most frequent genetic syndromes, such as Turner, Noonan, Williams or Marfan syndromes, and in Down syndrome, it is virtually absent.*

**1538. The only genetic syndrome with a strong relation with TGA is?**
*Front Pediatr. 2013;1:11*

A. Kartagener syndrome
B. Heterotaxy syndrome
C. Patau syndrome
D. Edward syndrome

*The only genetic syndrome with a strong relation with TGA is the Heterotaxy. Heterotaxy is defined as an abnormality where the internal thoraco-abdominal organs demonstrate abnormal arrangement across the left-right axis of the body.*

**1539. Which of the following is a form of trisomy?**
*Front Pediatr. 2013;1:11*

A. Down syndrome
B. Edward syndrome
C. Patau syndrome
D. All of the above

*Trisomy 21 (Down syndrome), Trisomy 18 (Edward syndrome) and Trisomy 13 (Patau syndrome).*

**1540. The incidence of Coarctation of the aorta is?**
*Harrison's 20th Ed. Chapter 271 Page 1899*

A. 0.1–4 per 1000 live births
B. 0.8–4 per 1000 live births
C. 1–8 per 1000 live births
D. 5–18 per 1000 live births

*Coarctation of the aorta was first described by Morgagni in 1760.*

**1541. Coarctation of the aorta occurs in what percentage of patients with congenital heart disease?**
*World J Cardiol. 2015;7(11):765-775*

A. 1%
B. 3%
C. 7%
D. 9%

*Narrowing or constriction of the lumen of the aorta may occur anywhere along its length but is most common distal to the origin of the left subclavian artery near the insertion of the ligamentum arteriosum. Coarctation of the aorta occurs in 7% of patients with congenital heart disease and is more common in males than females.*

**1542. Coarctation less commonly involves which of the following?**
*Harrison's 20th Ed. Chapter 264 Page 1837*

A. Ascending aortic arch
B. Transverse aortic arch
C. Abdominal aorta
D. None of the above

Coarctation less commonly involves the transverse aortic arch.

**1543. Which of the following is most common concomitant lesion with coarctation of the aorta?**
*Harrison's 20th Ed. Chapter 264 Page 1839 Figure 264-10*

A. Aortic regurgitation
B. Bicuspid aortic valve
C. ASD
D. VSD

Bicuspid aortic valve is most common concomitant lesion with coarctation of the aorta.

**1544. Which of the following is commonly associated with coarctation of the aorta?**
*Harrison's 20th Ed. Chapter 264 Page 1837, 1899*

A. Turner syndrome
B. Bicuspid aortic valve
C. Circle of Willis aneurysms
D. All of the above

Coarctation of the aorta is frequent in patients with gonadal dysgenesis (Turner syndrome) and is associated with bicuspid aortic valve (75%) and Circle of Willis aneurysms. Coarctation of the aorta is usually sporadic but occurs in 35% of children with Turner's syndrome.

**1545. Blood pressure difference in both arms is > 10 mm Hg in?**
*Harrison's 20th Ed. Chapter 234 Page 1669*

A. Supravalvular aortic stenosis
B. Aortic coarctation
C. Aortic dissection
D. All of the above

Blood pressure difference in both arms should be <10 mm Hg. A blood pressure differential that exceeds this threshold may be associated with atherosclerotic or inflammatory subclavian artery disease, supravalvular aortic stenosis, aortic coarctation, or aortic dissection.

**1546. In aortic coarctation, a blowing systolic murmur may be heard in?**
*Harrison's 20th Ed. Chapter 271 Page 1899*

A. Posterior right interscapular area
B. Posterior left interscapular area
C. Left axilla
D. Left occiput

In aortic coarctation, a blowing systolic murmur may be heard in the posterior left interscapular areas or along the course of one or more ribs.

**1547. In coarctation of the aorta, enlarged and pulsatile collateral vessels may be palpated in?**
*World J Cardiol. 2015;7(11):765-775*

A. Intercostal spaces
B. Axillae
C. Interscapular area
D. All of the above

In coarctation of the aorta, enlarged and pulsatile collateral vessels may be palpated in the intercostal spaces anteriorly, in the axillae, or posteriorly in the interscapular area.

**1548. In Chest X-ray, "3" sign relates to which of the following?**
*World J Cardiol. 2015;7(11):765-775*

A. Patent ductus arteriosus
B. Supravalvular Aortic Stenosis
C. Coarctation of the aorta
D. Tetralogy of Fallot

Chest X-ray in coarctation of the aorta shows a dilated left subclavian artery high on the left mediastinal border and a dilated ascending aorta. Indentation of the aorta at the site of coarctation with pre- and poststenotic dilatation ("3" sign) along left paramediastinal shadow are pathognomonic.

**1549. In coarctation of the aorta, radiographic notching of which of the following ribs is seen?**
*World J Cardiol. 2015;7(11):765-775*

A. 3rd to 5th ribs
B. 3rd to 7th ribs
C. 3rd to 9th ribs
D. 3rd to 12th ribs

In coarctation of the aorta, notching of the third to ninth ribs is an important radiographic sign. This is due to inferior rib erosion by dilated collateral vessels.

**1550. Which of the following is the hazard of coarctation of aorta?**
*Harrison's 20th Ed. Chapter 264 Page 1839 Figure 264-10*

A. Cerebral aneurysms and hemorrhage
B. Aortic dissection and rupture
C. Premature coronary arteriosclerosis
D. All of the above

In coarctation of the aorta, the chief hazards of proximal aortic severe hypertension include cerebral aneurysms and hemorrhage, aortic dissection and rupture, premature coronary arteriosclerosis, and LV failure.

**1551. Which of the following best relates to Fontan circulation?**
*Harrison's 20th Ed. Chapter 264 Page 1837*

A. Surgical removal of RV outflow tract obstruction
B. Surgical removal of the atrial septum
C. Absence of a pumping chamber to pulmonary artery
D. Physiologically corrected transposition of the great arteries

**1552. Which of the following relates to single ventricle heart disease?**
*Harrison's 20th Ed. Chapter 264 Page 1837*

A. Tricuspid atresia
B. Double inlet LV
C. Hypoplastic left heart syndrome
D. All of the above

**1553. In Eisenmenger's syndrome, a large communication between systemic and pulmonary circulation exists at?**
*Harrison's 20th Ed. Chapter 264 Page 1838*

A. Aortopulmonary level
B. Ventricular level
C. Atrial level
D. Any of the above

Eisenmenger's syndrome refers to a large communication between systemic and pulmonary circulations at the aortopulmonary, ventricular, or atrial levels. Flow is bidirectional or predominantly right-to-left because of high resistance and obstructive pulmonary hypertension.

### 1554. In Eisenmenger syndrome, symptoms in adult life consist of?
*N Engl J Med. 2000;342(5):334-342*

A. Chest pain
B. Syncope
C. Hemoptysis
D. All of the above

*In patients with Eisenmenger syndrome, symptoms in adult life consist of exertional dyspnea, chest pain, syncope, and hemoptysis. Hemoptysis occurs as a result of pulmonary infarction or rupture of dilated pulmonary arteries, arterioles, or aortocopulmonary collateral vessels.*

### 1555. In patients with Eisenmenger syndrome, right-to-left shunt leads to?
*N Engl J Med. 2000;342(5):334-342*

A. Cyanosis
B. Clubbing
C. Erythrocytosis
D. All of the above

*In patients with Eisenmenger syndrome, right-to-left shunt leads to cyanosis, clubbing, and erythrocytosis.*

### 1556. The murmur of which of the following disappears when Eisenmenger's syndrome develops?
*N Engl J Med. 2000;342(5):334-342*

A. Ventricular septal defect
B. Patent ductus arteriosus
C. Atrial septal defect
D. All of the above

*The murmur caused by a ventricular septal defect, patent ductus arteriosus, or atrial septal defect disappears when Eisenmenger's syndrome develops.*

### 1557. Which of the following can occur in Eisenmenger's syndrome?
*N Engl J Med. 2000;342(5):334-342*

A. Decrescendo diastolic murmur of pulmonary regurgitation
B. Holosystolic murmur of tricuspid regurgitation
C. Right-sided fourth heart sound
D. None of the above

*Many patients of Eisenmenger's syndrome have a decrescendo diastolic murmur of pulmonary regurgitation or a holosystolic murmur of tricuspid regurgitation. A right-sided S4 is usually present. The lungs are clear.*

### 1558. Pulmonary vascular disease does not progress after operative correction of shunt, if pulmonary vascular resistance is less than systemic vascular resistance by?
*N Engl J Med. 2000;342(5):334-342*

A. One-third
B. One-half
C. Two-third
D. Three-fourth

*The degree to which pulmonary vascular resistance is elevated before operation is a critical factor determining prognosis. If the pulmonary vascular resistance is one-third or less of the systemic value, progression of pulmonary vascular disease after operation is unusual.*

### 1559. Which of the following pulmonary vascular morphologic changes is irreversible in Eisenmenger's syndrome?
*N Engl J Med. 2000;342(5):334-342*

A. Plexiform lesions
B. Medial hypertrophy of pulmonary arterioles
C. Intimal proliferation and fibrosis
D. Occlusion of capillaries & small arterioles

### 1560. Which of the following is a pulmonary vasodilator?
*N Engl J Med. 2000;342(5):334-342*

A. Oxygen
B. Intravenous adenosine
C. Intravenous epoprostenol
D. All of the above

*Pulmonary vasodilators such as oxygen, inhaled nitrous oxide, or intravenous adenosine or epoprostenol are administered to assess the reversibility of pulmonary hypertension.*

### 1561. Eisenmenger's syndrome, which of the following portend a poor outcome?
*N Engl J Med. 2000;342(5):334-342*

A. A history of syncope
B. Clinically evident right ventricular systolic dysfunction
C. Severe hypoxemia
D. All of the above

*A history of syncope, clinically evident right ventricular systolic dysfunction, low cardiac output, and severe hypoxemia portend a poor outcome in Eisenmenger's syndrome.*

### 1562. Which of the following should be avoided in Eisenmenger syndrome?
*N Engl J Med. 2000;342(5):334-342*

A. Anticoagulants
B. Antiplatelet agents
C. Vasodilators
D. All of the above

*Anticoagulants and antiplatelet agents should be avoided in Eisenmenger syndrome, since they exacerbate the hemorrhagic diathesis.*

### 1563. Which of the following is a consequence of chronic hypoxemia in cyanotic CHD?
*N Engl J Med. 2000;342(5):334-342*

A. Secondary erythrocytosis
B. Abnormal hemostasis
C. Hyperviscosity
D. All of the above

### 1564. Which of the following is a symptom of hyperviscosity?
*N Engl J Med. 2000;342(5):334-342*

A. Visual disturbances
B. Fatigue, headache, dizziness
C. Paresthesias
D. All of the above

### 1565. Cerebrovascular accidents in Eisenmenger syndrome may occur as a result of?
*N Engl J Med. 2000;342(5):334-342*

A. Paradoxical embolization
B. Venous thrombosis of cerebral vessels
C. Intracranial hemorrhage
D. All of the above

**1566. Which of the following is aortic root - to - right-heart shunt?**
*Harrison's 19th Ed. 1523*

A. Congenital aneurysm of aortic sinus of Valsalva with fistula
B. Coronary arteriovenous fistula
C. Anomalous origin of LCA from pulmonary trunk
D. All of the above

The three most common causes of aortic root–to-right-heart shunts are congenital aneurysm of an aortic sinus of Valsalva with fistula, coronary arteriovenous fistula, and anomalous origin of the left coronary artery (LCA) from the pulmonary trunk.

**1567. Which of the following is not a feature of Williams-Beuren syndrome?**
*N Engl J Med. 2010;362:239-52*

A. "Elfin" facies
B. Mental retardation with retained language skills
C. Supravalvular aortic stenosis
D. Transient hyperkalemia

Supravalvular aortic stenosis is associated cardiac defect in Williams-Beuren syndrome, typically comprising of "elfin" facies, low nasal bridge, cheerful demeanor, mental retardation with retained language skills and love of music, and transient hypercalcemia.

**1568. Genetic defect for Williams-Beuren syndrome is located on which chromosome?**
*N Engl J Med. 2010;362:239-52*

A. 5
B. 6
C. 7
D. 8

In most patients, a genetic defect for Williams-Beuren syndrome is located in the same chromosomal region as elastin on chromosome 7. Williams syndrome is associated with interstitial deletions of the long arm of chromosome 7 (7ql 1 .23).

**1569. Which of the following is a microdeletion disorder?**
*N Engl J Med. 2010;362:239-52*

A. DiGeorge syndrome
B. Williams-Beuren syndrome
C. Pseudohypoparathyroidism IB (PHP-IB)
D. All of the above

PHP-Ib is caused by microdeletions within or upstream of the GNAS locus located on chromosome 20q 13.3. Men with oligospermia/azoospermia frequently have microdeletions on the long arm of tbe Y chromosome that involve one more of the azoospermla factor (AZF) genes. DiGeorge/velocardiofacial syndromes is associated with interstitial deletions of the long arm of chromosome 22 (22q 1 1 .2). Genetic mutations involving microdeletions at the elastin locus gene on chromosome 7 may play a role in the pathogenesis of Williams-Beuren syndrome.

**1570. Which of the following is a facial feature of Williams–Beuren syndrome children?**
*N Engl J Med. 2010;362:239-52*

A. Flat nasal bridge, short upturned nose
B. Periorbital puffiness & full cheeks
C. Long philtrum and delicate chin
D. All of the above

Facial feature of Williams–Beuren syndrome children include a flat nasal bridge, short upturned nose, periorbital puffiness, long philtrum, and delicate chin. Older patients have slightly coarse features, with full lips, a wide smile, and a full nasal tip.

**1571. Which of the following is a finding in Williams–Beuren syndrome?**
*N Engl J Med. 2010;362:239-52*

A. Hypercalcemia
B. Supravalvular aortic stenosis
C. Premature graying of the hair
D. All of the above

**1572. Which of the following is a finding in Williams–Beuren syndrome?**
*N Engl J Med. 2010;362:239-52*

A. Diverticulosis
B. Diabetes mellitus
C. Sensorineural hearing loss
D. All of the above

**1573. Which of the following gene is implicated in Williams–Beuren syndrome?**
*N Engl J Med. 2010;362:239-52*

A. SH
B. ELN
C. STAT1
D. HRP2

**1574. No endocarditis prophylaxis is required in which of the following CHD?**
*British Medical Bulletin. 2008;85:151-180, N Engl J Med. 2000;342:256-263*

A. Mitral valve prolapse without regurgitation
B. Pulmonary stenosis
C. Isolated secundum atrial septal defect
D. All of the above

Prophylaxis against infective endocarditis is not recommended for patients with atrial septal defects (repaired or unrepaired) unless a concomitant valvular abnormality is present.

**1575. Endocarditis prophylaxis indicated in which of the following CHD?**
*British Medical Bulletin. 2008;85:151-180*

A. Tetralogy of Fallot
B. Transposition of the great arteries (TGA)
C. Prosthetic heart valves
D. All of the above

**1576. Heritable syndromes with associated ASD include?**
*Circ Res. 2013;112:707-720*

A. Patau
B. Holt-Oram
C. Ellis-van Creveld
D. All of the above

**1577. Heritable syndromes with associated VSD include?**
*Circ Res. 2013;112:707-720*

A. Cri-Du-Chat
B. Okihiro syndrome
C. Kabuki syndrome
D. All of the above

1578. Heritable syndromes with associated PDA include?
*Circ Res. 2013;112:707-720*

   A. Char
   B. 1p36 Deletion
   C. Cri-Du-Chat
   D. All of the above

1579. Heritable syndromes that are associated with Tetralogy of Fallot include?
*Circ Res. 2013;112:707-720*

   A. 22q11 Deletion
   B. Cat Eye
   C. CHARGE
   D. All of the above

1580. Heritable syndrome with associated supravalvular aortic stenosis is?
*Circ Res. 2013;112:707-720*

   A. Kartagener
   B. Laurence-Moon-Biedl-Bardet
   C. Williams
   D. Crouzon

1581. Chromosomal abnormalities with associated VSD include?
*Circ Res. 2013;112:707-720*

   A. Cri du chat
   B. Holt-Oram
   C. Okihiro syndrome
   D. All of the above

1582. Which of the following heritable syndromes is associated with ASD?
*Circ Res. 2013;112:707-720*

   A. Ellis-van Creveld syndrome
   B. Patau
   C. Holt-Oram syndrome
   D. All of the above

1583. Which of the following heritable syndromes is associated with PDA?
*Circ Res. 2013;112:707-720*

   A. Char
   B. 1p36 Deletion
   C. Cri-Du-Chat
   D. All of the above

1584. Which of the following connective tissue disorders is associated with supravalvular aortic stenosis?
*Harrison's 20th Ed. Chapter 406 Page 2976*

   A. Marfan's
   B. Osteogenesis imperfecta
   C. Pseudoxanthoma elasticum
   D. Cutis laxa

1585. Which of the following chromosomal disorders is associated with Tetralogy of Fallot?
*Circ Res. 2013;112:707-720*

   A. 22q11 Deletion
   B. CHARGE
   C. Okihiro syndrome
   D. All of the above

1586. Which of the following chromosomal disorders is associated with coarctation of aorta?
*Circ Res. 2013;112:707-720*

   A. Turner syndrome
   B. Down syndrome
   C. Trisomy 18
   D. Cri du chat syndrome

1587. Which of the following heritable syndromes is associated with supravalvular aortic stenosis?
*Circ Res. 2013;112:707-720*

   A. Turner syndrome
   B. Catch-22 syndrome
   C. Shprintzen syndrome
   D. Williams syndrome

1588. Which genetic condition has clinical features overlapping those of Noonan syndrome?
*Circ Res. 2013;112:707-720*

   A. Turner syndrome
   B. LEOPARD syndrome
   C. Ellis-van Creveld syndrome
   D. Holt-Oram syndrome

## Pericardial Disease

**1589. Cardiac tamponade occurs when fluid in pericardial space reaches a pressure exceeding?**
*Cleveland Clinic Journal of Medicine. 2013;80(2):109*

A. Lymphatic pressure
B. Intrapleural pressure
C. Central venous pressure
D. Pulmonary artery wedge pressure

*Cardiac tamponade occurs when fluid in pericardial space reaches a pressure that exceeds central venous pressure (CVP).*

**1590. Pericardial cavity normally contains how much fluid?**
*Harrison's 20th Ed. Chapter 265 Page 1841*

A. 5 to 10 mL of fluid
B. 10 to 20 mL of fluid
C. 15 to 50 mL of fluid
D. 50 to 100 mL of fluid

*Normal pericardium is a double-layered sac. Visceral pericardium is a serous membrane that is separated by a small quantity (15 to 50 mL) of fluid, an ultrafiltrate of plasma, from the fibrous parietal pericardium.*

**1591. Which of the following is a function of normal pericardium?**
*Harrison's 20th Ed. Chapter 265 Page 1841*

A. Prevents sudden dilation of the cardiac chambers
B. Restricts anatomic position of the heart
C. Retards spread of infections from lungs & pleural cavities
D. All of the above

**1592. In partial left pericardial defects, which of the following may bulge through the defect?**
*Harrison's 20th Ed. Chapter 265 Page 1841*

A. Aorta
B. Left atrium
C. Left ventricle
D. Pulmonary vein

*In partial left pericardial defects, main pulmonary artery & left atrium may bulge through the defect.*

**1593. Effusive-constrictive pericarditis is a type of?**
*Harrison's 20th Ed. Chapter 265 Page 1841 Table 265-1*

A. Acute pericarditis
B. Subacute pericarditis
C. Chronic pericarditis
D. All of the above

**1594. Which of the following is a type of chronic pericarditis?**
*Harrison's 20th Ed. Chapter 265 Page 1841 Table 265-1*

A. Constrictive pericarditis
B. Effusive pericarditis
C. Adhesive (nonconstrictive) pericarditis
D. All of the above

**1595. Which of the following is a type of familial pericarditis?**
*Harrison's 20th Ed. Chapter 265 Page 1841 Table 265-1*

A. Wolman disease
B. Vici syndrome
C. Mulibrey nanism
D. Stauffer's syndrome

*Mulibrey nanism is an autosomal recessive syndrome characterized by growth failure, muscle hypotonia, hepatomegaly, ocular changes, enlarged cerebral ventricles, mental retardation, ventricular hypertrophy and chronic constrictive pericarditis.*

**1596. Dressler's syndrome best relates to?**
*Harrison's 20th Ed. Chapter 265 Page 1841 Table 265-1*

A. Post-myocardial infarction
B. Post-pericardiotomy
C. Post-traumatic
D. All of the above

**1597. Most common cause of acute pericarditis is?**
*N Engl J Med. 2004;351:2195-202*

A. Viral or unknown (idiopathic)
B. Trauma to the chest
C. Neoplastic invasion of the pericardium
D. Tuberculosis

**1598. Pain of pleural pericarditis is referred to the shoulder and neck is related to?**
*Harrison's 20th Ed. Chapter 265 Page 1841*

A. Sensory fibers originating in the first cervical segment
B. Sensory fibers originating in the second cervical segment
C. Sensory fibers originating in the third cervical segment
D. Sensory fibers originating in the fourth cervical segment

*Owing to the overlapping sensory supply of the central diaphragm via the phrenic nerve with somatic sensory fibers originating in the third to fifth cervical segments, the pain of pleural pericarditis is often referred to the shoulder and neck. Involvement of the pleural surface of the lateral diaphragm can lead to pain in the upper abdomen. Radiation to the trapezius ridge is characteristic of pericardial pain and does not usually occur with angina.*

**1599. Which of the following mainly influences the clinical presentation of cardiac tamponade?**
*Cleveland Clinic Journal of Medicine. 2013;80(2):109*

A. Quantity of pericardial fluid
B. Rate at which pericardial fluid accumulates
C. Left ventricular ejection fraction
D. All of the above

**1600. Rapid accumulation of pericardial fluid is characterized more by?**
*Cleveland Clinic Journal of Medicine. 2013;80(2):109*

A. Edema
B. Hypotension
C. Dyspnea
D. All of the above

*Rate at which pericardial fluid accumulates influences the clinical presentation of cardiac tamponade, particularly edema. Thus, edema & dyspnea are more prominent clinical presentations of cardiac tamponade, when there is a slow accumulation and hence slow rise in pericardial pressure. Rapid accumulation is characterized more by hypotension than by edema.*

**1601. Which of the following favors the diagnosis of cardiac tamponade?**
*Cleveland Clinic Journal of Medicine. 2013;80(2):109*

A. Hypotension
B. Tachycardia
C. Jugular venous distention
D. All of the above

**1602. Chest pain is often absent in which of the following?**
*Harrison's 20th Ed. Chapter 265 Page 1841*

A. Postirradiation pericarditis
B. Neoplastic pericarditis
C. Uremic pericarditis
D. All of the above

*Chest pain is absent in slowly developing TB, postirradiation, neoplastic & uremic pericarditis.*

**1603. Which of the following statements about chest pain of acute pericarditis is false?**
*Harrison's 20th Ed. Chapter 265 Page 1841*

A. Retrosternal and left precordial
B. Exacerbated by inspiration
C. Worse when the patient sits upright and leans forward and improves in supine position
D. Pain may radiate to one or both trapezius muscle ridges

*Pain of acute pericarditis is often severe, retrosternal & left precordial, referred to neck, arms, or left shoulder. Often pain is pleuritic, aggravated by inspiration, coughing & changes in body position. Pericardial pain is relieved by sitting up & leaning forward & is intensified by lying supine.*

**1604. Pericardial friction rub is best heard at?**
*Harrison's 20th Ed. Chapter 265 Page 1841*

A. Apex
B. Left lower sternal border
C. Right sternal border
D. All of the above

*Pericardial friction rub is high-pitched, elicited sometimes only at the left lower sternal border at end-expiration with the patient upright & leaning forward throughout the respiratory cycle.*

**1605. "Triphasic" pericardial friction rub is heard in about?**
*N Engl J Med. 2004;351:2195-202*

A. 100% of patients
B. 75% of patients
C. 50% of patients
D. 25% of patients

**1606. Which of the following is a component of "triphasic" pericardial friction rub?**
*N Engl J Med. 2004;351:2195-202*

A. Ventricular systole
B. Rapid early diastolic filling
C. Late presystolic filling after atrial contraction
D. All of the above

*The three components of "Triphasic" pericardial friction rub are ventricular systole, rapid early diastolic filling and late presystolic filling after atrial contraction in patients in sinus rhythm.*

**1607. Atrial repolarization (STa and Ta) may become apparent in?**
*N Engl J Med. 2004;351:2195-202*

A. Atrial infarction
B. Pre-excitation syndrome
C. Constrictive pericarditis
D. STEMI

*Atrial repolarization (STa and Ta) is usually too low in amplitude to be detected, but it may become apparent in conditions such as acute pericarditis and atrial infarction.*

**1608. PR-segment depression is seen in which stage of acute pericarditis?**
*Harrison's 20th Ed. Chapter 265 Page 1841*

A. Stage I
B. Stage II
C. Stage III
D. Stage IV

*PR-segment deviation (opposite in polarity to the ST segment) due to a concomitant atrial injury current.*

**1609. Widespread T-wave inversions are found in which stage of acute pericarditis?**
*Harrison's 20th Ed. Chapter 265 Page 1842*

A. Stage I
B. Stage II
C. Stage III
D. Stage IV

*ECG in acute pericarditis evolves through 4 stages. In stage 1, there is widespread elevation of ST segments with upward concavity, involving two or three standard limb leads and V2 to V6, as well as PR-segment depression with no significant changes in QRS. In stage 2, ST segments return to normal and then T waves become inverted (stage 3). Weeks or months later, ECG returns to normal in stage 4.*

**1610. In acute pericarditis, reciprocal depression is seen in?**
*Harrison's 20th Ed. Chapter 265 Page 1842*

A. aVR
B. aVL
C. aVF
D. All of the above

*ECG in stage 1 of acute pericarditis shows widespread elevation of ST segments, with upward concavity, involving two or three standard limb leads and V2 to V6, with reciprocal depressions only in aVR and sometimes V1, as well as depression of the PR segment below the TP segment reflecting atrial involvement without significant changes in QRS complexes.*

**1611. The most reliable ECG distinguishing feature between acute pericarditis and acute myocardial infarction is?**
*N Engl J Med. 2004;351:2195-202*

A. Ratio of ST segment elevation to T-wave height in $V_6$ of > 0.16
B. Ratio of ST segment elevation to T-wave height in $V_6$ of > 0.20
C. Ratio of ST segment elevation to T-wave height in $V_6$ of > 0.24
D. Ratio of ST segment elevation to T-wave height in $V_6$ of > 0.28

*In early repolarization, T waves are usually tall and the ST/T ratio is <0.25, this ratio is higher in acute pericarditis.*

1612. **Which of the following about ECG changes in pericarditis is false?**
*Harrison's 20th Ed. Chapter 265 Page 1842*

A. ST-segment elevation
B. Diffuse lead involvement not corresponding to a specific coronary anatomic distribution
C. PR-segment depression
D. None of the above

*In patients with ST-segment elevation, the presence of diffuse lead involvement not corresponding to a specific coronary anatomic distribution and PR-segment depression can aid in distinguishing pericarditis from acute MI.*

1613. **Auenbrugger's sign in cases of pericardial effusion best relates to?**
*American Review of Respiratory Disease. 1961;84(3):458*

A. Retraction of thoracic wall, synchronous with cardiac systole
B. Epigastric prominence
C. Percussion dullness in fifth right intercostal space
D. Dullness on auscultation beneath angle of left scapula

*Named after Joseph Leopold Auenbrugger, Auenbrugger's sign is a bulging of epigastrium noticed cases of severe pericardial effusion. Compression of this bulge may cause hemodynamic compromise & cardiac tamponade.*

1614. **Patch of dullness on auscultation beneath angle of left scapula in pericardial effusion is called?**
*Harrison's 20th Ed. Chapter 265 Page 1842*

A. Auenbrugger's sign
B. Ewart's Sign
C. Broadbent's sign
D. Ebstein's sign

*Patch of dullness on auscultation with egophony and bronchial breathing beneath angle of left scapula due to compressive atelectasis of left lung base by pericardial fluid is called Ewart's Sign (William Ewart, UK). Also known as Bamberger-Pins-Ewart Sign or Pins' Syndrome. Ewart's second sign - A large pericardial effusion makes the first rib more prominent along sternal border. Conner's sign - Dullness at the right lower lung field. Bamberger's sign - Disappearance of Ewart's or Conner's signs when patient sits up & leans forward. Dressler's sign - dullness to percussion of lower one half of sternum. Sansom's sign - Percussible dullness in left third intercostal space. Greene's sign - Lateral displacement of percussed cardiac border with expiration. Auenbrugger's sign - epigastric prominence seen in marked pericardial effusion. Broadbent's sign - retraction of thoracic wall, synchronous with cardiac systole, visible in left posterior axillary line is a sign of adherent pericardium. Ebstein's sign - obtuseness of the cardio-hepatic angle on percussion. Friedreich's sign - sudden collapse of previously distended veins of neck at each diastole. Rotch's sign - percussion dullness in fifth intercostal space on the right. Heim-Kreysig sign - in drawing of the intercostal spaces, synchronous with cardiac systole.*

1615. **Which of the following is not a part of Moschcowitz triad?**
*JAMA. 1933;100(21):1663-1664*

A. Widening of the area of cardiac flatness
B. Abrupt transition from pulmonary resonance to cardiac flatness
C. Widening of cardiac dulness in second intercostal space
D. Percussion dullness in fifth right intercostal space

1616. **Which of the following is the name given to the configuration of the cardiac silhouette in pericardial effusion?**
*Harrison's 20th Ed. Chapter 265 Page 1842*

A. Hour glass
B. Water bottle
C. Dust bin
D. Tear drop

*Chest roentgenogram in pericardial effusion may show a "water bottle" configuration of the cardiac silhouette but may be normal.*

1617. **Which of the following is concentrated in and interferes with the migration of neutrophils?**
*Harrison's 20th Ed. Chapter 265 Page 1843*

A. Aspirin
B. Indomethacin
C. Colchicine
D. Glucocorticoids

*Colchicine is concentrated in and interferes with the migration of neutrophils. In acute idiopathic pericarditis, colchicine should be administered for 3 months.*

1618. **In acute idiopathic pericarditis, full-dose corticosteroids should be given for what length of time?**
*Harrison's 20th Ed. Chapter 265 Page 1843*

A. 2–4 days
B. 2 weeks
C. 1 month
D. 3 months

*In acute idiopathic pericarditis, if the patient does not respond to or cannot tolerate NSAIDs and colchicine, glucocorticoids are indicated. However, since they increase the risk of subsequent recurrence, full-dose corticosteroids should be given for only 2–4 days and then tapered.*

1619. **Which of the following is an IL-1β receptor antagonist?**
*Harrison's 20th Ed. Chapter 265 Page 1843*

A. Anakinra
B. Azathioprine
C. Colchicine
D. None of the above

1620. **Which of the following drugs is not indicated in treatment of idiopathic acute pericarditis?**
*Harrison's 20th Ed. Chapter 265 Page 1843*

A. Phenylbutazone
B. Colchicine
C. Prednisone
D. Ibuprofen

*If treatment with aspirin is ineffective, colchicine is used. Colchicine may prevent recurrences.*

1621. **Azathioprine or anakinra is used in acute idiopathic pericarditis when?**
*Harrison's 20th Ed. Chapter 265 Page 1843*

A. Multiple, frequent, disabling recurrences for > 2 years
B. No response with continuing NSAIDs & colchicine
C. No response with glucocorticoids
D. All of the above

1622. **Which out of the following is the less common cause of cardiac tamponade?**
*Harrison's 20th Ed. Chapter 265 Page 1843*

A. Neoplastic disease
B. Tuberculosis
C. Idiopathic pericarditis
D. Renal failure

*3 commonest causes of tamponade are neoplastic disease, idiopathic pericarditis & renal failure.*

### 1623. In cardiac tamponade, Beck's triad consists of all except?
*Harrison's 20th Ed. Chapter 265 Page 1843*

A. Hypotension
B. Soft or absent heart sounds
C. Pulsus paradoxus
D. Jugular venous distention with a prominent "x" descent but an absent "y" descent

Three main features of acute cardiac tamponade (Beck's triad) are hypotension, soft, muffled or absent heart sounds, and jugular venous distention (JVD) with a prominent "x" descent but an absent "y" descent. Beck triad for chronic tamponade consists of increased CVP (JVD), ascites, and a small quiet heart (muffled heart sounds).

### 1624. Presence of which of the following should raise suspicion of cardiac tamponade?
*Harrison's 20th Ed. Chapter 265 Page 1843*

A. Reduction in amplitude of QRS complexes
B. Electrical alternans of P wave
C. Electrical alternans of QRS or T waves
D. All of the above

### 1625. In ECG, electrical alternans may be present in?
*Harrison's 20th Ed. Chapter 265 Page 1844 Table 265-2*

A. Cardiac tamponade
B. Constrictive pericarditis
C. Restrictive cardiomyopathy
D. Right ventricular myocardial infarction (RVMI)

### 1626. Kussmaul's sign is absent in which of the following?
*Harrison's 20th Ed. Chapter 265 Page 1844 Table 265-2*

A. Cardiac tamponade
B. Constrictive pericarditis
C. Restrictive cardiomyopathy
D. Right ventricular myocardial infarction (RVMI)

When jugular veins are distended and venous pressure fails to decline during inspiration is called Kussmaul's sign. It is absent in cardiac tamponade and is seen in chronic pericarditis, tricuspid stenosis, right ventricular infarction, and restrictive cardiomyopathy.

### 1627. Right ventricular size is small in which of the following?
*Harrison's 20th Ed. Chapter 265 Page 1844 Table 265-2*

A. Cardiac tamponade
B. Constrictive pericarditis
C. Restrictive cardiomyopathy
D. Right ventricular myocardial infarction (RVMI)

### 1628. On echocardiography, right atrial collapse and right ventricular diastolic collapse (RVDC) is present in which of the following?
*Harrison's 20th Ed. Chapter 265 Page 1844 Table 265-2*

A. Cardiac tamponade
B. Constrictive pericarditis
C. Restrictive cardiomyopathy
D. Right ventricular myocardial infarction (RVMI)

### 1629. Prominent "y" descent is usually present in which of the following condition?
*Harrison's 20th Ed. Chapter 265 Page 1844 Table 265-2*

A. Cardiac tamponade
B. Constrictive pericarditis
C. Restrictive cardiomyopathy
D. Right ventricular myocardial infarction (RVMI)

### 1630. Prominent "x" descent is rare in?
*Harrison's 20th Ed. Chapter 265 Page 1844 Table 265-2*

A. Cardiac tamponade
B. Constrictive pericarditis
C. Restrictive cardiomyopathy
D. Right ventricular myocardial infarction (RVMI)

In constrictive pericarditis, right & left atrial pressure pulses display an M-shaped contour, with prominent x and y descents. y descent, which is absent or diminished in cardiac tamponade, is the most prominent deflection in constrictive pericarditis. It reflects rapid early filling of the ventricles. y descent is interrupted by a rapid rise in atrial pressure during early diastole, when ventricular filling is impeded by constricting pericardium. In constrictive pericarditis, ventricular pressure pulses in both ventricles exhibit characteristic "square root" signs during diastole.

### 1631. Pericardial knock is often present in?
*Harrison's 20th Ed. Chapter 265 Page 1844 Table 265-2*

A. Cardiac tamponade
B. Constrictive pericarditis
C. Restrictive cardiomyopathy
D. RVMI

An early third heart sound i.e., a pericardial knock, occurring at the cardiac apex 0.09–0.12 s after aortic valve closure, is often conspicuous in constrictive pericarditis. It is due to an abrupt cessation of ventricular filling.

### 1632. Pulsus paradoxus is defined as a decrease in systolic arterial pressure of?
*Harrison's 20th Ed. Chapter 265 Page 1843*

A. > 10 mm Hg with inspiration
B. > 20 mm Hg with inspiration
C. > 30 mm Hg with inspiration
D. > 40 mm Hg with inspiration

The presence of cardiac tamponade consists of a greater than normal (10 mm Hg) inspiratory decline in systolic arterial pressure.

### 1633. Pulsus paradoxus is most common in?
*Harrison's 20th Ed. Chapter 265 Page 1843*

A. Cardiac tamponade
B. Constrictive pericarditis
C. Restrictive cardiomyopathy
D. All of the above

Paradoxical pulse occurs not only in cardiac tamponade but also in approximately one-third of patients with constrictive pericarditis.

### 1634. Pulsus paradoxus is observed in which of the following condition?
*Harrison's 20th Ed. Chapter 265 Page 1843*

A. Hypovolemic shock
B. Acute and chronic obstructive airways disease
C. Pulmonary embolus
D. All of the above

Pulsus paradoxus is not pathognomonic of pericardial disease as it may be observed in some cases of hypovolemic shock, acute & chronic obstructive airways disease & pulmonary embolus.

### 1635. The term pulsus paradoxus was coined by?
*Cleveland Clinic Journal of Medicine. 2013;80(2):109*

A. Korotkoff
B. Bainbridge
C. Kussmaul
D. Meyers

In 1873, term pulsus paradoxus was coined by Adolph Kussmaul. This was the time when physicians could even measure blood pressure.

### 1636. Factors that can oppose pulsus paradoxus include?
*Cleveland Clinic Journal of Medicine. 2013;80(2):109*

A. Positive pressure ventilation
B. Severe aortic regurgitation
C. Atrial septal defect
D. All of the above

### 1637. Factors that can oppose pulsus paradoxus include?
*Cleveland Clinic Journal of Medicine. 2013;80(2):109*

A. Severe left ventricular hypertrophy
B. Severe left ventricular dysfunction
C. Intravascular volume depletion
D. All of the above

### 1638. Doppler ultrasound in cardiac tamponade shows marked increase in flow velocities during inspiration across?
*Harrison's 20th Ed. Chapter 265 Page 1843*

A. Pulmonic valve
B. Pulmonic vein
C. Mitral valve
D. Aortic valve

In cardiac tamponade, Doppler ultrasound shows that tricuspid & pulmonic valve flow velocities increase markedly during inspiration, whereas pulmonic vein, mitral & aortic flow velocities diminish.

### 1639. Pericardiocentesis is done by which of the following approaches?
*Harrison's 20th Ed. Chapter 265 Page 1844*

A. Apical
B. Parasternal
C. Subxiphoid
D. Any of the above

### 1640. Which of the following about pericardiocentesis in cardiac tamponade is false?
*Harrison's 20th Ed. Chapter 265 Page 1844*

A. Pericardiocentesis must not be delayed
B. Pericardial fluid should be drained as completely as possible
C. Small, multiholed catheter may be left in place
D. None of the above

### 1641. Viral or idiopathic acute pericarditis occurs most commonly in?
*Harrison's 20th Ed. Chapter 265 Page 1845*

A. Infants
B. Young adult males
C. Menopausal females
D. Elderly males

Viral or idiopathic acute pericarditis occurs at all ages but is most common in young adult males.

### 1642. In viral or idiopathic acute pericarditis, fever & precordial pain develop how many days after a presumed viral illness?
*Harrison's 20th Ed. Chapter 265 Page 1845*

A. 3–5 days
B. 10–12 days
C. 14–21 days
D. 21–30 days

In viral or idiopathic acute pericarditis, almost simultaneous development of fever & precordial pain occurs 10 - 12 days after a presumed viral illness.

### 1643. Recurrent pericarditis after acute idiopathic pericarditis occurs in what percentage of patients?
*Harrison's 20th Ed. Chapter 265 Page 1845*

A. 5%
B. 10%
C. 25%
D. 50%

The most frequent complication of acute idiopathic pericarditis is recurrent (relapsing) pericarditis, which occurs in about one-fourth of patients.

### 1644. Abnormal T waves may persist for what length of time after acute idiopathic pericarditis?
*Harrison's 20th Ed. Chapter 265 Page 1845*

A. 3 months
B. 1 year
C. 3 years
D. Several years

### 1645. Which of the following is false about postcardiac injury syndrome?
*Harrison's 20th Ed. Chapter 265 Page 1845*

A. Clinical picture mimics acute viral or idiopathic pericarditis
B. Usually develops 1–4 weeks after the cardiac injury
C. Cardiac tamponade is rare
D. None of the above

Postcardiac injury syndrome results from a hypersensitivity reaction to antigens originating from injured myocardial tissue and/or pericardium.

### 1646. Which out of the following collagen vascular diseases is commonly complicated by pericarditis?
*Harrison's 20th Ed. Chapter 265 Page 1845*

A. Systemic lupus erythematosus (SLE)
B. Rheumatoid arthritis
C. Scleroderma
D. Polyarteritis nodosa

### 1647. In which of the following conditions, pericarditis may be of the fibrinous variety?
*Harrison's 20th Ed. Chapter 265 Page 1845*

A. Postcardiac injury syndrome
B. Uremic pericarditis
C. Dialysis-associated pericarditis
D. All of the above

**1648. In rheumatoid arthritis, pericardial fluid has which of the following features?**
*Harrison's 20th Ed. Chapter 265 Page 1845*

A. Exudate
B. Decreased concentrations of complement and glucose
C. Elevated cholesterol
D. All of the above

**1649. In constrictive pericarditis, right & left atrial pressure pulses display a contour of the shape of?**
*Harrison's 20th Ed. Chapter 265 Page 1846*

A. A - shape
B. M - shape
C. V - shape
D. W - shape

*In constrictive pericarditis, right & left atrial pressure pulses show M-shaped contour, with prominent x and y descents. The y descent, reflects rapid early filling of ventricles (absent or diminished in cardiac tamponade) is the most prominent deflection in constrictive pericarditis. The y descent is interrupted by a rapid rise in atrial pressure during early diastole, when ventricular filling is impeded by the constricting pericardium.*

**1650. Kussmaul's sign is not seen in?**
*Harrison's 20th Ed. Chapter 265 Page 1846*

A. Tricuspid stenosis
B. Right ventricular infarction
C. Restrictive cardiomyopathy
D. Cor pulmonale

*Kussmaul's sign refers to failure of venous pressure to decline during inspiration. It is common in chronic pericarditis but may occur in tricuspid stenosis, right ventricular infarction & restrictive cardiomyopathy. In cor pulmonale, Kussmaul's sign is negative.*

**1651. Broadbent's sign is a feature of?**
*Harrison's 20th Ed. Chapter 265 Page 1846*

A. Cardiac tamponade
B. Constrictive pericarditis
C. Restrictive cardiomyopathy
D. Right ventricular myocardial infarction (RVMI)

*In chronic constrictive pericarditis, apical pulse is reduced & may retract in systole - Broadbent's sign.*

**1652. Pericardial calcification is most common in?**
*Harrison's 20th Ed. Chapter 265 Page 1846*

A. Dialysis-associated pericarditis
B. Tuberculous pericarditis
C. Pericarditis due to systemic lupus erythematosus
D. Scleroderma

*Pericardial calcification is most common in tuberculous pericarditis.*

**1653. Which of the following is a feature of chronic constrictive pericarditis?**
*Harrison's 20th Ed. Chapter 265 Page 1846*

A. Jaundice
B. Intractable ascites
C. Splenomegaly
D. All of the above

**1654. Which of the following is less accurate to definitively establish or exclude the diagnosis of constrictive pericarditis?**
*Harrison's 20th Ed. Chapter 265 Page 1846*

A. Doppler echocardiography
B. CT
C. MRI
D. All of the above

**1655. Which of the following may simulate chronic constrictive pericarditis?**
*Harrison's 20th Ed. Chapter 265 Page 1846*

A. Cor pulmonale
B. Tricuspid stenosis
C. Restrictive cardiomyopathy
D. All of the above

**1656. Which of the following can cause subacute effusive-constrictive pericarditis?**
*Harrison's 20th Ed. Chapter 265 Page 1846*

A. Tuberculosis
B. Multiple attacks of acute idiopathic pericarditis
C. Renal failure
D. All of the above

**1657. Tuberculous pericarditis may present as?**
*Harrison's 20th Ed. Chapter 265 Page 1846*

A. Pericardial effusion
B. Chronic constrictive pericarditis
C. Subacute effusive constrictive pericarditis
D. Any of the above

**1658. The possible sequelae of pericarditis include?**
*N Engl J Med. 2004;351:2195-202*

A. Cardiac tamponade
B. Recurrent pericarditis
C. Pericardial constriction
D. All of the above

**1659. The presence of which of the following is most sensitive indicator of cardiac tamponade?**
*N Engl J Med. 2004;351:2195-202*

A. Systemic arterial hypotension
B. Tachycardia
C. Elevated jugular venous pressure
D. Pulsus paradoxus

**1660. The appearance of cardiomegaly on chest radiography indicates a pericardial effusion of?**
*N Engl J Med. 2004;351:2195-202*

A. > 150 mL
B. > 250 mL
C. > 350 mL
D. > 450 mL

**1661. Drugs implicated in the causation of pericarditis include?**
*N Engl J Med. 2004;351:2195-202*

A. Dantrolene
B. Doxorubicin
C. Hydralazine
D. All of the above

**1662. Drugs implicated in the causation of pericarditis include?**
*N Engl J Med. 2004;351:2195-202*

A. Isoniazid
B. Methysergide
C. Pergolide
D. All of the above

**1663. Drugs implicated in the causation of pericarditis include?**
*N Engl J Med. 2004;351:2195-202*

A. Phenylbutazone
B. Phenytoin
C. Procainamide
D. All of the above

*Procainamide, hydralazine, phenytoin, isoniazid, minoxidil, anticoagulants, methysergide can cause pericarditis.*

**1664. Plasma troponin concentrations are elevated in what percent of patients with pericarditis?**
*N Engl J Med. 2004;351:2195-202*

A. 10 to 15 percent
B. 20 to 25 percent
C. 35 to 50 percent
D. 50 to 60 percent

**1665. Which of the following is a complication of rapid pericardiocentesis?**
*Cleveland Clinic Journal of Medicine. 2013;80(2):109*

A. Hypotension
B. Pulmonary embolism
C. Pulmonary edema
D. All of the above

*The mechanism of pulmonary edema occuring after rapid pericardiocentesis is a sudden increase in right ventricular stroke volume and resultant left ventricular filling after excess pericardial fluid is removed, before systemic arteries, which constrict to keep the systemic blood pressure up during cardiac tamponade, have had time to relax.*

**1666. A large pericardial effusion is diagnosed if the echo-free space on 2D echocardiography is?**
*N Engl J Med. 2004;351:2195-202*

A. > 10 mm
B. > 20 mm
C. > 30 mm
D. > 40 mm

**1667. Which of the following endocrine diseases can cause cardiac tamponade?**
*Cleveland Clinic Journal of Medicine. 2013;80(2):109*

A. Hyperthyroidism
B. Hypothyroidism
C. Conn's syndrome
D. Addison's syndrome

**1668. Pericardial fluid is turbid, like gold paint in which of the following conditions?**
*Cleveland Clinic Journal of Medicine. 2013;80(2):109*

A. Mycobacterial infection
B. Rheumatoid arthritis
C. Myxedema
D. All of the above

**1669. Interferon alpha is reported to be beneficial in pericarditis caused by?**
*Cleveland Clinic Journal of Medicine. 2013;80(2):109*

A. Cytomegalovirus
B. Coxsackie B
C. Adenovirus
D. Parvovirus

**1670. Hyperimmune globulin is reported to be beneficial in pericarditis caused by?**
*Cleveland Clinic Journal of Medicine. 2013;80(2):109*

A. Cytomegalovirus
B. Adenovirus
C. Parvovirus
D. All of the above

*Hyperimmune globulin is beneficial in cytomegalovirus, adenovirus & parvovirus pericarditis, while interferon alpha has been reported to be so in coxsackie B pericarditis.*

**1671. Cardiac manifestation of systemic lupus erythematosus is?**
*Harrison's 20th Ed. Chapter 349 Page 2520*

A. Pericarditis
B. Libman-Sacks endocarditis
C. Myocarditis
D. All of the above

*Pericarditis, Libman-Sacks endocarditis, myocarditis, arterial and venous thrombosis are the cadriac manifestation of systemic lupus erythematosus.*

# Atrial Myxoma and Other Cardiac Tumors

**1672. Cardiac masses include which of the following?**
*Harrison's 20th Ed. Chapter 266 Page 1847*

A. Vegetation
B. Thrombus
C. Myocardial hypertrophy
D. All of the above

**1673. Which of the following imaging modality may differentiate tumor from thrombus?**
*Harrison's 20th Ed. Chapter 266 Page 1847 Table 266-1*

A. Transesophageal echocardiography (TEE)
B. Cardiac MRI with gadolinium contrast
C. Gated cardiac CT
D. FDG-PET

**1674. Which of the following imaging modality allows better assessment of cardiac calcified lesions?**
*Harrison's 20th Ed. Chapter 266 Page 1847 Table 266-1*

A. Transesophageal echocardiography (TEE)
B. Cardiac MRI with gadolinium contrast
C. Gated cardiac CT
D. FDG-PET

**1675. Which of the following imaging modality allows better assessment of cardiac neuroendocrine tumors?**
*Harrison's 20th Ed. Chapter 266 Page 1847 Table 266-1*

A. Transesophageal echocardiography (TEE)
B. Cardiac MRI with gadolinium contrast
C. Gated cardiac CT
D. FDG-PET

**1676. Which of the following is the most common primary tumor of heart in adults?**
*Harrison's 20th Ed. Chapter 266 Page 1847*

A. Myxoma
B. Rhabdomyoma
C. Fibroma
D. Hemangioma

*Myxomas are the most common type of primary cardiac tumor in all age groups, most commonly in third to sixth decade, with a female predilection.*

**1677. Which of the following is the most common primary tumor of heart in adults?**
*Harrison's 20th Ed. Chapter 266 Page 1847*

A. Lipoma
B. Myocytic hamartoma
C. Myxoma
D. Inflammatory psuedotumor

**1678. Which of the following statements is false?**
*Harrison's 20th Ed. Chapter 266 Page 1847*

A. 75% of primary tumors of heart are benign
B. Almost all primary cardiac malignant tumors are sarcomas
C. All cardiac tumors have life-threatening complications
D. None of the above

**1679. Which of the following statements about cardiac myxoma is false?**
*Harrison's 20th Ed. Chapter 266 Page 1847, J Thorac Dis 2014;6(S1):S32-S38*

A. Most common in third and sixth decades of life
B. Female predilection
C. Myxomas can originate from any of the heart chambers
D. Most myxomas are familial

*Myxomas represent the most common primary cardiac tumors. They can appear in almost all age groups but most commonly between III & VI decades of life with a female predilection. Myxomas can originate from any of the heart chambers, most commonly from left atrium. Right atrial myxomas and heart valve myxomas are rare. Most myxomas are single and sporadic although familiar cases are also well known.*

**1680. Which of the following statements about familial cardiac myxoma is false?**
*Harrison's 20th Ed. Chapter 266 Page 1847, J Thorac Dis 2014;6(S1):S32-S38*

A. Tend to occur in elderly individuals
B. Often multiple
C. May be ventricular in location
D. More likely to recur after initial resection

*Familial myxomas tend to occur in younger individuals, are often multiple, may be ventricular in location, and are more likely to recur after initial resection. Myxomas recur in 12–22% of familial cases but in only 1–2% of sporadic cases.*

**1681. Cardiac myxoma in the left atrium originate from?**
*Harrison's 20th Ed. Chapter 266 Page 1847, J Thorac Dis 2014;6(S1):S32-S38*

A. Left atrial appendage
B. Mitral valve annulus
C. Interatrial septum near or on the fossa ovalis
D. Any of the above

*Cardiac myxoma most commonly occurs in the left atrium, originating from the interatrial septum near or on the fossa ovalis.*

**1682. Which of the following statements about sporadic cardiac myxoma is false?**
*Harrison's 20th Ed. Chapter 266 Page 1847, J Thorac Dis 2014;6(S1):S32-S38*

A. Solitary
B. Often pedunculated on a fibrovascular stalk
C. Arise from interatrial septum in the vicinity of fossa ovalis
D. None of the above

*Most sporadic tumors are solitary, arise from the interatrial septum in the vicinity of the fossa ovalis (particularly in the left atrium), and are often pedunculated on a fibrovascular stalk.*

**1683. Carney syndrome is characterized by all except?**
*Harrison's 20th Ed. Chapter 266 Page 1847*

A. Spotty skin pigmentation
B. Myxomas
C. Cataract
D. Pituitary adenomas

Carney complex comprises of myxomas (cardiac, skin, and/or breast), lentigines and/or pigmented nevi and endocrine overactivity (primary nodular adrenal cortical disease with or without Cushing's syndrome, testicular tumors, and/or pituitary adenomas with gigantism or acromegaly).

**1684. NAME syndrome includes all except?**
*Harrison's 20th Ed. Chapter 266 Page 1847*

A. Nevi
B. Atrial myxoma
C. Myxoedema
D. Ephelides

NAME syndrome consists of nevi, atrial myxoma, myxoid neurofibroma and ephelides.

**1685. LAMB syndrome includes all except?**
*Harrison's 20th Ed. Chapter 266 Page 1847*

A. Lentigines
B. Atrial myxoma
C. Melanoma
D. Blue nevi

LAMB syndrome consists of lentigines, atrial myxoma and blue nevi.

**1686. Myxoma can occur in?**
*Harrison's 20th Ed. Chapter 266 Page 1847*

A. Left atrium
B. Left ventricle
C. Right ventricle
D. All of the above

Myxomas most commonly arise from left atrium, usually from a stalk attached to the atrial septum, 75% in the left atrium, up to 20% in the right atrium, and around 8% in the ventricles.

**1687. Which of the following gene best relates to Carney complex?**
*Harrison's 20th Ed. Chapter 266 Page 1847*

A. MEN1
B. NF1
C. PRKAR1A
D. VHL

The genetic basis of Carney complex is inactivating mutations in the tumor-suppressor gene PRKAR1A, which encodes protein kinase A type I-α regulatory subunit.

**1688. Which of the following statements about "tumor plop" is false?**
*Harrison's 20th Ed. Chapter 266 Page 1848, N Engl J Med. 2018; 379:e26*

A. Low-pitched sound on cardiac auscultation
B. Early or mid-diastole
C. Due to impact of tumor against mitral valve or ventricular wall
D. None of the above

**1689. Mechanism of symptoms of cardiac tumors is?**
*J Thorac Dis 2014;6(S1):S32-S38*

A. Intracardiac obstruction
B. Systematic embolization of tumor fragments
C. Constitutional symptoms
D. All of the above

**1690. The most common presenting symptom of myxoma is?**
*J Thorac Dis 2014;6(S1):S32-S38*

A. Dyspnoea
B. Chest pain
C. Pain and paraesthesia of the limbs
D. Weight loss

The most common presenting symptom of myxoma is dyspnoea.

**1691. Differential diagnosis of myxoma include?**
*Harrison's 20th Ed. Chapter 266 Page 1848*

A. Endocarditis
B. Collagen vascular disease
C. Paraneoplastic syndrome
D. All of the above

Constitutional signs and symptoms in myxoma include fever, weight loss, cachexia, malaise, arthralgias, rash, clubbing and Raynaud's phenomenon.

**1692. Most common tumor of the cardiac valves is?**
*Harrison's 20th Ed. Chapter 266 Page 1848*

A. Lipoma
B. Papillary fibroelastoma
C. Sarcoma
D. Cardiac metastases

Papillary fibroelastomas are the most common tumors of the cardiac valves.

**1693. Which of the following best relates to papillary fibroelastoma?**
*Harrison's 20th Ed. Chapter 266 Page 1848*

A. Cardiac trauma
B. Irradiation
C. Cytomegalovirus
D. Folic acid deficiency

Remnants of cytomegalovirus have been recovered from papillary fibroelastoma, raising the possibility that they arise as a result of chronic viral endocarditis.

**1694. Which of the following is the most common primary tumor of heart in infants and children?**
*Harrison's 20th Ed. Chapter 266 Page 1848*

A. Myxoma
B. Rhabdomyoma
C. Lipoma
D. Hemangioma

Rhabdomyomas and fibromas are the most common cardiac tumors in infants and children and usually occur in ventricles. Rhabdomyomas are strongly associated with tuberous sclerosis.

**1695. Which of the following about cardiac rhabdomyoma is false?**
*Harrison's 20th Ed. Chapter 266 Page 1848*

A. Multiple in 90% of cases
B. Strongly associated with tuberous sclerosis
C. Have a tendency to regress completely or partially
D. None of the above

**1696. Which of the following cardiac tumors are universally ventricular in location?**
*Harrison's 20th Ed. Chapter 266 Page 1849*

A. Fibroma
B. Rhabdomyoma
C. Lipoma
D. Hemangioma

*Fibromas are usually single, universally ventricular in location, often calcified, tend to grow and cause arrhythmias and obstructive symptoms, and should be completely resected when possible.*

**1697. Which of the following heart tumor is located in the roof of the left atrium?**
*Harrison's 20th Ed. Chapter 266 Page 1849*

A. Chemodectoma
B. Neurilemoma
C. Granular cell myoblastoma
D. Paraganglioma

*Paragangliomas represent extra-adrenal pheochromocytomas. Most are located in roof of left atrium. They are highly vascular and may be hormonally active, resulting in uncontrolled hypertension.*

**1698. Which of the following heart tumour is intramyocardial in location?**
*Harrison's 20th Ed. Chapter 266 Page 1849*

A. Myxoma
B. Rhabdomyoma
C. Lipoma
D. Hemangioma

*Hemangiomas and mesotheliomas most often are intramyocardial in location, and may cause atrioventricular (AV) conduction disturbances.*

**1699. Which of the following about cardiac sarcoma is false?**
*Harrison's 20th Ed. Chapter 266 Page 1849*

A. Almost all malignant primary cardiac tumors are sarcomas
B. Angiosarcomas are the most common type in adults
C. Rhabdomyosarcomas are the most common type in children
D. None of the above

**1700. Which of the following cardiac sarcoma may respond to a combination of chemo- and radiotherapy?**
*Harrison's 20th Ed. Chapter 266 Page 1849*

A. Angiosarcoma
B. Lymphosarcoma
C. Rhabdomyosarcoma
D. None of the above

**1701. Relative incidence of cardiac metastases is highest in which of the following malignancies?**
*Harrison's 20th Ed. Chapter 266 Page 1849*

A. Leukemia
B. Lymphoma
C. Malignant melanoma
D. None of the above

*Relative incidence of cardiac metastases is high in malignant melanoma.*

**1702. Most common primary originating site of cardiac metastases is?**
*Harrison's 20th Ed. Chapter 266 Page 1849*

A. Carcinoma breast
B. Carcinoma thyroid
C. Carcinoma pancreas
D. Carcinoma testes

*Most common primary originating sites of cardiac metastases are carcinoma of breast & lung.*

**1703. In cardiac metastases, which of the following is least involved?**
*Harrison's 20th Ed. Chapter 266 Page 1849*

A. Pericardium
B. Myocardium
C. Endocardium
D. Any of the above

*Cardiac metastases occur via hematogenous or lymphangitic spread or by direct tumor invasion. Pericardium is most often involved, followed by myocardial and rarely by involvement of endocardium or cardiac valves.*

**1704. Which of the following investigation is most useful in diagnostic evaluation of cardiac metastases & cardiac tumors?**
*Harrison's 20th Ed. Chapter 266 Page 1849*

A. Echocardiography
B. CT
C. Cardiac MRI
D. Angiography

*Cardiac MRI plays a central role in diagnostic evaluation of cardiac metastases & cardiac tumors.*

**1705. Characteristic endocardial lesions of SLE (Libman & Sacks) are most often located at?**
*Harrison's 16th Ed. 1424*

A. Atria
B. Ventricular surface of mitral valve
C. Left ventricular outflow tract
D. Right ventricular outflow tract

**1706. What is meant by "commotio cordis"?**
*N Engl J Med. 2010;362:917-27*

A. Impact to chest wall overlying heart
B. Torsion injury of heart
C. Kinking of coronary artery
D. Aneurysmal rupture of coronary artery

*Blunt, nonpenetrating injuries to chest that trigger ventricular fibrillation is referred to as commotio cordis (Latin: agitation of the heart). Impact to chest wall overlying heart during the susceptible phase of repolarization just prior to peak of T wave is the cause. Prompt defibrillation saves life.*

**1707. In Commotio Cordis, which of the following is injured?**
*N Engl J Med. 2010;362:917-27*

A. Ribs
B. Sternum
C. Heart
D. None of the above

*In Commotio Cordis, there is no damage to the ribs, sternum, or heart. Also, there is no underlying cardiovascular disease in the patient. In cardiac contusion, high-impact blows result in traumatic damage to myocardial tissue and the overlying thorax.*

**1708. Which of the following is the most frequent cardiovascular cause of sudden death in young athletes?**
*N Engl J Med. 2010;362:917-27*

A. Hypertrophic cardiomyopathy
B. Congenital coronary-artery anomalies

C. Commotio Cordis
D. Cardiac contusion

*Commotio Cordis is among the most frequent cardiovascular causes of sudden death in young athletes, after hypertrophic cardiomyopathy and congenital coronary-artery anomalies.*

**1709. Which of the following about Commotio cordis is false?**
*N Engl J Med. 2010;362:917-27*

A. Predilection for children and adolescents
B. Rarely been reported in blacks or in girls or women
C. Most victims are white
D. None of the above

**1710. Broken-Heart Syndrome refers to?**
*Tex Heart Inst J. 2007;34(1):76-79*

A. Commotio cordis
B. Takotsubo syndrome
C. Cardiac contusion
D. Any of the above

*Takotsubo cardiomyopathy mimics acute coronary syndrome and is accompanied by reversible left ventricular apical ballooning in the absence of angiographically significant coronary artery stenosis. In Japanese, "Takotsubo" means "fishing pot for trapping octopus," and the left ventricle of a patient diagnosed with this condition resembles that shape. Takotsubo cardiomyopathy, which is transient and typically precipitated by acute emotional stress, is also known as "stress cardiomyopathy" or "broken-heart syndrome" or Gebrochenes-Herz syndrome.*

**1711. Which of the following is false about Takotsubo syndrome?**
*Tex Heart Inst J. 2007;34(1):76-79*

A. Sudden emotional trauma
B. Hyperdynamic function at ventricular base
C. Anterior ST-segment elevation
D. None of the above

*Takotsubo syndrome or apical ballooning syndrome is due to sudden emotional or physiologic trauma leading to dysfunction of mid-portion & apex of LV with hyperdynamic function at ventricular base. More common in women, it presents with chest pain, anterior ST-segment elevation & mildly elevated cardiac enzymes without significant epicardial coronary artery disease. Prognosis is favorable & complete & spontaneous resolution of ventricular dysfunction occurs within weeks.*

**1712. Which of the following is the most common vascular deceleration injury?**
*Scand J Trauma Resusc Emerg Med. 2009;17:42*

A. Post-pericardiotomy syndrome
B. Takotsubo syndrome
C. Commotio cordis
D. Rupture of the aorta

*Rupture of aorta, usually just above aortic valve or at the site of ligamentum arteriosum, is the most common vascular deceleration injury with clinical presentation similar to that of aortic dissection.*

# Non-ST-Segment Elevation Acute Coronary Syndrome (Non-ST-Segment Elevation Myocardial Infarction and Unstable Angina)

**1713. Acute coronary syndrome (ACS) includes?**
*Harrison's 20th Ed. Chapter 268 Page 1866*

A. ST-segment elevation MI (STEMI)
B. Non-ST-segment elevation MI (NSTEMI)
C. Unstable angina (UA)
D. All of the above

Patients with IHD fall into two large groups — those with stable angina secondary to chronic coronary artery disease and patients with acute coronary syndromes (ACS). ACS include patients with acute myocardial infarction with ST-segment elevation (STEMI) on their presenting ECG and those with non-ST-segment elevation acute coronary syndrome (NSTE-ACS). NSTE-ACS include patients with non-ST-segment elevation myocardial infarction (NSTEMI), who have evidence of myocyte necrosis and those with unstable angina (UA), who do not have evidence of myocyte necrosis.

**1714. Which of the following about non-ST-segment elevation myocardial infarction (NSTEMI) is false?**
*Harrison's 20th Ed. Chapter 268 Page 1866*

A. Acute coronary syndrome (ACS)
B. Non-ST-segment ↑ acute coronary syndrome (NSTE-ACS)
C. Evidence of myocyte necrosis
D. None of the above

**1715. Which of the following about unstable angina (UA) is false?**
*Harrison's 20th Ed. Chapter 268 Page 1866*

A. Acute coronary syndrome (ACS)
B. Non-ST-segment ↑ acute coronary syndrome (NSTE-ACS)
C. No evidence of myocyte necrosis
D. None of the above

**1716. Which of the following statements is false?**
*Harrison's 20th Ed. Chapter 268 Page 1866*

A. Relative incidence of NSTEMI is rising
B. Relative incidence of STEMI is declining
C. Relative incidence of UA is declining
D. None of the above

The relative incidence of NSTEMI is rising due to increasing burden of diabetes & chronic kidney disease in an aging population. Relative incidence of STEMI is declining due to greater use of aspirin, statins, and less smoking. Among patients with NSTE-ACS, the proportion with NSTEMI is rising while that with UA is falling because of the wider use of troponin assays with higher sensitivity to detect myocyte necrosis, thereby reclassifying UA as NSTEMI.

**1717. Which of the following is the most common pathophysiologic process in the development of UA?**
*Harrison's 20th Ed. Chapter 268 Page 1866*

A. Plaque rupture with superimposed nonocclusive thrombus
B. Dynamic obstruction
C. Progressive mechanical obstruction
D. Increased myocardial oxygen demand &/or decreased supply

UA/NSTEMI can be caused by a reduction in oxygen supply and/or by an increase in myocardial oxygen demand (tachycardia or severe anemia) superimposed on a coronary obstruction. Pathophysiologic processes leading to UA are plaque rupture or erosion with superimposed nonocclusive thrombus (most common cause), dynamic obstruction (coronary spasm, as in Prinzmetal's variant angina), progressive mechanical obstruction [rapidly advancing coronary atherosclerosis or restenosis following percutaneous coronary intervention (PCI)] & secondary UA related to increased myocardial oxygen demand and/or decreased supply (anemia). More than one of these processes may be involved in many patients.

**1718. Among patients with NSTE-ACS, what percentage would have left main stenosis coronary artery disease?**
*Harrison's 20th Ed. Chapter 268 Page 1866*

A. 10%
B. 20%
C. 30%
D. 40%

**1719. Among patients with NSTE-ACS, what percentage would have three-vessel coronary artery disease?**
*Harrison's 20th Ed. Chapter 268 Page 1866*

A. 5%
B. 15%
C. 35%
D. 40%

**1720. Among patients with NSTE-ACS, what percentage would have two-vessel coronary artery disease?**
*Harrison's 20th Ed. Chapter 268 Page 1866*

A. 10%
B. 20%
C. 30%
D. 40%

**1721. Among patients with NSTE-ACS, what percentage would have single-vessel coronary artery disease?**
*Harrison's 20th Ed. Chapter 268 Page 1866*

A. 5%
B. 20%
C. 30%
D. 40%

**1722. Among patients with UA/NSTEMI, what percentage would have no critical coronary artery stenosis?**
*Harrison's 20th Ed. Chapter 268 Page 1866*

A. 5%
B. 15%
C. 30%
D. 40%

Among patients with NSTE-ACS studied angiographically, ~10% have stenosis of left main coronary artery, 35% have three-vessel CAD, 20% have two-vessel disease, 20% have single-vessel disease and 15% have no apparent critical epicardial coronary artery stenosis.

**1723. Vulnerable plaques are composed of?**
*Harrison's 20th Ed. Chapter 268 Page 1866*

A. Rich lipid core and thin fibrous cap
B. Rich lipid core and thick fibrous cap
C. Poor lipid core and thin fibrous cap
D. Poor lipid core and thick fibrous cap

Histologic studies indicate that the coronary plaques prone to disruption are those with a rich lipid core and a thin fibrous cap.

### 1724. Which of the following is true for unstable angina (UA)?
*Harrison's 20th Ed. Chapter 268 Page 1868*

A. Occurs at rest lasting > 10 minutes
B. Relatively recent onset angina pectoris
C. Occurs with a crescendo pattern
D. All of the above

*UA is defined as angina pectoris or equivalent ischemic discomfort with at least one of three features: it occurs at rest usually lasting > 10 minutes, it is severe and of relatively recent onset (previous 2 weeks), and/or it occurs with a crescendo pattern. The diagnosis of NSTEMI is established if a patient with the clinical features of UA develops evidence of myocardial necrosis, as reflected in elevated cardiac biomarkers.*

### 1725. The clinical hallmark of NSTE-ACS is chest pain that is?
*Harrison's 20th Ed. Chapter 268 Page 1868*

A. Substernal
B. Retrosternal
C. Suprasternal
D. Any of the above

*Clinical hallmark of UA/NSTEMI is chest pain, typically located in the substernal region or sometimes in epigastrium, that radiates to the neck & jaw, left shoulder, and/or the left arm.*

### 1726. Which of the following is considered as anginal equivalent?
*Harrison's 20th Ed. Chapter 268 Page 1868*

A. Dyspnea
B. Epigastric discomfort
C. Nausea
D. All of the above

*Anginal equivalents are dyspnea, epigastric discomfort, nausea, or weakness. They may occur instead of chest discomfort.*

### 1727. Anginal equivalents are more frequent in?
*Harrison's 20th Ed. Chapter 268 Page 1868*

A. Women
B. Elderly
C. Patients with diabetes mellitus
D. All of the above

*Anginal equivalents are more frequent in women, the elderly, and patients with diabetes mellitus.*

### 1728. T-wave inversions in NSTE-ACS have more specificity for myocardial ischemia if they are?
*Harrison's 20th Ed. Chapter 268 Page 1868*

A. ≥ 0.1 mV deep
B. ≥ 0.2 mV deep
C. ≥ 0.3 mV deep
D. ≥ 0.4 mV deep

*T-wave changes in NSTE-ACS are more common but are less specific signs of ischemia, unless they are new and deep T-wave inversions (≥ 0.3 mV).*

### 1729. Minor troponin elevations can be caused by?
*Harrison's 20th Ed. Chapter 268 Page 1868*

A. Heart failure
B. Myocarditis
C. Pulmonary embolism
D. All of the above

*Minor troponin elevations are due to congestive heart failure, myocarditis or pulmonary embolism.*

### 1730. Which of the following is a cause of elevated cardiac troponin?
*Harrison's 20th Ed. Chapter 268 Page 1868 Table 268-1*

A. Tachyarrhythmias
B. Aortic stenosis
C. Aortic dissection
D. All of the above

### 1731. Which of the following is a cause of elevated cardiac troponin?
*Harrison's 20th Ed. Chapter 268 Page 1868 Table 268-1*

A. Pericarditis
B. Takotsubo cardiomyopathy
C. Coronary spasm
D. All of the above

### 1732. Which of the following is a cause of elevated cardiac troponin?
*Harrison's 20th Ed. Chapter 268 Page 1868 Table 268-1*

A. Hypertensive emergencies
B. Amyloidosis
C. Hemochromatosis
D. All of the above

### 1733. Which of the following is a cause of elevated cardiac troponin?
*Harrison's 20th Ed. Chapter 268 Page 1868 Table 268-1*

A. Snake venom
B. Hypo or hyperthyroidism
C. Stroke
D. All of the above

### 1734. Which of the following improves the accuracy & speed of the diagnostic evaluation in NSTEMI-ACS?
*Harrison's 20th Ed. Chapter 268 Page 1868*

A. ECG
B. Cardiac biomarkers
C. Stress testing
D. Coronary computed tomographic angiography (CCTA)

### 1735. ECG & cardiac markers are typically obtained at what timings after presentation?
*Harrison's 20th Ed. Chapter 268 Page 1868*

A. Baseline, at 1 hour & at 3 hours
B. Baseline, at 3 hour & at 6 hours
C. Baseline, at 4–6 hours & at 12 hours
D. Baseline, at 6 hours & 24 hours

*ECGs and cardiac markers are typically obtained at baseline and at 4-6 hours and 12 hours after presentation.*

### 1736. What percentage of patients with documented NSTE-ACS carry a risk of early death (30 days)?
*Harrison's 20th Ed. Chapter 268 Page 1868*

A. 1 to 2%
B. 1 to 4%
C. 1 to 6%
D. 1 to 10%

### 1737. What percentage of patients with documented NSTE-ACS carry a risk of recurrent ACS?
*Harrison's 20th Ed. Chapter 268 Page 1868*

A. 1–4% during the first year
B. 3–8% during the first year
C. 5–15% during the first year
D. 9–35% during the first year

*1 to 10% patients with documented NSTE-ACS carry a risk of early death (30 days). 5 - 15% patients with documented NSTE-ACS carry a risk of recurrent ACS during the first year.*

### 1738. Number of independent risk factors included in clinical risk scoring system developed from Thrombolysis in Myocardial Infarction (TIMI) Trials is?
*Harrison's 20th Ed. Chapter 268 Page 1868*

A. 5
B. 7
C. 9
D. 11

*Clinical risk scoring system developed from the Thrombolysis in Myocardial Infarction (TIMI) Trials includes seven independent risk factors. They are age ≥ 65 years, 3 or more of the traditional risk factors for coronary heart disease, known history of coronary artery disease or coronary stenosis of at least 50%, daily aspirin use in the prior week, more than one anginal episode in the past 24 hour, ST segment deviation of at least 0.5 mm, and an elevated cardiac specific biomarker above the upper limit of normal.*

### 1739. Risk factor for CAD include?
*Harrison's 20th Ed. Chapter 268 Page 1868*

A. Elevated levels of creatinine
B. Brain natriuretic peptides
C. C-reactive protein
D. All of the above

*Besides the seven independent risk factors in Thrombolysis in Myocardial Infarction (TIMI) Trials, other risk factors are diabetes mellitus, left ventricular dysfunction & elevated levels of creatinine, brain natriuretic peptides & C-reactive protein.*

### 1740. B-type natriuretic peptide is a marker of?
*Harrison's 20th Ed. Chapter 268 Page 1868*

A. Vascular inflammation
B. Increased myocardial wall tension
C. Plaque rupture
D. All of the above

*C-reactive protein is a marker of vascular inflammation and B-type natriuretic peptide is a marker of increased myocardial wall tension.*

### 1741. According to which study, early invasive strategy conferred a 40% reduction in recurrent cardiac events in patients with an elevated cTn level?
*Harrison's 20th Ed. Chapter 268 Page 1868*

A. TRITON-TIMI 38 Trial
B. TACTICS-TIMI 18 Trial
C. FREEDOM Trial
D. SYNTAX Trial

*TACTICS-TIMI 18 Trial, an early invasive strategy conferred a 40% reduction in recurrent cardiac events in patients with an elevated cTn level, whereas no benefit was observed in those without detectable troponin.*

### 1742. Inhaled oxygen is given in patients of NSTE-ACS who have arterial $O_2$ saturation of?
*Harrison's 20th Ed. Chapter 268 Page 1869*

A. < 100%
B. < 96%
C. < 90%
D. < 86%

*Inhaled oxygen is given in patients of NSTE-ACS who have arterial $O_2$ saturation of <90%, and/or in those with heart failure and rales.*

### 1743. Instead of sublingual nitrates, intravenous nitroglycerin is recommended if ischemic pain persists after?
*Harrison's 20th Ed. Chapter 268 Page 1869*

A. Three doses given 5 minutes apart
B. Three doses given 15 minutes apart
C. Three doses given 30 minutes apart
D. Three doses given 60 minutes apart

*Nitrates should first be given sublingually or by buccal spray (0.3-0.6 mg) if the patient is having ischemic pain. If pain persists after three doses given 5 minutes apart, intravenous nitroglycerin (5–10 μg/minute using nonabsorbing tubing) is recommended. The rate of infusion may be increased by 10 μg/minute every 3–5 minute until symptoms are relieved, systolic arterial pressure falls to <100 mm Hg or the dose reaches 200 μg/minute.*

### 1744. Nitrates must not be administered if sildenafil (Viagra) has been used by the patient within the previous?
*Harrison's 20th Ed. Chapter 268 Page 1869*

A. 3 hours
B. 6 hours
C. 12 hours
D. 24 hours

*Absolute contraindications to the use of nitrates are hypotension or the recent use of a phosphodiesterase type 5 (PDE-5) inhibitor, sildenafil or vardenafil (within 24 hours), or tadalafil (within 48 hours).*

### 1745. In ACS, oral beta blockade is recommended to being heart rate to?
*Harrison's 20th Ed. Chapter 268 Page 1869*

A. 40 - 50 beats / minute
B. 50 - 60 beats / minute
C. 60 - 70 beats / minute
D. 70 - 80 beats / minute

*In patients with acute coronary syndrome (ACS), oral beta blockade targeted to a heart rate of 50–60 beats/minute is recommended.*

### 1746. In NSTE-ACS, verapamil or diltiazem, are recommended for patients who have?
*Harrison's 20th Ed. Chapter 268 Page 1869*

A. Lack of improvement after full-dose of nitrates
B. Lack of improvement after full-dose of beta blockers
C. Contraindications to nitrates or beta blockers
D. All of the above

*Heart rate slowing calcium channel blockers (verapamil or diltiazem) are recommended for patients who have persistent symptoms or ECG signs of ischemia after treatment with full-dose nitrates & beta blockers and in patients with contraindications to either class of these agents.*

### 1747. Administration of statins prior to percutaneous coronary intervention (PCI) reduces?
*Harrison's 20th Ed. Chapter 268 Page 1869*

A. Arrhythmias
B. Peri-procedural MI
C. Hypotension
D. All of the above

Early administration of intensive HMG-CoA reductase inhibitors (statins) prior to percutaneous coronary intervention (PCI), and continued thereafter, reduces peri-procedural MI and recurrences of ACS.

### 1748. Inadequate lipid lowering response to maximally tolerated statin is?
*Harrison's 20th Ed. Chapter 268 Page 1869*

A. < 10% decrease in LDL-C from untreated baseline
B. < 20% decrease in LDL-C from untreated baseline
C. < 40% decrease in LDL-C from untreated baseline
D. < 50% decrease in LDL-C from untreated baseline

Inadequate lipid lowering response to maximally tolerated statin is <50% decrease in LDL-C from untreated baseline or LDL-C on treatment >70 mg/dL.

### 1749. In patients with acute coronary syndrome (ACS), typical initial dose of aspirin is?
*Harrison's 20th Ed. Chapter 268 Page 1869*

A. 75 mg / day
B. 162 mg / day
C. 325 mg / day
D. 1000 mg / day

In patients with acute coronary syndrome (ACS), the typical initial dose of aspirin is 325 mg/day, with lower doses (75 - 100 mg/day) recommended thereafter.

### 1750. "Aspirin resistance" has been noted what percentage of patients?
*Harrison's 19th Ed. Page 1596*

A. 0.2 - 0.8%
B. 1 - 1.6%
C. 1.6 - 2%
D. 2 - 8%

"Aspirin resistance" has been noted in 2-8% of patients.

### 1751. Letter "C" in CURE trial stands for?
*Harrison's 19th Ed. Page 1596*

A. Coronary
B. Carotid
C. Clopidogrel
D. Cardiac

CURE is CURE trial stands for Clopidogrel in Unstable Angina to Prevent Recurrent Events.

### 1752. Prasugrel is contraindicated in patients with?
*Harrison's 20th Ed. Chapter 268 Page 1870*

A. Peripheral artery disease
B. Prior stroke or transient ischemic attack
C. Tuberculosis
D. Hypertension

Thienopyridine drug prasugrel has a more rapid onset, and higher level of platelet inhibition than clopidogrel. Dose is 60 mg load followed by 10 mg/day for up to 15 months. It is contraindicated in patients with prior stroke or transient ischemic attack.

### 1753. With prasugrel therapy, which of the following was prone to serious bleeding?
*N Engl J Med. 2009;361:941*

A. Elderly
B. Underweight
C. Patients with previous stroke or transient ischemic attack
D. All of the above

With prasugrel therapy, three subgroups appeared to be particularly prone to serious bleeding—the elderly, the underweight, and patients with a previous stroke or transient ischemic attack.

### 1754. Which of the following is a reversible platelet P2Y12 inhibitor?
*Harrison's 20th Ed. Chapter 268 Page 1870*

A. Clopidogrel
B. Prasugrel
C. Ticagrelor
D. All of the above

Ticagrelor is a reversible and direct-acting oral antagonist of the adenosine diphosphate receptor P2Y12. It reduces the risk of cardiovascular death, MI, or stroke by 16% compared with clopidogrel in ACS patients without increasing the risk of total bleeding.

### 1755. Dual antiplatelet therapy (DAPT) should continue for how long in patients with NSTE-ACS?
*Harrison's 20th Ed. Chapter 268 Page 1870*

A. At least 3 months
B. At least 6 months
C. At least 1 year
D. At least 2 years

Dual antiplatelet therapy (DAPT) should continue for at least 1 year in patients with NSTE-ACS, especially those with a drug-eluting stent, to prevent stent thrombosis.

### 1756. Which of the following is an intravenous P2Y12 inhibitor?
*Harrison's 20th Ed. Chapter 268 Page 1871*

A. Cangrelor
B. Ticlopidine
C. Clopidogrel
D. Ticagrelor

Cangrelor is an intravenous, direct and rapidly acting, P2Y12 inhibitor.

### 1757. Besides aspirin & clopidogrel, triple antiplatelet therapy uses which of the following as the third drug?
*Harrison's 20th Ed. Chapter 268 Page 1871*

A. Cangrelor
B. Bivalirudin
C. Glycoprotein IIb/IIIa inhibitors
D. Prasugrel

The addition of intravenous glycoprotein IIb/IIIa inhibitors to aspirin and a P2Y12 inhibitor (triple antiplatelet therapy) should be reserved for unstable patients undergoing PCI. These include patients with recurrent rest pain, elevated cTn, and ECG changes, & those who have a coronary thrombus evident on angiography.

### 1758. Which of the following is a direct thrombin inhibitor?
*Harrison's 20th Ed. Chapter 268 Page 1871*

A. Heparin
B. Bivalirudin
C. Fondaparinux
D. Enoxaparin

Fondaparinux is a Factor Xa inhibitor. Bivalirudin is a direct thrombin inhibitor. Enoxaparin is a low molecular weight heparin (LMWH).

**1759. Laboratory test used to measure the antiplatelet effects of aspirin is?**
*Biomark Med. 2011 Feb;5(1):31-42*

A. Optical platelet aggregation
B. Skin bleeding time
C. Urinary 11-dehydrothromboxane B2
D. All of the above

*The direct measurement of inhibition of thromboxane-forming capacity is the most specific pharmacological assay for aspirin. Measurement of urinary levels of the TXB(2) metabolite, 11-dehydro-thromboxane B(2), represents an index of TXA(2) biosynthesis in vivo.*

**1760. Which of the following is an intravenous antiplatelet agent?**
*Harrison's 20th Ed. Chapter 268 Page 1870 Table 268-3*

A. Abciximab
B. Tirofiban
C. Cangrelor
D. All of the above

**1761. The Global Registry of Acute Coronary Events (GRACE) risk score estimates probability of death within how many months of hospital discharge in patients with ACS?**
*Am J Cardiol. 2016;118(8):1105-1110*

A. 3 months
B. 6 months
C. 1 year
D. 2 years

*The Global Registry of Acute Coronary Events (GRACE) risk score provides an estimate of the probability of death within 6 months of hospital discharge in patients with acute coronary syndrome (ACS).*

**1762. The Global Registry of Acute Coronary Events (GRACE) risk score 2.0 estimates probability of death within how many months of hospital discharge in patients with ACS?**
*Am J Cardiol. 2016;118(8):1105-1110*

A. 3 months
B. 6 months
C. 1 year
D. 2 years

*GRACE Risk Score 2.0 simplified algorithm for predicting 1-year mortality in ACS patients.*

**1763. Immediate invasive strategy in patients with NSTE-ACS is recommended in all except?**
*Harrison's 20th Ed. Chapter 268 Page 1871 Table 268-4*

A. Refractory angina
B. Hemodynamic instability
C. Temporal change in troponin
D. Sustained ventricular tachycardia or ventricular fibrillation

**1764. Patients at high ischemic risk include?**
*Harrison's 20th Ed. Chapter 268 Page 1871*

A. Prior MI
B. Diabetes mellitus
C. Congestive heart failure
D. All of the above

**1765. Patients at high ischemic risk should continue DAPT for?**
*Harrison's 20th Ed. Chapter 268 Page 1871*

A. 1 year
B. 2 years
C. 3 years
D. 5 years

*Patients at high ischemic risk (those with prior MI, diabetes mellitus, vein graft stent, congestive heart failure) who are also at low risk of bleeding, continuation of DAPT for 3 years is beneficial.*

**1766. Prinzmetal's variant angina is due to?**
*Harrison's 20th Ed. Chapter 268 Page 1871*

A. Focal spasm of an epicardial coronary artery
B. Focal spasm of an intramyocardial coronary artery
C. Diffuse spasm of an epicardial coronary artery
D. Diffuse spasm of an intramyocardial coronary artery

*Described by Prinzmetal in 1959, Prinzmetal's variant angina is due to focal spasm of an epicardial coronary artery, leading to severe myocardial ischemia. It may be related to hypercontractility of vascular smooth muscle due to vasoconstrictor mitogens, leukotrienes, or serotonin.*

**1767. Prinzmetal's variant angina may be associated with?**
*Harrison's 20th Ed. Chapter 268 Page 1872*

A. Migraine
B. Raynaud's phenomenon
C. Aspirin-induced asthma
D. All of the above

*Prinzmetal's variant angina is a manifestation of a vasospastic disorder and is associated with migraine, Raynaud's phenomenon or aspirin-induced asthma.*

**1768. In Prinzmetal's variant angina, focal spasm is most common in?**
*N Engl J Med. 2017; 376:e52*

A. Right coronary artery
B. Left anterior descending coronary artery
C. Left circumflex coronary artery
D. Posterior descending coronary artery

*Focal spasm is most common in right coronary artery, and it may occur at one or more sites in one artery or in multiple arteries simultaneously. Atherosclerotic plaques in at least one proximal coronary artery occur in ~ half of patients & in these patients, spasm usually occurs within 1 cm of plaque.*

**1769. Which of the following can be used to provoke focal coronary spasm in Prinzmetal's variant angina?**
*Harrison's 20th Ed. Chapter 268 Page 1872*

A. Ergonovine
B. Acetylcholine
C. Hyperventilation
D. All of the above

*Ergonovine, acetylcholine & hyperventilation can provoke focal coronary stenosis. It is used to establish the diagnosis of Prinzmetal's variant angina.*

**1770. Which of the following is false regarding Prinzmetal's variant angina?**
*Harrison's 20th Ed. Chapter 268 Page 1872*

A. Nitrates and $Ca^{++}$ channel blockers are main treatments
B. $Ca^{++}$ channel blockers given in maximally tolerated doses
C. Aspirin is of therapeutic value
D. Aspirin may increase the severity of ischemic episodes

*Nitrates & calcium channel blockers are the main treatments for Prinzmetal's variant angina. Calcium antagonists are extremely effective in preventing coronary artery spasm of variant angina & they should be prescribed in maximally tolerated doses. Prazosin, a selective alpha adrenoreceptor blocker, has also been found to be of value in some patients, while aspirin may increase the severity of ischemic episodes. The response to beta blockers is variable.*

## Ischemic Heart Disease

**1771. Which of the following is a determinant of myocardial oxygen demand (MVO$_2$)?**
*Harrison's 20th Ed. Chapter 267 Page 1850*

A. Heart rate
B. Myocardial contractility
C. Myocardial wall tension (stress)
D. All of the above

*The major determinants of myocardial oxygen demand (MVO$_2$) are heart rate, myocardial contractility, and myocardial wall tension (stress).*

**1772. Oxygen-carrying capacity of the blood is determined by?**
*Harrison's 20th Ed. Chapter 267 Page 1850*

A. Inspired level of oxygen
B. Pulmonary function
C. Hemoglobin concentration and function
D. All of the above

*An adequate supply of oxygen to the myocardium requires a satisfactory level of oxygen-carrying capacity of the blood. Apart from adequate level of coronary blood flow it is determined by inspired level of oxygen, pulmonary function and hemoglobin concentration and function.*

**1773. Majority of blood flow through coronary arteries is during?**
*Harrison's 20th Ed. Chapter 267 Page 1850*

A. Systole
B. Diastole
C. Presystole
D. Prediastole

*Blood flows through coronary arteries in a phasic fashion, with majority occurring during diastole.*

**1774. In the absence of significant flow-limiting atherosclerotic obstructions, major determinant of total coronary resistance is found in?**
*Harrison's 20th Ed. Chapter 267 Page 1850*

A. Large epicardial arteries (R$_1$)
B. Prearteriolar vessels (R$_2$)
C. Arteriolar and intramyocardial capillary vessels (R$_3$)
D. R$_2$ & R$_3$

*About 75% of the total coronary resistance to flow occurs across three sets of arteries: (1) large epicardial arteries (Resistance 1 = R$_1$), (2) prearteriolar vessels (R$_2$), and (3) arteriolar and intramyocardial capillary vessels (R$_3$). In the absence of significant flow-limiting atherosclerotic obstructions, R$_1$ is trivial. The major determinant of coronary resistance is found in R$_2$ and R$_3$.*

**1775. Which of the following statements is false?**
*Harrison's 20th Ed. Chapter 267 Page 1850*

A. Large epicardial coronary arteries are conductance vessels
B. Intramyocardial arterioles are resistance vessels
C. Abnormal constriction of conductance vessels can cause Prinzmetal's angina
D. Abnormal constriction of resistance vessels can cause Prinzmetal's angina

*Although the large epicardial coronary arteries are capable of constriction and relaxation, in healthy persons they serve as conduits and are referred to as conductance vessels, while the intramyocardial arterioles normally exhibit changes in tone and are therefore referred to as resistance vessels. Abnormal constriction of the conductance vessels can cause severe ischemia in Prinzmetal's angina. Abnormal constriction or failure of normal dilation of coronary resistance vessels causes ischemia termed as microvascular angina.*

**1776. What is the size of the epicardial coronary arteries?**
*Harrison's 20th Ed. Chapter 267 Page 1851 Figure 267-1*

A. > 100 μm
B. > 200 μm
C. > 300 μm
D. > 400 μm

**1777. What is the size of the arterioles in the coronary microcirculation?**
*Harrison's 20th Ed. Chapter 267 Page 1851 Figure 267-1*

A. < 10 μm
B. < 40 μm
C. < 80 μm
D. < 100 μm

**1778. Which of the following offers maximum percentage of total resistance to flow?**
*Harrison's 20th Ed. Chapter 267 Page 1851 Figure 267-1*

A. Epicardial arteries
B. Small arteries
C. Arterioles
D. Capillaries

**1779. Principal function of small arteries & arterioles is?**
*Harrison's 20th Ed. Chapter 267 Page 1851 Figure 267-1*

A. Transport
B. Regulation
C. Exchange
D. All of the above

**1780. Which of the following is part of the coronary microcirculation?**
*Harrison's 20th Ed. Chapter 267 Page 1851 Figure 267-1*

A. Small arteries
B. Arterioles
C. Capillaries
D. All of the above

**1781. Main stimulus for vasomotion in epicardial arteries is?**
*Harrison's 20th Ed. Chapter 267 Page 1851 Figure 267-1*

A. Flow
B. Pressure
C. Metabolites
D. All of the above

**1782. Coronary blood flow can be limited compromised by?**
*Harrison's 20th Ed. Chapter 267 Page 1850*

A. Spasm
B. Arterial thrombi
C. Coronary emboli
D. All of the above

*Coronary blood flow also can be limited by spasm (Prinzmetal's angina, vasoconstrictors), arterial thrombi, coronary emboli and ostial narrowing due to aortitis.*

**1783. Microvascular angina best relates to which of the following?**
*Harrison's 20th Ed. Chapter 267 Page 1851*

A. Failure of normal dilation of coronary resistance vessels
B. Coronary emboli
C. Coronary ostial narrowing
D. All of the above

*Abnormal constriction or failure of normal dilation of the coronary resistance vessels also can cause ischemia. When it causes angina, this condition is referred to as microvascular angina.*

**1784. Which of the following is a normal function of the vascular endothelium?**
*Harrison's 20th Ed. Chapter 267 Page 1851*

A. Local control of vascular tone
B. Maintenance of an antithrombotic surface
C. Control of inflammatory cell adhesion & diapedesis
D. All of the above

*Normal functions of the vascular endothelium include local control of vascular tone, maintenance of an antithrombotic surface and control of inflammatory cell adhesion and diapedesis.*

**1785. Which of the following define the atherosclerotic plaque?**
*Harrison's 20th Ed. Chapter 267 Page 1851*

A. Subintimal collections of fat
B. Subintimal collections of smooth muscle cells
C. Subintimal collections of fibroblasts
D. All of the above

*Subintimal collections of fat, smooth muscle cells, fibroblasts and intercellular matrix define the atherosclerotic plaque.*

**1786. Which of the following contribute to a state of "vulnerable blood"?**
*Harrison's 20th Ed. Chapter 267 Page 1851*

A. Increased concentrations of platelet microparticles
B. Increased concentrations of von Willebrand factor
C. Increased concentrations of coagulation factor VII
D. All of the above

*Alterations in the nature of the circulating blood like hyperglycemia, increased concentrations of LDL cholesterol, tissue factor, fibrinogen, von Willebrand factor, coagulation factor VII and platelet microparticles lead to a state of "vulnerable blood". The combination of a "vulnerable vessel" in a patient with "vulnerable blood" promotes a state of hypercoagulability and hypofibrinolysis. This is especially true in patients with diabetes mellitus.*

**1787. Which of the following sites has the most predilection for atherosclerotic plaques to develop?**
*Harrison's 20th Ed. Chapter 267 Page 1851*

A. Origin of epicardial arteries
B. Branch points in epicardial arteries
C. Terminal regions of epicardial arteries
D. Any of the above

*Atherosclerotic plaques have a predilection to develop at sites of increased turbulence in coronary flow like branch points in the epicardial arteries.*

**1788. Coronary blood flow at rest may be reduced, when the diameter is reduced by?**
*Harrison's 20th Ed. Chapter 267 Page 1851*

A. 50%
B. 60%
C. 70%
D. 80%

*When a stenosis reduces the diameter of an epicardial coronary artery by 50%, there is a limitation of the ability to increase flow to meet increased myocardial demand. When the diameter is reduced by ~80%, blood flow at rest may be reduced.*

**1789. Gregg effect best relates to which of the following?**
*Z Kardiol. 2001;90(5):319-26*

A. Congenital cataracts among infants
B. Increase in myocardial oxygen consumption with increase in coronary perfusion pressure
C. Failure of aldosterone to suppress
D. Disruption of adrenal androgen secretion

*In 1958, Gregg reported that myocardial oxygen consumption increased when coronary perfusion pressure was increased.*

**1790. Which of the following collateral vessels is false?**
*Harrison's 20th Ed. Chapter 267 Page 1851*

A. Promoted by chronic severe coronary narrowing
B. Promoted by myocardial ischemia
C. May sustain viability of myocardium at rest but not during conditions of increased demand
D. None of the above

**1791. Which of the following occur when a proximal epicardial artery is stenosed?**
*Harrison's 20th Ed. Chapter 267 Page 1851*

A. Pressure gradient develops across the proximal stenosis
B. Poststenotic pressure falls
C. Myocardial blood flow becomes dependent on pressure in the coronary artery distal to stenosis
D. All of the above

**1792. Myocardial ischemia causes disturbance in which of the following?**
*Harrison's 20th Ed. Chapter 267 Page 1851*

A. Mechanical functions of the myocardium
B. Biochemical functions of the myocardium
C. Electrical functions of the myocardium
D. All of the above

**1793. Which of the following about coronary atherosclerosis is false?**
*Harrison's 20th Ed. Chapter 267 Page 1852*

A. Focal process
B. Causes nonuniform ischemia
C. Causes loss of endothelial control of dilation
D. None of the above

**1794. Normal myocardium metabolizes which of the following?**
*Harrison's 20th Ed. Chapter 267 Page 1852*

A. Fatty acids
B. Amino acids
C. Lactate
D. All of the above

*Normal myocardium metabolizes fatty acids and glucose to carbon dioxide and water.*

### 1795. Which of the following occurs during myocardial ischemia?
*Harrison's 20th Ed. Chapter 267 Page 1852*

A. Intracellular pH is reduced
B. Intracellular creatine phosphate is reduced
C. Intracellular glucose is converted to lactate
D. All of the above

*With severe oxygen deprivation, fatty acids cannot be oxidized and glucose is converted to lactate. Intracellular pH and myocardial stores of high-energy phosphates (ATP, creatine phosphate) are reduced.*

### 1796. During myocardial ischemia, impairment of cell membrane function leads to?
*Harrison's 20th Ed. Chapter 267 Page 1852*

A. Leakage of potassium from myocytes
B. Uptake of sodium by myocytes
C. Increase in cytosolic calcium
D. All of the above

*Impaired myocyte cell membrane function due to ischemia leads to leakage of potassium and uptake of sodium by myocytes as well as an increase in cytosolic calcium.*

### 1797. Minimum duration of total occlusion of epicardial vessel in absence of collaterals for development of myocardial necrosis is?
*Harrison's 20th Ed. Chapter 267 Page 1852*

A. > 20 minutes
B. > 25 minutes
C. > 30 minutes
D. > 35 minutes

*Severity & duration of imbalance between myocardial oxygen supply & demand determine whether damage is reversible (≤20 minutes for total occlusion in the absence of collaterals) or whether it is permanent, with subsequent myocardial necrosis (>20 minutes).*

### 1798. In ECG, transient ST-segment depression reflects?
*Harrison's 20th Ed. Chapter 267 Page 1852*

A. Subendocardial ischemia
B. Transmural ischemia
C. Epicardial ischemia
D. All of the above

### 1799. In ECG, transient ST-segment elevation reflects?
*Harrison's 20th Ed. Chapter 267 Page 1852*

A. Subendocardial ischemia
B. Transmural ischemia
C. Epicardial ischemia
D. All of the above

*Ischemia also causes characteristic changes in ECG such as repolarization abnormalities in the form of inversion of T waves and, when more severe, by displacement of ST segments. Transient ST-segment depression reflects patchy subendocardial ischemia, while ST-segment elevation is caused by more severe transmural ischemia.*

### 1800. Coronary atherosclerosis begins to develop at what age?
*Harrison's 20th Ed. Chapter 267 Page 1852*

A. < 20 years
B. 20 - 30 years
C. 30 - 40 years
D. > 40 years

*Postmortem studies have shown that coronary atherosclerosis often begins to develop prior to age 20 and is widespread even among adults who were asymptomatic during life.*

### 1801. Which of the following statements about angina pectoris is false?
*Harrison's 20th Ed. Chapter 267 Page 1852*

A. Males constitute ~70% of all patients with angina pectoris
B. Angina pectoris in women is often atypical in presentation
C. Angina pectoris only rarely presents as frank pain
D. None of the above

### 1802. Squeezing, central, substernal discomfort in angina pectoris is termed?
*Harrison's 20th Ed. Chapter 267 Page 1853*

A. Landolfi's sign
B. Levine's sign
C. Lhermitte's sign
D. Carvolo's sign

*Squeezing, central, substernal discomfort indicative of angina pectoris is termed as Levine's sign.*

### 1803. Which of the following statements about angina is false?
*Harrison's 20th Ed. Chapter 267 Page 1853*

A. Angina is usually crescendo-decrescendo in nature
B. Typically lasts for 10 to 15 minutes
C. Pain can radiate to both arms
D. Rarely localized below umbilicus or above mandible

*Angina is usually crescendo-decrescendo in nature, typically lasts 2 to 5 minutes, and can radiate to left shoulder and to both arms, especially to the ulnar surfaces of forearm and hand. It can also arise in or radiate to the back, interscapular region, root of the neck, jaw, teeth, and epigastrium. Angina is rarely localized below the umbilicus or above the mandible.*

### 1804. Radiation of chest pain towards which of the following is more typical of pericarditis?
*Harrison's 20th Ed. Chapter 267 Page 1853*

A. Interscapular region
B. Jaw
C. Epigastrium
D. Trapezius muscles

*Chest discomfort due to myocardial ischemia does not radiate to the trapezius muscles; such a radiation pattern is more typical of pericarditis.*

### 1805. "Angina decubitus" refers to anginal pain occuring when the patient is in which of the following positions?
*Harrison's 20th Ed. Chapter 267 Page 1853*

A. Squatting
B. Sitting with legs hanging
C. Recumbent
D. Any of the above

*Episodes of angina that occur at night while the patient is recumbent is termed as angina decubitus.*

### 1806. Nocturnal angina may be due to?
*Harrison's 20th Ed. Chapter 267 Page 1853*

A. Episodic tachycardia
B. Changes in respiratory pattern during sleep
C. Expansion of intrathoracic blood volume
D. All of the above

*Nocturnal angina may be due to episodic tachycardia, diminished oxygenation as the respiratory pattern changes during sleep or expansion of intrathoracic blood volume that occurs with recumbency.*

**1807. Expansion of the intrathoracic blood volume during recumbency leads to?**
*Harrison's 20th Ed. Chapter 267 Page 1853*

A. Increase in end-diastolic volume
B. Increase in wall tension
C. Increase in myocardial oxygen demand
D. All of the above

**1808. Atypical presentations of angina pectoris are more frequent in?**
*Harrison's 20th Ed. Chapter 267 Page 1853, N Engl J Med. 2005;352:2524-33*

A. Older patients
B. Diabetics
C. Women
D. All of the above

**1809. Anginal "equivalents" are all except?**
*Harrison's 20th Ed. Chapter 267 Page 1853*

A. Dyspnea
B. Fatigue
C. Palpitation
D. Faintness

**1810. Anginal "equivalents" are more common in?**
*Harrison's 20th Ed. Chapter 267 Page 1853*

A. Women
B. Smoker
C. Hypertension
D. Diabetes mellitus

*Anginal "equivalents" are symptoms of myocardial ischemia other than angina. These include dyspnea, fatigue and faintness and are more common in the elderly and in diabetic patients.*

**1811. Which of the following point towards an unstable anginal syndrome?**
*Harrison's 20th Ed. Chapter 267 Page 1853*

A. Angina occurring with less exertion than in the past
B. Angina occurring at rest
C. Angina awakening the patient from sleep
D. All of the above

**1812. Coronary reactivity testing can be done by which of the following vasoactive agents?**
*Harrison's 20th Ed. Chapter 267 Page 1853*

A. Adenosine
B. Acetylcholine
C. Nitroglycerin
D. All of the above

*Coronary reactivity testing can be done by vasoactive agents such as intracoronary adenosine, acetylcholine and nitroglycerin.*

**1813. Abnormal cardiac nociception may be ameliorated by?**
*Harrison's 20th Ed. Chapter 267 Page 1853*

A. Calcium antagonists
B. Statins
C. Nicorandil
D. Imipramine

*Abnormal cardiac nociception is more difficult to manage and may be ameliorated in some cases by imipramine.*

**1814. Disorders that may cause angina in absence of coronary atherosclerosis are all except?**
*Harrison's 20th Ed. Chapter 267 Page 1854*

A. Hypertrophic cardiomyopathy
B. Aortic regurgitation
C. Pulmonary hypertension
D. Systemic hypertension

*Aortic stenosis, aortic regurgitation, pulmonary hypertension and hypertrophic cardiomyopathy may cause angina in the absence of coronary atherosclerosis.*

**1815. Which of the following statements is false?**
*Harrison's 20th Ed. Chapter 391 Page 2825*

A. Angina is the commonest initial symptom of CHD in women
B. Myocardial infarction is the commonest initial symptom of CHD in men
C. Women with MI are more likely to present with cardiac arrest or cardiogenic shock
D. None of the above

*In the Framingham study, angina was the most common initial symptom of CHD in women, whereas myocardial infarction (MI) was the most common initial presentation in men. Women more often have atypical symptoms such as nausea, vomiting, indigestion, and upper back pain. Women with MI are more likely to present with cardiac arrest or cardiogenic shock, whereas men are more likely to present with ventricular tachycardia. Younger women with MI are more likely to die than are men of similar age.*

**1816. Poor exercise tolerance is defined as?**
*Harrison's 20th Ed. Chapter 467 Page 3447*

A. Inability to walk four blocks
B. Inability to climb two flights of stairs at normal pace
C. Meet a metabolic equivalent (MET) level of 4
D. All of the above

*Poor exercise tolerance is defined as inability to walk four blocks or climb two flights of stairs at a normal pace or to meet a metabolic equivalent (MET) level of 4 because of the development of dyspnea, angina or excessive fatigue.*

**1817. Which of the following can closely mimic angina?**
*Harrison's 20th Ed. Chapter 11 Page 76*

A. Esophageal reflux
B. Esophageal spasm
C. Peptic ulcer
D. Gall bladder disease

*The pain of esophageal spasm is commonly an intense squeezing discomfort that is retrosternal in location and like angina may be relieved by nitroglycerin or dihydropyridine calcium channel antagonists.*

**1818. Cardiac cephalgia best relates to?**
*Harrison's 20th Ed. Chapter 422 Page 3106*

A. Primary cough headache
B. Primary exercise headache
C. Primary thunderclap headache
D. Primary sex headache

*Cardiac cephalgia refers exertional headache. Pain from angina may be referred to the head, probably by central connections of vagal afferents. The link to exercise is the main clinical clue that headache is of cardiac origin.*

**1819. Which of the following makes it unlikely that the chest pain is caused by myocardial ischemia?**
*Harrison's 20th Ed. Chapter 267 Page 1854*

A. Tenderness of the chest wall
B. Localization of discomfort with a single fingertip on chest
C. Reproduction of the pain with palpation of chest
D. All of the above

**1820. Which of the following is useful in therapeutic decision-making about the initiation of hypolipidemic treatment?**
*Harrison's 20th Ed. Chapter 267 Page 1854*

A. Lp(a)
B. CRP
C. Homocysteine
D. All of the above

*Evidence exists that ↑ level of high-sensitivity C-reactive protein (CRP) (between 0 - 3 mg/dL) is an independent risk factor for IHD and is useful in therapeutic decision-making about initiation of hypolipidemic treatment.*

**1821. Which of the following ECG change is more specific for the diagnosis of angina pectoris?**
*Harrison's 20th Ed. Chapter 267 Page 1854*

A. Dynamic ST-segment and T-wave changes
B. Disturbances of cardiac rhythm
C. Intraventricular conduction defect
D. All of the above

*Dynamic ST-segment and T-wave changes that accompany episodes of angina pectoris and disappear thereafter are more specific in patients with angina pectoris.*

**1822. All of the following are indications of discontinuing exercise stress testing except?**
*Harrison's 20th Ed. Chapter 267 Page 1854*

A. Chest discomfort
B. Severe shortness of breath
C. Dizziness
D. Rise in systolic blood pressure > 40 mm Hg

**1823. All of the following are indications of discontinuing exercise stress testing except?**
*Harrison's 20th Ed. Chapter 267 Page 1854*

A. ST-segment depression > 0.2 mV (2 mm)
B. Fall in systolic blood pressure > 10 mm Hg
C. Development of supraventricular tachyarrhythmia
D. Development of ventricular tachyarrhythmia

*Treadmill exercise stress test is discontinued upon evidence of chest discomfort, severe shortness of breath, dizziness, severe fatigue, ST-segment depression > 0.2 mV (2 mm), a fall in systolic blood pressure >10 mm Hg, or the development of a ventricular tachyarrhythmia.*

**1824. Which of the following represents baseline in ECG?**
*Harrison's 20th Ed. Chapter 267 Page 1854*

A. PR segment
B. ST segment
C. QT segment
D. TP segment

*The PR segment is considered as the baseline in ECG.*

**1825. Ischemic ST-segment response on standard exercise treadmill testing (ETT) is?**
*Harrison's 20th Ed. Chapter 267 Page 1854*

A. Flat or downsloping depression of the ST segment
B. > 0.1 mV below baseline
C. Lasting longer than 0.08 seconds
D. All of the above

*The ischemic ST-segment response on standard exercise treadmill testing (ETT) is defined as flat or downsloping depression of the ST segment >0.1 mV below baseline (PR segment) and lasting longer than 0.08 seconds.*

**1826. On standard exercise treadmill testing (ETT), which of the following is not considered characteristic of ischemia or is not diagnostic?**
*Harrison's 20th Ed. Chapter 267 Page 1854*

A. Upsloping or junctional ST-segment changes
B. Conduction disturbances
C. Ventricular arrhythmias
D. All of the above

*On standard exercise treadmill testing (ETT), upsloping or junctional ST-segment changes are not considered characteristic of ischemia and do not constitute a positive test. Although T-wave abnormalities, conduction disturbances, and ventricular arrhythmias that develop during exercise should be noted, they are also not diagnostic.*

**1827. In standard exercise treadmill testing (ETT), target heart rate (THR) is defined as?**
*Harrison's 20th Ed. Chapter 267 Page 1854*

A. 65% of maximal predicted heart rate for age and sex
B. 75% of maximal predicted heart rate for age and sex
C. 85% of maximal predicted heart rate for age and sex
D. 95% of maximal predicted heart rate for age and sex

*Negative exercise tests in which the target heart rate (85% of maximal predicted heart rate for age and sex) is not achieved are considered nondiagnostic.*

**1828. The standard Bruce treadmill protocol begins at what speed and gradient?**
*Harrison's 20th Ed. Chapter 267 Page 1857 Table 267-2*

A. 1.7 miles per hour and 0% gradient
B. 1.7 miles per hour and 5% gradient
C. 1.7 miles per hour and 10% gradient
D. 1.7 miles per hour and 12% gradient

*The standard Bruce treadmill protocol begins at 1.7 MPH and 10% gradient and progresses every 3 min to a higher speed and elevation.*

**1829. In standard Bruce treadmill protocol, what is the maximum speed and maximum gradient?**
*Harrison's 20th Ed. Chapter 267 Page 1857 Table 267-2*

A. 5 miles per hour and 18% gradient
B. 5 miles per hour and 22% gradient
C. 6 miles per hour and 18% gradient
D. 6 miles per hour and 22% gradient

**1830. The standard Bruce treadmill protocol progresses to a higher speed and elevation every?**
*Harrison's 20th Ed. Chapter 267 Page 1857 Table 267-2*

A. 1 minute
B. 2 minutes
C. 3 minutes
D. 4 minutes

*The standard Bruce treadmill protocol progresses to a higher speed and elevation every 3 minutes.*

**1831.** Methoxyisobutyl isonitrite (MIBI) best relates to?
*Harrison's 20th Ed. Chapter 267 Page 1855 Figure 267-3*

A. 2D echocardiography
B. Nuclear perfusion scan
C. Cardiac MR scan
D. Cardiac PET scan

**1832.** False-positive or false negative results occur in what proportion of ECG stress tests?
*Harrison's 20th Ed. Chapter 267 Page 1854*

A. 25%
B. 33%
C. 50%
D. 75%

*Pretest probability of ECG stress tests being false-positive or false negative for coronary artery disease (CAD) exists in the patient or population is 33%.*

**1833.** Likelihood of CAD in a positive ECG stress test is increased in?
*Harrison's 20th Ed. Chapter 267 Page 1854*

A. Males who are > 50 years
B. History of typical angina pectoris
C. Who develop chest discomfort during the test
D. All of the above

*A positive result on exercise indicates that the likelihood of CAD is 98% in males who are > 50 years with a history of typical angina pectoris and who develop chest discomfort during the test. The likelihood decreases if the patient has atypical or no chest pain by history and/or during the test.*

**1834.** Incidence of false-positive exercise stress electrocardiography is significantly increased in?
*Harrison's 20th Ed. Chapter 267 Page 1854*

A. Patients taking digitalis and antiarrhythmic agents
B. Patients with ventricular hypertrophy
C. Patients with abnormal serum potassium levels
D. All of the above

*Incidence of false-positive tests is significantly increased in patients with low probabilities of IHD like asymptomatic men <40 years or in premenopausal women with no risk factors for premature atherosclerosis. It is also increased in patients taking cardioactive drugs like digitalis & antiarrhythmic agents, or in those with intraventricular conduction disturbances, resting ST-segment & T-wave abnormalities, ventricular hypertrophy, or abnormal serum potassium levels.*

**1835.** False-negative stress test is usual in obstructive disease limited to which coronary artery?
*Harrison's 20th Ed. Chapter 267 Page 1854*

A. Left anterior descending coronary artery
B. Left circumflex coronary artery
C. Right coronary artery
D. Posterior descending artery

*Obstructive disease limited to circumflex coronary artery results in a false-negative stress test since lateral portion of heart which it supplies is not well represented on the surface 12-lead ECG.*

**1836.** Overall sensitivity of exercise stress electrocardiography is?
*Harrison's 20th Ed. Chapter 267 Page 1854*

A. ~ 55%
B. ~ 65%
C. ~ 75%
D. ~ 85%

*Overall sensitivity of exercise stress electrocardiography is only ~75%.*

**1837.** Modified (heart rate limited) exercise stress tests can be earliest performed safely in patients of uncomplicated MI after how many days?
*Harrison's 20th Ed. Chapter 267 Page 1854*

A. 3 days
B. 6 days
C. 9 days
D. 12 days

*Modified (heart rate limited rather than symptom-limited) exercise tests can be performed safely in patients as early as 6 days after uncomplicated MI.*

**1838.** Contraindications to exercise stress testing include all except?
*Harrison's 20th Ed. Chapter 267 Page 1854*

A. Rest angina within 48 hours
B. Unstable rhythm
C. Severe aortic stenosis
D. Severe mitral stenosis

**1839.** Contraindications to exercise stress testing include all except?
*Harrison's 20th Ed. Chapter 267 Page 1854*

A. Acute myocarditis
B. Uncontrolled heart failure
C. Hypertension
D. Active infective endocarditis

*Contraindications to exercise stress testing include rest angina within 48 hours, unstable rhythm, severe aortic stenosis, acute myocarditis, uncontrolled heart failure, severe pulmonary hypertension and active infective endocarditis.*

**1840.** Adverse prognostic signs in exercise stress testing include all except?
*Harrison's 20th Ed. Chapter 267 Page 1854*

A. Failure of blood pressure to increase
B. Development of angina
C. Severe ST-segment depression at low workload
D. ST-segment depression persisting for > 3 minutes after termination of exercise

*Failure of BP to increase or an actual decrease with signs of ischemia during the exercise test is an important adverse prognostic sign, since it may reflect ischemia induced global left ventricular dysfunction. Development of angina and/or severe (>0.2 mV) ST-segment depression at a low workload (before completion of stage II of Bruce protocol), and/or ST-segment depression that persists for ">5 minutes" after the termination of exercise increases the specificity of the test and suggests severe IHD and a high risk of future adverse events.*

**1841.** Stress myocardial perfusion imaging is more informative than exercise test in all of the following conditions except?
*Harrison's 20th Ed. Chapter 267 Page 1854*

A. Wolff-Parkinson-White syndrome
B. Left bundle branch block
C. Right bundle branch block
D. Paced ventricular rhythm

*When resting ECG is abnormal (Wolff-Parkinson-White syndrome, >1 mm of resting ST segment depression, left bundle branch block, paced ventricular rhythm), information gained from an exercise test can be enhanced by stress myocardial perfusion imaging.*

**1842.** Which of the following drugs can be used in place of exercise for noninvasive stress testing?
*Harrison's 20th Ed. Chapter 267 Page 1854*

A. Intravenous nitroglycerine
B. Intravenous dopamine
C. Intravenous adenosine
D. Intravenous phenylephrine

*Intravenous dipyridamole or adenosine can be used in place of exercise for noninvasive stress testing to create a coronary "steal" by temporarily increasing flow in nondiseased segments of the coronary vasculature at the expense of diseased segments. Graded incremental infusion of dobutamine may be administered to increase $MVO_2$.*

**1843. Agatston score is used for?**
*Harrison's 20th Ed. Chapter 267 Page 1857*

A. Regional wall motion abnormalities
B. Myocardial ischemia quantification
C. Coronary calcium quantification
D. Collateral blood flow quantification

*Coronary calcium detected by electron beam computed tomography (EBCT) & multidetector computed tomography (MDCT) is quantified using the Agatston score which is based on the area & density of calcification.*

**1844. Glagov effect, or positive remodeling refers to?**
*N Engl J Med. 2005;352:2524-33*

A. As coronary plaque burden increases, atherosclerotic mass tends to stay external to lumen, which allows diameter of lumen to be maintained
B. Coronary plaque tends to produce different levels of coronary obstruction at different times
C. Coronary plaque is unduly unstable
D. All of the above

*Coronary arteriography outlines the lumina of the coronary arteries. It provides no information about the arterial wall, and severe atherosclerosis that does not encroach on the lumen may go undetected.*

**1845. Which of the following is associated with coronary artery aneurysms?**
*Circulation. 2004;110:2747-2771*

A. Kawasaki disease
B. Antiphospholipid antibody syndrome
C. Syphilis
D. Bacterial endocarditis

*Vasculitis of the coronary arteries (intimal proliferation and infiltration of the vessel wall with mononuclear cells) occurs in Kawasaki disease leading to beadlike aneurysms and thromboses, myocardial ischemia and infarction. Coronary artery aneurysms or ectasia develop in ~15% to 25% of untreated children and may lead to ischemic heart disease or sudden death.*

**1846. Which of the following about Kawasaki disease is false?**
*Circulation. 2004;110:2747-2771*

A. Acute, self-limited vasculitis
B. Unknown etiology
C. Occurs predominantly in infants and young children
D. None of the above

*Kawasaki disease is an acute, self-limited vasculitis of unknown etiology that occurs predominantly in infants and young children. It is characterized by fever, bilateral nonexudative conjunctivitis, erythema of the lips and oral mucosa, strawberry tongue, changes in the extremities, rash, and cervical lymphadenopathy.*

**1847. The principal prognostic indicator in patients with IHD is?**
*Harrison's 20th Ed. Chapter 267 Page 1858*

A. Age
B. Functional state of the left ventricle
C. Location and severity of coronary artery narrowing
D. All of the above

*The principal prognostic indicators in patients with IHD are age, functional state of left ventricle, location(s) and severity of coronary artery narrowing, and the severity or activity of myocardial ischemia.*

**1848. Which of the following indicate an increased risk for adverse coronary events?**
*Harrison's 20th Ed. Chapter 267 Page 1858*

A. Angina pectoris of recent onset
B. Unstable angina
C. Early postmyocardial infarction angina
D. All of the above

*Angina pectoris of recent onset, unstable angina, early postmyocardial infarction angina, angina unresponsive or poorly responsive to medical therapy, and angina accompanied by symptoms of congestive heart failure all indicate an increased risk for adverse coronary events.*

**1849. Which of the following indicate an increased risk for adverse coronary events?**
*Harrison's 20th Ed. Chapter 267 Page 1858*

A. Episodes of pulmonary edema
B. Mitral regurgitation
C. LVEF <0.40 by echocardiography
D. All of the above

*Physical signs of heart failure, episodes of pulmonary edema, transient S3, and mitral regurgitation, cardiac enlargement and reduced (<0.40) LV ejection fraction indicate an ↑ risk for adverse coronary events.*

**1850. Which of the following indicates a high risk for coronary events?**
*Harrison's 20th Ed. Chapter 267 Page 1858*

A. Inability to exercise for 6 minutes (stage II of Bruce protocol)
B. ST-segment ↓ for >5 minutes after cessation of exercise
C. A decline in systolic pressure >10 mm Hg during exercise
D. All of the above

*Indicators of a high risk for coronary events are inability to exercise for 6 minutes (stage II of Bruce protocol) of ETT; onset of myocardial ischemia at low workloads (≥0.1 mV ST segment depression before completion of stage II, ≥0.2 mV ST-segment depression at any stage, ST-segment depression for >5 minutes after cessation of exercise, a decline in systolic pressure >10 mm Hg during exercise, or the development of ventricular tachyarrhythmias during exercise).*

**1851. On cardiac catheterization, which of the following is associated with a poor prognosis?**
*Harrison's 20th Ed. Chapter 267 Page 1858*

A. Elevations of LV end-diastolic pressure
B. Elevations of LV end-diastolic volume
C. Reduced LV ejection fraction
D. All of the above

*On cardiac catheterization, elevations of LV end-diastolic pressure and ventricular volume and reduced ejection fraction are the most important signs of LV dysfunction and are associated with a poor prognosis.*

**1852. Obstructive lesions of which of the following coronary artery is associated with a greater risk?**
*Harrison's 20th Ed. Chapter 267 Page 1858*

A. Left anterior descending coronary artery
B. Right coronary artery
C. Left circumflex coronary artery
D. Posterior descending artery

*Obstructive lesions of the left main (>50% luminal diameter) or left anterior descending coronary artery proximal to the origin of the first septal artery are associated with a greater risk than are lesions of the right or left circumflex coronary artery because of the greater quantity of myocardium at risk.*

**1853. Which of the following reflect episodes of rapid progression in coronary lesions?**
*Harrison's 20th Ed. Chapter 267 Page 1858*

A. Recent onset of symptoms
B. Development of severe ischemia during stress testing
C. Unstable angina pectoris
D. All of the above

*The recent onset of symptoms, development of severe ischemia during stress testing, and unstable angina pectoris reflect episodes of rapid progression in coronary lesions.*

**1854. Which of the following indicates an increased risk of coronary events?**
*Harrison's 20th Ed. Chapter 267 Page 1858*

A. Elevated levels of plasma CRP
B. Extensive coronary calcification on electron beam CT
C. Increased carotid intimal thickening on ultrasound
D. All of the above

**1855. Advanced age refers to?**
*Harrison's 20th Ed. Chapter 267 Page 1858*

A. > 65 years
B. > 70 years
C. > 75 years
D. > 80 years

**1856. Obesity often is accompanied by which of the following risk factors?**
*Harrison's 20th Ed. Chapter 267 Page 1859*

A. Diabetes mellitus
B. Hypertension
C. Hyperlipidemia
D. All of the above

*Obesity often is accompanied by three other risk factors: diabetes mellitus, hypertension, and hyperlipidemia.*

**1857. Target LDL cholesterol level in diabetes mellitus is?**
*Harrison's 20th Ed. Chapter 267 Page 1859*

A. < 70 mg/dL
B. < 100 mg/dL
C. < 150 mg/dL
D. < 180 mg/dL

**1858. Which of the following markedly lowers LDL-C levels?**
*Harrison's 20th Ed. Chapter 267 Page 1860*

A. Monoclonal antibodies against PCSK9
B. Monoclonal antibodies against IL-5
C. Monoclonal antibodies against LFA-1
D. Monoclonal antibodies against CD15s

*The proprotein convertase subtilisin/kexin type 9 (PCSK9) is a secreted protein that binds to LDL receptor & targets it for lysosomal degradation. Normally, after LDL binds to LDL receptor, it is internalized along with the receptor, and in the low pH of the endosome, the LDL receptor dissociates from the LDL and recycles to the cell surface. When circulating PCSK9 binds LDL receptor, the complex is internalized and the receptor is directed to lysosome, rather than to cell surface, reducing the number of active LDL receptors. Loss-of-function mutations in PCSK9 markedly lower LDL-C levels. Injectable monoclonal antibodies against PCSK9 are capable of producing dramatic lowering of LDL cholesterol beyond that achieved with a statin alone.*

**1859. Nitroglycerin deteriorates with exposure to?**
*Can Med Assoc J. 1974;110(7):788-791*

A. Air
B. Moisture
C. Sunlight
D. All of the above

*Nitroglycerin deteriorates with exposure to air, moisture, and sunlight.*

**1860. Increase in which of the following causes relaxation of vascular smooth muscle?**
*Harrison's 20th Ed. Chapter 267 Page 1861*

A. Guanosine diphosphate (GDP)
B. Guanosine triphosphate (GTP)
C. Cyclic guanosine monophosphate
D. Platelet guanylyl cyclase

*When metabolized, organic nitrates release nitric oxide (NO) that binds to guanylyl cyclase in vascular smooth muscle cells, leading to an increase in cyclic guanosine monophosphate, which causes relaxation of vascular smooth muscle. Nitroglycerin and related nitrates used to treat angina produce vasodilation by elevating cyclic GMP.*

**1861. To minimize nitrate tolerance, patient should be kept free of the drug for a minimum of how many hours each day?**
*Harrison's 20th Ed. Chapter 267 Page 1861*

A. 2 hours
B. 4 hours
C. 6 hours
D. 8 hours

*In order to minimize the effects of nitrate tolerance, minimum effective dose should be used and a minimum of 8 hours each day kept free of the drug.*

**1862. β-adrenergic blocker can be discontinued with doses tapered over?**
*Harrison's 20th Ed. Chapter 267 Page 1861*

A. 1 week
B. 2 weeks
C. 3 weeks
D. 4 weeks

*Since sudden discontinuation of β-adrenergic blockers can intensify ischemia, its doses should be tapered over 2 weeks.*

**1863. Asymptomatic persons with severe coronary atherosclerosis include?**
*Harrison's 17th Ed. 1526*

A. Patients with higher pain thresholds
B. Patients with higher endorphin levels
C. Diabetics with autonomic dysfunction
D. All of the above

*Asymptomatic persons with severe coronary atherosclerosis who exhibit ST-segment changes during activity include those who exhibit higher thresholds to electrically induced pain, higher endorphin levels and diabetics with autonomic dysfunction.*

**1864. Which of the following drug is useful in the management of angina pectoris?**
*Harrison's 20th Ed. Chapter 267 Page 1862, Table 267-7*

A. Betaxolol
B. Ranolazine
C. Pentaerythritol tetranitrate
D. All of the above

*Betaxolol is a selective beta 1 blocker. Ranolazine casts its antianginal effect through blockage of late inward sodium current. Pentaerythritol tetranitrate is used sublingually for its antianginal effect.*

### 1865. Sildenafil was initially developed as?
*Harrison's 19th Ed. Page 43*

A. Mast cell stabilizer
B. Bronchodilator
C. Antianginal drug
D. Antipletelet drug

Sildenafil was initially developed as an antianginal, but its effects to alleviate erectile dysfunction not only led to a new drug indication but also to increased understanding of the role of type 5 phosphodiesterase in erectile tissue. Sildenafil leads to inhibition of phosphodiesterase type 5 isoform that inactivates cyclic guanosine monophosphate (GMP) in the vasculature.

### 1866. Which of the following is a second-generation dihydropyridine calcium antagonist?
*Harrison's 20th Ed. Chapter 267 Page 1861*

A. Nicardipine
B. Isradipine
C. Felodipine
D. All of the above

### 1867. Which of the following is not a dihydropyridine calcium channel blocker?
*Harrison's 20th Ed. Chapter 267 Page 1860, Table 267-6*

A. Amlodipine
B. Felodipine
C. Diltiazem
D. Isradipine

### 1868. Which of the following is a nondihydropyridine calcium channel blocker?
*Harrison's 20th Ed. Chapter 267 Page 1860, Table 267-6*

A. Nicardipine
B. Nifedipine
C. Nisoldipine
D. Verapamil

### 1869. Which of the following calcium channel blocker has the longest duration of action?
*Harrison's 20th Ed. Chapter 267 Page 1860, Table 267-6*

A. Amlodipine
B. Isradipine
C. Nisoldipine
D. Nicardipine

### 1870. Which of the following calcium channel blocker may be associated with increased risk of mortality if administered during acute myocardial infarction?
*Harrison's 20th Ed. Chapter 267 Page 1860, Table 267-6*

A. Amlodipine
B. Diltiazem (Immediate release)
C. Nifedipine (Immediate release)
D. Verapamil (Immediate release)

Nifedipine (Immediate release) may be associated with increased risk of mortality if administered during acute myocardial infarction. In general, short-acting dihydropyridines should be avoided because of the risk of precipitating infarction, particularly in the absence of beta blockers.

## ST-Segment Elevation Myocardial Infarction

**1871. Who coined the term angina pectoris?**
*American Journal of Clinical Medicine. 2011;8(1):15*

A. Carl Weigert
B. William Heberden
C. William Osler
D. George Dock

*William Heberden coined the term angina pectoris in 1768. Carl Weigert in 1880 clearly correlated myocardial infarction as a disease of the coronary arteries. In 1910, Russian clinicians, Obraztsov and Strazhesko, actually documented clinical features of myocardial infarction in a living patient. In 1918, James Herrick was one of the first to encourage electrocardiography, which had been created by Einthoven in 1902.*

**1872. Acute coronary syndrome refers to?**
*N Engl J Med. 2006; 354:1524-1527*

A. Myocardial infarction with ST-segment elevation
B. Myocardial infarction without ST-segment elevation
C. Unstable angina
D. All of the above

*Acute coronary syndromes is defined as myocardial infarction with ST-segment elevation, myocardial infarction without ST-segment elevation, and unstable angina. They share a common pathophysiology i.e. atherosclerotic plaque rupture, erosion, or both with superimposed intracoronary thrombosis, commonly known as atherothrombosis.*

**1873. What percentage of acute myocardial infarction related deaths occur before the stricken individual reaches the hospital?**
*Harrison's 20th Ed. Chapter 269 Page 1872*

A. ~ 10%
B. ~ 20%
C. ~ 30%
D. ~ 50%

*About half of acute myocardial infarction (AMI)-related deaths occur before the stricken individual reaches the hospital.*

**1874. The in-hospital mortality rate after admission for acute myocardial infarction (AMI) is?**
*Harrison's 20th Ed. Chapter 269 Page 1873*

A. ~ 1%
B. ~ 5%
C. ~ 10%
D. ~ 15%

*The in-hospital mortality rate after admission for AMI is ~5%.*

**1875. The 1-year mortality rate after AMI is?**
*Harrison's 20th Ed. Chapter 269 Page 1873*

A. ~ 1%
B. ~ 5%
C. ~ 10%
D. ~ 15%

*The 1-year mortality rate after AMI is about 15%.*

**1876. AMI-related mortality is how many times higher in elderly patients (>75 years) as compared with younger patients?**
*Harrison's 20th Ed. Chapter 269 Page 1873*

A. ~ 1 x
B. ~ 2 x
C. ~ 3 x
D. ~ 4 x

*AMI-related mortality is ~ 4 times higher in elderly patients (>75 years) as compared with younger patients.*

**1877. Which of the following statements about acute coronary syndromes is false?**
*Harrison's 20th Ed. Chapter 269 Page 1873 Figure 269-1*

A. Majority of patients with ST-segment elevation ultimately develop Q-wave on ECG (QwMI)
B. Majority of patients without ST-segment elevation (NSTEMI) ultimately develop Q-wave on ECG (QwMI)
C. Patients without ST-segment elevation are suffering from either unstable angina or a non-ST-segment elevation MI (NSTEMI)
D. None of the above

*Of patients with ST-segment elevation, the majority ultimately develop a Q-wave on the ECG (QwMI). Majority of patients presenting with NSTEMI do not develop a Q-wave on the ECG.*

**1878. Histologically, coronary plaques prone to disruption are those with?**
*Harrison's 20th Ed. Chapter 269 Page 1873*

A. Rich lipid core and thin fibrous cap
B. Rich lipid core and thick fibrous cap
C. Poor lipid core and thin fibrous cap
D. Poor lipid core and thick fibrous cap

*Histologic studies indicate that the coronary plaques prone to disruption are those with a rich lipid core and a thin fibrous cap.*

**1879. Agonists that promote platelet activation at the site of ruptured plaque include all except?**
*Harrison's 20th Ed. Chapter 269 Page 1873*

A. Collagen
B. ATP
C. Epinephrine
D. Serotonin

*After an initial platelet monolayer forms at the site of the ruptured plaque, various agonists like collagen, ADP, epinephrine and serotonin promote platelet activation.*

**1880. Which of the following best describes thromboxane $A_2$?**
*Harrison's 20th Ed. Chapter 269 Page 1873*

A. Adhesive protein
B. Local vasoconstrictor
C. Resistance to fibrinolysis
D. Platelet aggregator

*At the site of disrupted plaque, agonists like collagen, ADP, epinephrine, serotonin promote platelet activation and from them thromboxane $A_2$ - a potent local vasoconstrictor is released and potential resistance to fibrinolysis develops.*

**1881. Fibrinogen can bind to how many platelets simultaneously?**
*Harrison's 20th Ed. Chapter 269 Page 1873*

A. 1
B. 2
C. 3
D. 4

Fibrinogen is a multivalent molecule and can bind to two different platelets simultaneously, resulting in platelet cross-linking & aggregation.

**1882. Cyclooxygenase is also known as?**
*N Engl J Med. 2001; 345:1809-1817*

A. Prostaglandin G/H synthase
B. Prostaglandin D/E synthase
C. Prostaglandin M/N synthase
D. Prostaglandin U/V synthase

Aspirin acts by irreversibly acetylating a serine residue at position 529 in platelet prostaglandin G/H synthase, an enzyme colloquially known as cyclooxygenase.

**1883. Out of the following, which is the least likely condition that increases risk of developing STEMI?**
*Harrison's 20th Ed. Chapter 269 Page 1874*

A. Collagen vascular disease
B. Unstable angina
C. Cocaine abuse
D. Alcohol abuse

Patients at increased risk of developing STEMI include those with multiple coronary risk factors and those with unstable angina or Prinzmetal's variant angina. Less common underlying medical conditions predisposing patients to STEMI include hypercoagulability, collagen vascular disease, cocaine abuse, and intracardiac thrombi or masses that can produce coronary emboli.

**1884. Which of the following best relates to management of STEMI?**
*Harrison's 20th Ed. Chapter 269 Page 1874*

A. The linking theory
B. Attention to time
C. Chain of survival
D. The weak link

Management of STEMI aims at providing expeditious implementation of a reperfusion strategy through a highly integrated system termed as "chain of survival" which involves prehospital care that extends to early hospital management.

**1885. STEMI tends to occur most commonly at?**
*Harrison's 20th Ed. Chapter 269 Page 1874*

A. Early morning, few hours before awakening
B. Morning, within a few hours after awakening
C. After meals
D. Late evening, following return from work

Although STEMI may commence at any time of the day or night, circadian variations have been reported such that clusters are seen in the morning within a few hours of awakening.

**1886. Which of the following is false regarding 'pain' in STEMI?**
*Harrison's 20th Ed. Chapter 269 Page 1874*

A. Most common presenting complaint
B. Deep and visceral
C. Different in character to discomfort of angina pectoris
D. May radiate as high as occipital area

Pain is the most common presenting complaint in STEMI. Pain is deep & visceral. It is similar in character to discomfort of angina pectoris but is more severe, lasts longer and does not usually subside with cessation of activity. Typically, pain involves central portion of chest and/or epigastrium & on occasion it radiates to arms.

**1887. Which of the following is false regarding 'pain' in STEMI?**
*Harrison's 20th Ed. Chapter 269 Page 1874*

A. Does not radiate below umbilicus
B. May radiate to trapezius
C. Pain does not subside with cessation of activity
D. Painless STEMIs is greater in diabetics

Pain of STEMI may radiate as high as occipital area but not below umbilicus. Pain does not subside with cessation of activity, in contrast to angina pectoris. Radiation of discomfort to trapezius is not seen in patients with STEMI & distinguishes it from pericarditis. Painless STEMIs is more in diabetes mellitus, and it increases with age. In elderly, STEMI may present as sudden-onset breathlessness, which may progress to pulmonary edema.

**1888. Which of the following best relates to acute coronary syndrome?**
*Br Med J 1964;2:688*

A. Crum symnoni
B. Strum preci
C. Angor animi
D. Klent groci

Angor animi (also referred to as angina animi, Gardner's disease and also angina pectoris sine dolore), in medicine, is a symptom defined as a patient's perception that they are in fact dying.

**1889. Sympathetic nervous system hyperactivity is more common in?**
*Harrison's 20th Ed. Chapter 269 Page 1874*

A. Anterior infarction
B. Inferior infarction
C. Posterior infarction
D. Lateral infarction

**1890. Parasympathetic nervous system hyperactivity is more common in?**
*Harrison's 20th Ed. Chapter 269 Page 1874*

A. Anterior infarction
B. Inferior infarction
C. Posterior infarction
D. Lateral infarction

Combination of substernal chest pain lasting >30 minutes & diaphoresis suggests STEMI. 25% patients with anterior infarction have manifestations of sympathetic nervous system hyperactivity (tachycardia and/or hypertension), and up to one-half with inferior infarction show parasympathetic hyperactivity (bradycardia and/or hypotension).

**1891. Which of the following is not an auscultatory finding in myocardial infarction?**
*Harrison's 20th Ed. Chapter 269 Page 1874*

A. Decreased intensity of S1
B. Paradoxical splitting of S2
C. Early systolic apical systolic murmur
D. Pericardial friction rub

A transient midsystolic or late systolic apical systolic murmur due to dysfunction of the mitral valve apparatus may be present in myocardial infarction.

**1892. In most patients with transmural myocardial infarction, systolic pressure declines by how much from the preinfarction state?**
*Harrison's 20th Ed. Chapter 269 Page 1874*

A. ~ 5–10 mm Hg
B. ~ 10–15 mm Hg
C. ~ 15–20 mm Hg
D. ~ 20–25 mm Hg

*In most patients with transmural myocardial infarction, systolic pressure declines by ~ 10—15 mm Hg from the preinfarction state.*

**1893. In temporal staging of myocardial infarction, acute stage is?**
*Harrison's 20th Ed. Chapter 269 Page 1874*

A. First few hours
B. First few hours to 3 days
C. First few hours to 5 days
D. First few hours to 7 days

**1894. In temporal staging of myocardial infarction, healing stage is?**
*Harrison's 20th Ed. Chapter 269 Page 1874*

A. 3 to 10 days
B. 7 to 15 days
C. 10 to 21 days
D. 7 to 28 days

*Myocardial infarction (MI) progresses through three temporal stages—acute (first few hours to 7 days), healing (7 to 28 days) and healed (≥ 29 days).*

**1895. Development of a Q wave on ECG is more dependent on?**
*Harrison's 20th Ed. Chapter 269 Page 1874*

A. Transmurality of myocardial infarction
B. Volume of infarcted myocardial tissue
C. Thickness of the opposite myocardial wall
D. All of the above

*Contemporary studies using MRI suggest that the development of a Q wave on the ECG is more dependent on the volume of infarcted myocardial tissue rather than transmurality of infarction.*

**1896. Which of the following was earliest to be used for diagnosis of patients with suspected myocardial infarction?**
*Chest 1997;111(1):1-3*

A. Serum glutamic-oxaloacetic transaminase (SGOT)
B. Lactic dehydrogenase (LDH)
C. Creatine kinase (CK)
D. Troponin T

*Serum glutamic-oxaloacetic transaminase (SGOT) assay was used for the diagnosis & management of patients with suspected myocardial infarction in 1954, followed by lactic dehydrogenase (LDH) isoenzymes in 1957, and creatine kinase (CK) in 1966 and CK isoenzyme analysis (CK-MB) in mid 70's.*

**1897. "I" in troponin I stands for?**
*J. Biol. Chem. 1973;248:2125-2133*

A. Interactive
B. Inhibitory
C. Increased
D. In-situ

*The nomenclature "troponin C (TnC), troponin I, and troponin T," for the three constituents of the troponin complex was coined in 1973, based on their functional properties ("C" for calcium binding, "I" for inhibitory, and "T" for tropomyosin binding). The inhibitory element within the troponin complex is TnI, which binds to actin-tropomyosin to inhibit actomyosin Mg++-ATPase in the absence of intracellular calcium.*

**1898. Which of the following about cardiac biomarkers is false?**
*Harrison's 20th Ed. Chapter 269 Page 1874*

A. Detected in serum
B. Cardiac biomarkers are proteins
C. Released from necrotic heart muscle
D. None of the above

*Serum cardiac biomarkers are proteins released from necrotic heart muscle after STEMI.*

**1899. Which of the following statements about troponins is false?**
*Chest 1997;111(1):1-3*

A. Troponin complex is not found in smooth muscle
B. Cardiac troponin I has smaller molecular weight than troponin T
C. Cardiac troponin T varies from skeletal troponin T by a unique set of amino acids
D. None of the above

**1900. Which of the following regulates muscle contraction in smooth muscle?**
*J. Biol. Chem. 1973;248:2125-2133*

A. Thrombomodulin
B. Uromodulin
C. Calmodulin
D. Oxyntomodulin

*Troponin complex is not found in smooth muscle, where calmodulin regulates muscle contraction.*

**1901. Levels of cTnI and cTnT may remain elevated for how many days after STEMI?**
*Harrison's 20th Ed. Chapter 269 Page 1875*

A. 1 to 3 days
B. 2 to 5 days
C. 7 to 10 days
D. 10 to 21 days

*Levels of cardiac-specific troponin T (cTnT) and cardiac-specific troponin I (cTnI) detected by highly specific monoclonal antibodies may remain elevated for 7 to 10 days after STEMI.*

**1902. After disruption of cardiomyocyte sarcolemmal membrane, biomarkers are released first from?**
*Harrison's 20th Ed. Chapter 269 Page 1873, Figure 269-3*

A. Sarcolemma
B. Cytoplasmic pool
C. Mitochondria
D. Endoplasmic reticulum

*After disruption of the sarcolemmal membrane of the cardiomyocyte, the cytoplasmic pool of biomarkers is released first.*

**1903. Cardiac biomarkers that are released into the interstitium are first cleared by?**
*Harrison's 20th Ed. Chapter 269 Page 1873, Figure 269-3*

A. Arterioles
B. Venules
C. Capillaries
D. Lymphatics

*Cardiac biomarkers that are released into the interstitium are first cleared by lymphatics followed subsequently by spillover into the venous system.*

1904. **Cardiac troponin levels rise to how many times the upper reference limit in "classic" acute myocardial infarction?**
*Harrison's 20th Ed. Chapter 269 Page 1873, Figure 269-3*

A. ~ 20-50 times
B. ~ 100-200 times
C. ~ 200-500 times
D. ~ 500-1000 times

Cardiac troponin levels rise to about 20–50 times the upper reference limit in "classic" acute myocardial infarction (MI). cTn are found as structural (bound) proteins and as a small free pool that exists in the cytosol, which is about 6–8% for cTnT and 3.5% for cTnI.

1905. **Cardiac troponins are particularly valuable in distinguishing?**
*Harrison's 20th Ed. Chapter 269 Page 1875*

A. Angina pectoris from UA
B. UA from NSTEMI
C. NSTEMI from STEMI
D. All of the above

Cardiac troponins are of particular value in distinguishing UA from NSTEMI.

1906. **Which of the following can elevate serum troponin concentrations?**
*Cleveland Clin J Med. 2018;85(4):274-277*

A. Sepsis
B. Chemotherapy
C. Stress cardiomyopathy
D. All of the above

Sepsis, stroke, chronic kidney disease, pulmonary disease, chemotherapy, heart failure, and stress cardiomyopathy can all raise serum troponin concentrations.

1907. **Which of the following chemotherapeutic agents is associated with cardiotoxicity?**
*Cleveland Clin J Med. 2018;85(4):274-277*

A. Anthracyclines
B. Trastuzumab
C. Mitomycin
D. All of the above

Chemotherapeutic agents associated with cardiotoxicity include anthracyclines, trastuzumab, chlormethine, and mitomycin.

1908. **In sepsis, troponin elevations are caused by?**
*Cleveland Clin J Med. 2018;85(4):274-277*

A. Decreased clearance of troponin fragments by kidneys
B. Cytokine-induced cardiac damage
C. Increased endogenous & exogenous catecholamines damage cardiac myocytes
D. All of the above

Patients with a troponin elevation at the time of diagnosis of sepsis had a risk of death almost twice that of patients without a troponin elevation.

1909. **Macrotroponin is composed of troponin I fragments and?**
*Cleveland Clin J Med. 2018;85(4):274-277*

A. IgM antibodies
B. IgG antibodies
C. IgA antibodies
D. IgE antibodies

Macrotroponin, a molecule found in patients with autoantibodies against troponin I, is composed of troponin I fragments and IgG antibodies and can also cause a false-positive troponin immunoassay.

1910. **Which of the following is a biomarker in acute myocardial infarction?**
*BMC Medicine 2010;8:34*

A. C-terminal-provasopressin (Copeptin)
B. Heart-Type Fatty Acid Binding Protein (H-FABP)
C. Troponin T
D. All of the above

1911. **Which of the following is a biomarker of plaque instability and inflammation?**
*BMC Medicine 2010;8:34*

A. HsCRP (High-sensitivity C-reactive Protein)
B. Myeloperoxidase (MPO)
C. Pregnancy associated Plasma Protein A (PaPPA)
D. All of the above

1912. **Which of the following biomarker is associated with cardiovascular death?**
*BMC Medicine 2010;8:34*

A. NTproBNP
B. TIMP1
C. MMP 9
D. All of the above

1913. **Which of the following about creatine kinase is false?**
*Clin Rheumatol. 2016;35(6):1541-1547*

A. Enzyme
B. Primarily found in muscle tissue
C. Catalyzes conversion of creatine & ATP into phosphocreatine & ADP
D. None of the above

Creatine kinase is an enzyme primarily found in muscle tissue that catalyzes the conversion of creatine and adenosine triphosphate (ATP) into phosphocreatine and adenosine diphosphate (ADP).

1914. **Which of the following about creatine kinase is false?**
*Cleveland Clin J Med. 2000;67(11):37-843*

A. Better for detecting reinfarctions soon after the first event
B. More reliable for estimating the size of myocardial infarction
C. Clearance of CK-MB is not affected by renal function
D. None of the above

1915. **Which of the following is true for levels of creatine phosphokinase (CK) in STEMI?**
*Harrison's 20th Ed. Chapter 269 Page 1875*

A. Rises within 10 to 30 minutes
B. Rises within 30 minutes to 1 hour
C. Rises within 1 to 4 hours
D. Rises within 4 to 8 hours

1916. **Which of the following is true for levels of creatine phosphokinase (CK) in STEMI?**
*Harrison's 20th Ed. Chapter 269 Page 1875*

A. Returns to normal within 24 hours
B. Returns to normal by 24 to 48 hours
C. Returns to normal by 48 to 72 hours
D. Returns to normal by 72 to 96 hours

CK rises within 4 to 8 hours and generally returns to normal by 48 to 72 hours.

**1917. What ratio (relative index) of CKMB mass : CK activity suggests myocardial infarction?**
*Harrison's 20th Ed. Chapter 269 Page 1875*

A. ≥ 1.2
B. ≥ 1.8
C. ≥ 2.2
D. ≥ 2.5

A ratio (relative index) of CKMB mass : CK activity ≥2.5 "suggests" myocardial rather than a skeletal muscle source for the CKMB elevation.

**1918. When patients with STEMI undergo reperfusion, which of the following is false about cardiac biomarkers?**
*Harrison's 20th Ed. Chapter 269 Page 1875*

A. Are detected sooner
B. Rise to a higher peak value
C. Decline more rapidly
D. None of the above

When patients with STEMI undergo reperfusion, cardiac biomarkers are detected sooner, rise to a higher peak value, but decline more rapidly.

**1919. Potential sources of total CK elevation are all except?**
*Cleve Clin J Med. 2016 ;83(1):37-42*

A. Muscular dystrophy
B. Myopathies
C. Polymyositis
D. Hyperthyroidism

Hyperthyroidism is typically associated with normal serum CK concentrations.

**1920. Potential sources of total CK elevation are all except?**
*Cleve Clin J Med. 2016 ;83(1):37-42*

A. Alcohol binge
B. Hypothyroidism
C. Stroke
D. Prolonged immobilization

Potential sources of total CK elevation are skeletal muscular diseases (muscular dystrophy, myopathies and polymyositis), electrical cardioversion, hypothyroidism, stroke, surgery, skeletal muscle damage secondary to trauma, convulsions and prolonged immobilization.

**1921. Mechanism of CK elevation in response to statins is?**
*Cleve Clin J Med. 2016 ;83(1):37-42*

A. Increased muscle membrane fragility due to decreased cholesterol content
B. Inhibition of isoprenoid production
C. Depletion of ubiquinone
D. All of the above

Mechanisms of CK elevation in response to statins include increased muscle membrane fragility due to decreased cholesterol content, inhibition of isoprenoid production (step in synthesis of membrane proteins), and depletion of ubiquinone, leading to mitochondrial dysfunction.

**1922. Macro CK type 1 is associated with?**
*Cleve Clin J Med. 2016 ;83(1):37-42*

A. Malignancies
B. Autoimmune diseases
C. Skeletal trauma
D. Renal failure

Macro CK type 1 is found in ~1.2% of the general population. The complexes are composed of CK & immunoglobulin and are associated with autoimmune diseases. Macro CK type 2 complexes consist of CK and an undetermined protein and are associated with malignancies.

**1923. Which of the following is false about myoglobin in STEMI?**
*Harrison's 20th Ed. Chapter 269 Page 1873, Figure 269-3*

A. First serum cardiac markers to rise after STEMI
B. High cardiac specificity
C. Rapidly excreted in urine
D. Blood levels return to normal within 24 hours

Myoglobin and CK isoforms are one of the first serum cardiac markers that rises after STEMI but it lacks cardiac specificity. It is rapidly excreted in urine therefore blood levels return to normal range within 24 hours of the onset of myocardial infarction.

**1924. Abnormalities of wall motion on 2D echocardiography are present in?**
*Harrison's 20th Ed. Chapter 269 Page 1875*

A. Acute STEMI
B. Acute severe ischemia
C. Old myocardial scar
D. All of the above

Abnormalities of wall motion on 2D echocardiography are almost universally present in acute STEMI. They are also found in old myocardial scar or from acute severe ischemia.

**1925. MI can be detected accurately with?**
*Harrison's 20th Ed. Chapter 269 Page 1876*

A. Myocardial perfusion imaging with [201$_{Tl}$]
B. Myocardial perfusion imaging with [99m$_{Tc}$]-sestamibi
C. Radionuclide ventriculography with [99m$_{Tc}$] - labeled RBCs
D. High-resolution cardiac MRI

**1926. Which of the following about high-resolution cardiac MRI is false?**
*Harrison's 20th Ed. Chapter 269 Page 1876*

A. Standard imaging agent is gadolinium
B. Little gadolinium enters normal myocardium
C. Produces bright signal in areas of infarction
D. None of the above

MI can be detected accurately with high-resolution cardiac MRI using a technique referred to as late enhancement. Infarct zone appears as a bright signal in areas of infarction that appears in stark contrast to the dark areas of normal myocardium.

**1927. Which of the following appears in the criteria for acute Myocardial infarction?**
*Harrison's 20th Ed. Chapter 269 Page 1876 Table 269-1*

A. RBBB
B. LBBB
C. CHB
D. All of the above

**1928. In percutaneous coronary intervention (PCI)-related MI, cTn levels (with normal baseline values) rise by?**
*Harrison's 20th Ed. Chapter 269 Page 1876 Table 269-1*

A. 2 times
B. 3 times
C. 4 times
D. 5 times

Percutaneous coronary intervention (PCI)-related MI is arbitrarily defined by elevation of cTn values >5 x 99th percentile URL in patients with normal baseline values.

**1929. In percutaneous coronary intervention (PCI)-related MI, cTn levels (with elevated baseline values) rise by?**
*Harrison's 20th Ed. Chapter 269 Page 1876 Table 269-1*

A. > 10%
B. > 20%
C. > 30%
D. > 40%

*Percutaneous coronary intervention (PCI)-related MI is arbitrarily defined by a rise of cTn values >20% if the baseline values are elevated.*

**1930. In myocardial infarction associated with CABG, cTn levels rise by?**
*Harrison's 20th Ed. Chapter 269 Page 1876 Table 269-1*

A. 3 times
B. 5 times
C. 10 times
D. 15 times

*In myocardial infarction associated with CABG, cTn levels rise by >10 x 99th percentile URL.*

**1931. Spontaneous myocardial infarction related to atherosclerotic plaque rupture is classified as?**
*Harrison's 20th Ed. Chapter 269 Page 1877 Table 269-2*

A. Type 1
B. Type 2
C. Type 3
D. Type 4a

**1932. Myocardial infarction secondary to an ischemic imbalance is classified as?**
*Harrison's 20th Ed. Chapter 269 Page 1877 Table 269-2*

A. Type 1
B. Type 2
C. Type 3
D. Type 4a

**1933. Myocardial infarction related to percutaneous coronary intervention (PCI) is classified as?**
*Harrison's 20th Ed. Chapter 269 Page 1877 Table 269-2*

A. Type 3
B. Type 4a
C. Type 4b
D. Type 5

**1934. Myocardial infarction related to stent thrombosis is classified as?**
*Harrison's 20th Ed. Chapter 269 Page 1877 Table 269-2*

A. Type 3
B. Type 4a
C. Type 4b
D. Type 5

**1935. Myocardial infarction related to coronary artery bypass grafting (CABG) is classified as?**
*Harrison's 20th Ed. Chapter 269 Page 1877 Table 269-2*

A. Type 3
B. Type 4a
C. Type 4b
D. Type 5

**1936. Most out-of-hospital deaths from STEMI are due to the sudden development of?**
*Harrison's 20th Ed. Chapter 269 Page 1876*

A. Ventricular asystole
B. Ventricular fibrillation
C. Complete heart block
D. Torsades de pointes

*Most out-of-hospital deaths from STEMI are due to the sudden development of ventricular fibrillation, mostly within the first 24 hours of the onset of symptoms, and of these, over half occur in the first hour.*

**1937. The greatest delay in obtaining hospital care in patients with suspected STEMI occurs in?**
*Harrison's 20th Ed. Chapter 269 Page 1876*

A. Between onset of pain & patient's decision to call for help
B. Transportation to the hospital
C. Emergency department
D. Cardiac catheterization laboratory

*The greatest delay usually occurs not during transportation to the hospital but, rather, between the onset of pain and the patient's decision to call for help. The goal is to minimize time from first medical contact (FMC) to initiation of reperfusion therapy within 120 minutes.*

**1938. In the Emergency department, the goals for the management of patients with suspected STEMI is?**
*Harrison's 20th Ed. Chapter 269 Page 1876*

A. Control of cardiac discomfort
B. Identification of patients for urgent reperfusion therapy
C. Avoidance of inappropriate discharge of patients with STEMI
D. All of the above

*In Emergency department, goals for management of patients with suspected STEMI include control of cardiac discomfort, rapid identification of patients who are candidates for urgent reperfusion therapy, triage of lower-risk patients to appropriate location in hospital, & avoidance of inappropriate discharge of patients with STEMI.*

**1939. Angiography & revascularization should not be performed within how many hours after administration of fibrinolytic therapy?**
*Harrison's 20th Ed. Chapter 269 Page 1878 Figure 269-4*

A. First half - 1 hour
B. First 1 - 2 hours
C. First 2 - 3 hours
D. First 3 - 6 hours

*Angiography and revascularization should not be performed within the first 2 - 3 hours after administration of fibrinolytic therapy.*

**1940. Who is credited for the concept of low doses of aspirin in myocardial infarction?**
*American Journal of Clinical Medicine. 2011;8(1):15*

A. Carl Weigert
B. Lawrence Craven
C. William Osler
D. George Dock

*In 1950, Lawrence Craven, a general practitioner in Glendale, California hypothesized that aspirin was preventive of coronary thrombosis. However, Craven's work languished in obscurity for decades.*

### 1941. Aspirin is effective in?
*Harrison's 20th Ed. Chapter 269 Page 1876*

A. Unstable angina
B. NSTEMI
C. STEMI
D. All of the above

*Aspirin is essential in the management of patients with suspected STEMI and is effective across the entire spectrum of acute coronary syndromes.*

### 1942. Aspirin should be given in a dose of?
*Harrison's 20th Ed. Chapter 269 Page 1876*

A. 75–162 mg
B. 160–325 mg
C. 325–625 mg
D. 625–1000 mg

*Aspirin must be given immediately in doses of 160-325 mg to inhibit cyclooxygenase-1 in platelets with reduction of thromboxane A2 levels. This should be followed by daily oral administration of aspirin in a dose of 75 - 162 mg.*

### 1943. In acute MI patients with hypoxemia, $O_2$ is administered by nasal prongs or face mask at the rate of?
*Harrison's 20th Ed. Chapter 269 Page 1877*

A. 2–4 L/minute
B. 4–6 L/minute
C. 6–8 L/minute
D. 8–10 L/minute

*In STEMI patients, whose arterial $O_2$ saturation is normal, supplemental $O_2$ is of limited clinical benefit. When hypoxemia is present, $O_2$ is given by nasal prongs or face mask @ 2 - 4 L/minute for the first 6 to 12 hours after infarction and then according to the situation.*

### 1944. In STEMI, three doses of sublingual nitroglycerin (0.4 mg) should be administered at an interval of?
*Harrison's 20th Ed. Chapter 269 Page 1877*

A. 5 minutes
B. 10 minutes
C. 30 minutes
D. One hour

*Sublingual nitroglycerin can be given safely to most patients with STEMI. Up to three doses of 0.4 mg should be administered at about 5 minute intervals.*

### 1945. Therapy with nitrates in STEMI should be avoided in?
*Harrison's 20th Ed. Chapter 269 Page 1877*

A. Low systolic arterial pressure (< 90 mm Hg)
B. When there is clinical suspicion of RV infarction
C. Who have taken 'sildenafil' within preceding 24 hours
D. All of the above

*Therapy with nitrates is avoided in MI patients who have low systolic arterial pressure (<90 mm Hg), if RV infarction is suspected, in patients who have taken phosphodiesterase-5 inhibitor sildenafil within the preceding 24 hours since it may potentiate the hypotensive effects of nitrates.*

### 1946. Which of the following raises clinical suspicion of right ventricular (RV) infarction?
*Harrison's 20th Ed. Chapter 269 Page 1877*

A. Inferior infarction on ECG
B. Elevated jugular venous pressure
C. Clear lungs
D. All of the above

*Clinical suspicion of RV infarction is indicated by inferior infarction on ECG, elevated jugular venous pressure, clear lungs & hypotension.*

### 1947. Idiosyncratic hypotensive reaction to nitrates is reversed promptly by?
*Harrison's 20th Ed. Chapter 269 Page 1877*

A. IV Calcium gluconate
B. IV Atropine
C. IV Norepinephrine
D. IV Fluids

*An idiosyncratic reaction to nitrates, consisting of sudden marked hypotension can be reversed promptly by the rapid administration of intravenous atropine.*

### 1948. Which of the following about morphine in acute MI is false?
*Harrison's 20th Ed. Chapter 269 Page 1877*

A. Morphine has a vagotonic effect
B. May cause advanced heart block particularly in patients with anterior wall infarction
C. Shoule be given IV rather than subcutaneously
D. None of the above

*Morphine has vagotonic effect & may cause bradycardia or advanced degrees of heart block particularly in patients with posteroinferior infarction. These side effects respond to atropine. Morphine is routinely administered by repetitive (every 5 min) intravenous injection of small doses (2–4 mg) rather than by subcutaneous administration of a larger quantity, because absorption may be unpredictable by subcutaneous route.*

### 1949. Which of the following about IV β-blockers in acute MI is false?
*Harrison's 20th Ed. Chapter 269 Page 1877*

A. Useful in the control of pain of STEMI
B. Reduce the risks of reinfarction
C. Reduce the risks of ventricular fibrillation
D. None of the above

*Intravenous beta blockers are useful in the control of pain of STEMI by diminishing myocardial O2 demand & ischemia. Intravenous beta blockers reduce risks of reinfarction & ventricular fibrillation.*

### 1950. In acute MI, IV metoprolol is given as?
*Harrison's 20th Ed. Chapter 269 Page 1877*

A. 5 mg every 2–5 minutes for a total of three doses
B. 10 mg every 2–5 minutes for a total of five doses
C. 5 mg every 10–15 minutes for a total of three doses
D. 5 mg every 10–15 minutes for a total of five doses

*A commonly employed regimen is metoprolol, 5 mg every 2-5 minutes for a total of three doses, provided the patient has a heart rate >60 beats/minute, systolic pressure > 100 mm Hg, a PR interval <0.24 seconds and rales that are no higher than 10 cm up from the diaphragm. Fifteen minutes after the last intravenous dose, an oral regimen is initiated of 50 mg every 6 hours for 48 hours, followed by 100 mg every 12 hours.*

### 1951. Which of the following has no role in the control of chest discomfort in STEMI?
*Harrison's 20th Ed. Chapter 269 Page 1877*

A. Sublingual nitroglycerin
B. Morphine
C. Beta blockers
D. Calcium antagonists

*Calcium antagonists are of little value in acute setting of STEMI. Short-acting dihydropyridines may be associated with an increased mortality risk.*

**1952. After fibrinolytic therapy, angiography & revascularization should not be performed for?**

*Harrison's 20th Ed. Chapter 269 Page 1878 Figure 269-4*

A. 1 to 2 hours
B. 2 to 3 hours
C. 3 to 4 hours
D. 4 to 6 hours

Angiography and revascularization should not be performed within the first 2 to 3 hours after administration of fibrinolytic therapy.

**1953. Reperfusion therapy is not helpful in?**

*Harrison's 20th Ed. Chapter 269 Page 1877*

A. ST-segment ↑ of ≥ 2 mm in 2 contiguous precordial leads
B. ST-segment ↑ of ≥ 1 mm in two adjacent limb leads
C. Absence of ST-segment elevation
D. None of the above

In the absence of ST-segment elevation, fibrinolysis is not helpful, and it may be harmful.

**1954. In STEMI, the goal is to keep total ischemic time within?**

*Harrison's 20th Ed. Chapter 269 Page 1878 Figure 269-4*

A. 30 minutes
B. 60 minutes
C. 90 minutes
D. 120 minutes

In STEMI, the goal is to keep total ischemic time within 120 minutes.

**1955. ECG finding in a patient of acute MI that makes a candidate suitable for reperfusion therapy is?**

*Harrison's 20th Ed. Chapter 269 Page 1877*

A. ST-segment elevation of at least 1 mm in two contiguous precordial leads
B. ST-segment elevation of at least 2 mm in two contiguous precordial leads
C. ST-segment elevation of at least 1 mm in three contiguous precordial leads
D. ST-segment elevation of at least 2 mm in three contiguous precordial leads

The primary tool for screening patients and making triage decisions is the initial 12-lead ECG. When ST-segment elevation of at least 2 mm in two contiguous precordial leads and 1 mm in two adjacent limb leads is present, a patient should be considered candidate for reperfusion therapy. In the absence of ST-segment elevation, fibrinolysis is not helpful, in fact harmful.

**1956. What proportion of patients with STEMI may achieve spontaneous reperfusion of infarct-related coronary artery within 24 hours?**

*Harrison's 20th Ed. Chapter 269 Page 1877*

A. One - fourth
B. One - third
C. One - half
D. Two - third

Up to one–third of patients with STEMI may achieve spontaneous reperfusion of the infarct-related coronary artery within 24 hours.

**1957. Which of the following extends the "window" of time for salvage of myocardium by reperfusion strategies?**

*Harrison's 20th Ed. Chapter 269 Page 1878*

A. Treatment of congestive heart failure (CHF)
B. Minimization of tachycardia
C. Control of hypertension
D. All of the above

Protection of the ischemic myocardium by maintenance of an optimal balance between myocardial $O_2$ supply & demand through pain control, treatment of congestive heart failure, and minimization of tachycardia & hypertension extends the "window" of time for salvage of myocardium by reperfusion strategies.

**1958. Which of the following drugs should be avoided in patients with STEMI?**

*Harrison's 20th Ed. Chapter 269 Page 1878*

A. Glucocorticoids
B. Nonsteroidal anti-inflammatory agents
C. Short-acting dihydropyridines calcium antagonists
D. All of the above

**1959. Glucocorticoids are deleterious in patients with STEMI due to?**

*Harrison's 20th Ed. Chapter 269 Page 1878*

A. They impair infarct healing & result in a larger infarct scar
B. They increase the risk of myocardial rupture
C. They increase coronary vascular resistance
D. All of the above

Glucocorticoids & nonsteroidal anti-inflammatory agents (other than aspirin), should be avoided in STEMI as they impair infarct healing resulting in a larger infarct scar & increase the risk of myocardial rupture. They also increase coronary vascular resistance, thereby potentially reducing flow to ischemic myocardium.

**1960. In STEMI, the golden hour refers to?**

*Am Heart J. 2010;160(6):1079-84*

A. First 15 minutes
B. First 30 minutes
C. First 60 minutes
D. First 180 minutes

**1961. The first description of the coronary care unit (CCU) was given by?**

*American Journal of Clinical Medicine. 2011;8(1):15*

A. Carl Weigert
B. Lawrence Craven
C. Desmond Julian
D. George Dock

The very first description of the coronary care unit (CCU) was presented to the British Thoracic Society in July 1961 by Desmond Julian.

**1962. A cardiologist is considered as an "experienced operator" if he has does how many percuteneous coronary intervention (PCI) cases per year?**

*Heart 2004;90:e37*

A. ≥ 15
B. ≥ 25
C. ≥ 50
D. ≥ 75

A cardiologist is considered as an "experienced operator" if he does ≥75 percutaneous coronary intervention (PCI) cases per year.

**1963. A cardiological unit is considered as a "dedicated medical center" if it does how many percuteneous coronary intervention (PCI) cases per year?**
*Heart 2004;90:e37*

A. ≥ 5
B. ≥ 15
C. ≥ 25
D. ≥ 33

*A cardiological unit is considered as a "dedicated medical center" if it does ≥33 percutaneous coronary intervention (PCI) cases per year.*

**1964. Primary PCI is preferred over fibrinolysis when?**
*Harrison's 20th Ed. Chapter 269 Page 1878*

A. Diagnosis is in doubt
B. Cardiogenic shock is present
C. Bleeding risk is increased
D. All of the above

*Primary PCI is preferred over fibrinolysis when the diagnosis is in doubt, cardiogenic shock is present, bleeding risk is increased, or symptoms have been present for at least 2 - 3 hours when the clot is more mature and less easily lysed by fibrinolytic drugs.*

**1965. In STEMI, fibrinolytic therapy should ideally be initiated within?**
*Harrison's 20th Ed. Chapter 269 Page 1878*

A. 10 minutes of presentation
B. 30 minutes of presentation
C. 60 minutes of presentation
D. 90 minutes of presentation

*In STEMI, fibrinolytic therapy should ideally be initiated within 30 minutes of presentation (door-to-needle time 30 minutes) with a principal goal to promptly restore full coronary arterial patency (TIMI grade 3).*

**1966. Value of reducing delay time between onset of symptoms and initiation of treatment was illustrated by?**
*American Journal of Clinical Medicine. 2011;8(1):15*

A. GISSI-2
B. ISIS-3
C. GUSTO-1
D. All of the above

*GISSI-2, ISIS-3, and GUSTO-1 concluded that the choice of thrombolytic therapy was much less important to ultimate survival than was the delay time between onset of symptoms and initiation of treatment.*

**1967. Which of the following is a characteristic of an ideal fibrinolytic agent?**
*American Journal of Clinical Medicine. 2011;8(1):15*

A. One that would achieve 100% patency in a short time period
B. Has minimal bleeding complications
C. Improves microvascular function and flow
D. All of the above

**1968. Which of the following fibrinolytic agent acts by promoting conversion of plasminogen to plasmin?**
*Harrison's 20th Ed. Chapter 269 Page 1878*

A. Tissue plasminogen activator (tPA)
B. Streptokinase
C. Tenecteplase (TNK)
D. All of the above

*Tissue plasminogen activator (tPA), streptokinase, tenecteplase (TNK) & reteplase (rPA) are fibrinolytic agents that act by promoting conversion of plasminogen to plasmin, which subsequently lyses fibrin thrombi.*

**1969. Which of the following is a 'bolus fibrinolytic' agent?**
*Harrison's 20th Ed. Chapter 269 Page 1878*

A. Streptokinase
B. Tenecteplase (TNK)
C. Urokinase
D. Tissue plasminogen activator (tPA)

**1970. Which of the following is a 'bolus fibrinolytic' agent?**
*Harrison's 20th Ed. Chapter 269 Page 1878*

A. Streptokinase
B. Reteplase (rPA)
C. Urokinase
D. Tissue plasminogen activator (tPA)

*Tenecteplase (TNK) & reteplase (rPA) are bolus fibrinolytics since their administration does not require a prolonged intravenous infusion.*

**1971. Angiographically flow in the culprit coronary artery is assessed by which of the following grading system?**
*Harrison's 20th Ed. Chapter 269 Page 1878*

A. TIMI
B. ISIS
C. CURE
D. CAPRIE

*When assessed angiographically, flow in the culprit coronary artery is described by a simple qualitative scale called the thrombolysis in myocardial infarction (TIMI) grading system.*

**1972. Method of angiographic assessment of the efficacy of fibrinolysis is?**
*Harrison's 20th Ed. Chapter 269 Page 1879*

A. TIMI flow grade
B. TIMI frame count
C. TIMI myocardial perfusion grade
D. All of the above

*Qualitative scale to angiographically assess flow in the culprit coronary artery is the thrombolysis in myocardial infarction (TIMI) grading system. Grade 0 - complete occlusion of infarct-related artery (IRA), grade 1 - some penetration of contrast material beyond the point of obstruction but without perfusion of distal coronary bed, grade 2 - perfusion of entire infarct vessel into distal bed, but with flow that is delayed compared with that of a normal artery and grade 3 - full perfusion of the infarct vessel with normal flow. Additional methods of angiographic assessment of efficacy of fibrinolysis include counting the number of frames on cine film required for dye to flow from the origin of the IRA to a landmark in distal vascular bed (TIMI frame count) and determining the rate of entry and exit of contrast dye from microvasculature in myocardial infarct zone (TIMI myocardial perfusion grade).*

**1973. Which TIMI flow grade indicates full perfusion of infarct vessel with normal flow following reperfusion therapy?**
*Harrison's 20th Ed. Chapter 269 Page 1879*

A. TIMI 1
B. TIMI 2
C. TIMI 3
D. TIMI 4

*TIMI grade 3 indicates full perfusion of the infarct vessel with normal flow which is the goal of reperfusion therapy.*

**1974. In STEMI, fibrinolytic therapy can reduce the relative risk of in-hospital death by up to?**
*N Engl J Med. 2013;368:1379-87*

A. 10%
B. 25%
C. 50%
D. 75%

*In STEMI, fibrinolytic therapy can reduce the relative risk of in-hospital death by up to 50% when administered within the first hour of the onset of symptoms. Benefit is maintained for at least 10 years.*

**1975. Which of the following is given as a "single" weight-based intravenous bolus?**
*Harrison's 20th Ed. Chapter 269 Page 1879*

A. Tissue plasminogen activator (tPA)
B. Reteplase (rPA)
C. Tenecteplase (TNK)
D. Streptokinase (STK)

*TNK is given as a "single" weight-based intravenous bolus of 0.53 mg/kg over 10 seconds.*

**1976. Which of the following fibrinolytic agent is administered in a double-bolus regimen?**
*Harrison's 20th Ed. Chapter 269 Page 1879*

A. Tissue plasminogen activator (tPA)
B. Reteplase (rPA)
C. Tenecteplase (TNK)
D. Streptokinase (STK)

*tPA is given as a 15 mg bolus followed by 50 mg intravenously over the first 30 minutes, followed by 35 mg over the next 60 minutes. Streptokinase is administered as 1.5 million units (MU) intravenously over 1 hour. rPA is administered in a double-bolus regimen consisting of a 10-MU bolus given over 2 - 3 minutes, followed by a second 10-MU bolus 30 minutes later.*

**1977. Combination reperfusion regimens involve giving a fibrinolytic agent with which of the following?**
*Harrison's 20th Ed. Chapter 269 Page 1879*

A. Aspirin
B. Clopidogrel
C. Intravenous glycoprotein IIb/IIIa inhibitor
D. Percutaneous coronary intervention (PCI)

*Combination reperfusion regimens for coronary reperfusion combine an intravenous glycoprotein IIb/IIIa inhibitor with a reduced dose of a fibrinolytic agent.*

**1978. Clear contraindications to the use of fibrinolytic agents are all except?**
*Harrison's 20th Ed. Chapter 269 Page 1879*

A. Cerebrovascular hemorrhage at any time
B. Nonhemorrhagic stroke at any time
C. Suspicion of aortic dissection
D. Active internal bleeding

*Clear contraindications to the use of fibrinolytic agents include a history of cerebrovascular hemorrhage at any time, a nonhemorrhagic stroke or other cerebrovascular event within the past year, marked hypertension (>180/110 mm Hg) at any time during acute presentation, suspicion of aortic dissection, and active internal bleeding (excluding menses).*

**1979. In STEMI, which of the following is a relative contraindication to fibrinolytic therapy?**
*Harrison's 20th Ed. Chapter 269 Page 1879*

A. Current use of anticoagulants (INR >=2)
B. Pregnancy
C. Hemorrhagic diabetic retinopathy
D. All of the above

*Relative contraindications to fibrinolytic therapy, which require clinical consideration of risk:benefit ratio include current use of anticoagulants (INR >=2), a recent (<2 weeks) invasive or surgical procedure or prolonged (>10 minute) cardiopulmonary resuscitation, known bleeding diathesis, pregnancy, a hemorrhagic ophthalmic condition (hemorrhagic diabetic retinopathy), active peptic ulcer disease, and a history of severe hypertension that is currently adequately controlled.*

**1980. For what period, streptokinase should not be given, if the patient has received it in past?**
*Harrison's 20th Ed. Chapter 269 Page 1879*

A. Never in life
B. 5 days to 2 years
C. 1 to 2 years
D. 3 to 5 years

*Because of the risk of an allergic reaction, patients should not receive streptokinase if that agent had been received within the preceding 5 days to 2 years.*

**1981. Allergic reactions to streptokinase occur in about what percentage of patients who receive it?**
*Harrison's 20th Ed. Chapter 269 Page 1879*

A. 1%
B. 2%
C. 3%
D. 4%

*Allergic reactions to streptokinase occur in ~2% of patients who receive it.*

**1982. Minor degree of hypotension occurs in what percentage of patients who receive streptokinase?**
*Harrison's 20th Ed. Chapter 269 Page 1879*

A. 4–10%
B. 10–16%
C. 16–30%
D. 30–40%

*Minor hypotension occurs in 4 - 10% of patients given STK, marked hypotension occurs rarely.*

**1983. Hemorrhagic stroke occurs in about what percentage of patients who receive streptokinase?**
*Harrison's 20th Ed. Chapter 269 Page 1879*

A. 0.1–0.5%
B. 0.5–0.9%
C. 0.9–1.5%
D. 1.5–2.4%

*Hemorrhagic stroke, the most serious complication, occurs in ~0.5 - 0.9% of patients receiving fibrinolytic agents. Rate of intracranial hemorrhage with tPA or rPA is slightly higher than with STK.*

**1984. Integrated approach in the management of STEMI addresses patients to receive?**
*Harrison's 20th Ed. Chapter 269 Page 1879*

A. Fibrinolytic therapy
B. Percutaneous coronary intervention (PCI)
C. Coronary artery bypass grafting (CABG)
D. All of the above

*Prior approaches that segregated pharmacologic and catheter-based approaches to reperfusion have been replaced with an integrated approach to triage & transfer of STEMI patients to receive PCI.*

1985. Failure of reperfusion refers to persistent chest pain & ST-segment elevation beyond?
*Harrison's 20th Ed. Chapter 269 Page 1879*

A. > 30 minutes
B. > 60 minutes
C. > 90 minutes
D. > 120 minutes

*Cardiac catheterization & coronary angiography should be carried out after fibrinolytic therapy if there is evidence of failure of reperfusion, which means persistent chest pain & ST-segment elevation >90 minutes. Rescue PCI should be considered in such a situation.*

1986. Development of recurrent ischemia is handled by?
*Harrison's 20th Ed. Chapter 269 Page 1879*

A. Rescue PCI
B. Urgent PCI
C. Elective PCI
D. Any of the above

1987. Patients with confirmed STEMI and low risk may be safely transferred out of the coronary care unit within?
*Harrison's 20th Ed. Chapter 269 Page 1879*

A. 6 hours
B. 12 hours
C. 24 hours
D. 48 hours

*Patients with confirmed STEMI & low risk (no prior MI & no persistent chest discomfort, CHF, hypotension or cardiac arrhythmias) may be safely transferred out of CCU within 24 hours.*

1988. Patients with STEMI should be kept at bed rest for the first?
*Harrison's 20th Ed. Chapter 269 Page 1879*

A. 3–6 hours
B. 6–12 hours
C. 12–24 hours
D. 24–48 hours

*Patients with STEMI should be at bed rest for the first 6–12 hours. In the absence of complications, patients should be encouraged, under supervision, to resume an upright posture by dangling their feet over the side of the bed & sitting in a chair within the first 24 hours. By day 3 after MI, patients should increase their ambulation progressively to a goal of 185 meters (600 ft) three times a day.*

1989. STEMI patients should receive either nothing or only clear liquids by mouth for the first?
*Harrison's 20th Ed. Chapter 269 Page 1879*

A. 4–6 hours
B. 4–8 hours
C. 4–10 hours
D. 4–12 hours

*STEMI patients should receive either nothing or only clear liquids by mouth for the first 4–12 hours.*

1990. The typical coronary care unit diet should provide?
*Harrison's 20th Ed. Chapter 269 Page 1879*

A. ≤ 30% of total calories as fat
B. Cholesterol content should be ≤ 300 mg/day
C. Complex carbohydrates should be 50—55% of total calories
D. All of the above

*The typical coronary care unit diet should provide ≤30% of total calories as fat and have a cholesterol content of ≤300 mg/day. Complex carbohydrates should make up 50–55% of total calories.*

1991. In STEMI, diet rich in which of the following is recommended?
*Harrison's 20th Ed. Chapter 269 Page 1879*

A. Potassium
B. Magnesium
C. Fiber
D. All of the above

*In STEMI, foods that are high in potassium, magnesium, and fiber, but low in sodium are recommended.*

1992. Which of the following drugs used in coronary care unit can produce delirium, particularly in the elderly?
*Harrison's 20th Ed. Chapter 269 Page 1880*

A. Atropine
B. $H_2$ blockers
C. Narcotics
D. All of the above

*Atropine, H2 blockers & narcotics can produce delirium, particularly in the elderly.*

1993. In STEMI, goal of treatment with antiplatelet and anticoagulant agents is?
*Harrison's 20th Ed. Chapter 269 Page 1880*

A. To maintain patency of infarct-related artery (IRA)
B. To reduce likelihood of mural thrombus formation
C. To reduce likelihood of deep venous thrombosis
D. All of the above

1994. Data from Antiplatelet Trialists' Collaboration shows a relative reduction in mortality of how much in patients with MI receiving antiplatelet agents?
*Harrison's 20th Ed. Chapter 269 Page 1880*

A. 12%
B. 21%
C. 27%
D. 34%

*Data from Antiplatelet Trialists' Collaboration patients with MI showed a relative reduction of 27% in mortality rate, from 14.2% in control patients to 10.4% in patients receiving antiplatelet agents.*

1995. In STEMI, the maximum recommended dose of unfractionated heparin (UFH) given as an initial bolus is?
*Harrison's 20th Ed. Chapter 269 Page 1880*

A. 2500 U
B. 4000 U
C. 5000 U
D. 7500 U

1996. In STEMI, the maximum recommended dose of unfractionated heparin (UFH) given after the initial bolus is?
*Harrison's 20th Ed. Chapter 269 Page 1880*

A. 500 U / hour
B. 1000 U / hour
C. 1500 U / hour
D. 2000 U / hour

1997. In STEMI, with the use of UFH, activated partial thromboplastin time during maintenance therapy should be?
*Harrison's 20th Ed. Chapter 269 Page 1880*

A. 1.5 times the control value
B. 1.5–2 times the control value
C. 2.5–3 times the control value
D. 3–3.5 times the control value

*In STEMI, the recommended dose of unfractionated heparin (UFH) is an initial bolus of 60 U/kg (maximum 4000 U) followed by an initial infusion of 12 U/kg per hour (maximum 1000 U/hour). Activated partial thromboplastin time during maintenance therapy should be 1.5 - 2 times the control value.*

**1998. In STEMI, which of the following can be used as an alternative to UFH for anticoagulation?**
*Harrison's 20th Ed. Chapter 269 Page 1880*

A. Fondaparinux
B. Bivalirudin
C. Enoxaparin
D. All of the above

*Advantages of low-molecular-weight heparin (LMWH) preparations include high bioavailability permitting subcutaneous administration, reliable anticoagulation without monitoring, and greater antiXa:IIa activity.*

**1999. Unique pentasaccharide sequence of heparin consists of?**
*The Journal of Biological Chemistry. 2009; 284(40):27054-27064*

A. D-fructosamine and hexosamine
B. D-nitrosamine and N-acetylglucosamine
C. D-glucosamine and uronic acid
D. D-glucuronic acid and N-acetyl-D-glucosamine

**2000. Which of the following is essential for heparin for binding and activating antithrombin?**
*The Journal of Biological Chemistry. 2009; 284(40):27054-27064*

A. 1-O-sulfo group
B. 2-O-sulfo group
C. 3-O-sulfo group
D. 4-O-sulfo group

*The key structural unit of heparin is a unique pentasaccharide sequence which consists of three D-glucosamine and two uronic acid residues. The central D-glucosamine residue contains a unique 3-O-sulfo moiety that is rare outside of this sequence. Removal of unique 3-O-sulfo group results in complete loss of the anticoagulant activity.*

**2001. Which of the following about fondaparinux is false?**
*N Engl J Med. 2006; 354:1524-1527*

A. Synthetic pentasaccharide
B. Inhibits factor Xa within clot, prevents thrombus progression
C. Does not inhibit platelet function
D. None of the above

**2002. Which of the following about fondaparinux is false?**
*Harrison's 20th Ed. Chapter 269 Page 1880*

A. Synthetic version of the pentasaccharide sequence of heparin
B. Should not be used alone during PCI
C. Does not cause heparin-induced thrombocytopenia
D. None of the above

**2003. The first LMW heparin was?**
*N Engl J Med. 2006; 354:1524-1527*

A. Enoxaparin
B. Dalteparin
C. Parnaparin
D. Tinzaparin

**2004. Which of the following about LMW heparin is false?**
*Harrison's 20th Ed. Chapter 269 Page 1880*

A. LMWH is prepared from unfractionated heparin
B. Mean molecular weight of LMWH is about 5000
C. LMWH is cleared almost exclusively by the kidneys
D. None of the above

**2005. Which of the following clinical trials evaluated fondaparinux in STEMI?**
*Harrison's 20th Ed. Chapter 269 Page 1880, N Engl J Med. 2006; 354:1524-1527*

A. OASIS-2
B. OASIS-4
C. OASIS-6
D. OASIS-8

*In Organization to Assess Strategies in Acute Ischemic Syndromes (OASIS-6) trial, fondaparinux was compared with a control group treated with UFH (N= 3221) & patients who had myocardial infarction with ST-segment elevation and who presented relatively late (N= 12,902). Primary end point of death or reinfarction at 30 days was significantly lower in the fondaparinux group.*

**2006. Which of the under mentioned myocardial infarction has an increased risk of systemic or pulmonary thromboembolism?**
*Harrison's 20th Ed. Chapter 269 Page 1880*

A. Anterior
B. Inferior
C. Posterior
D. Lateral

*Patients with anterior myocardial infarction, severe LV dysfunction, heart failure, history of embolism, 2D echocardiographic evidence of mural thrombus or atrial fibrillation are at increased risk of systemic or pulmonary thromboembolism.*

**2007. In STEMI, acute intravenous beta blockade leads to?**
*Harrison's 20th Ed. Chapter 269 Page 1880*

A. Improvement in the myocardial $O_2$ supply-demand relationship
B. Decrease in chest pain
C. Reduces infarct size
D. All of the above

*In STEMI, acute intravenous beta blockade improves the myocardial O2 supply-demand relationship, decreases pain, reduces infarct size, and decreases the incidence of serious ventricular arrhythmias.*

**2008. In STEMI patients who undergo fibrinolysis, beta blockers do not reduce?**
*Harrison's 20th Ed. Chapter 269 Page 1880*

A. Mortality rate
B. Recurrent ischemia
C. Reinfarction
D. None of the above

*In STEMI patients who undergo fibrinolysis soon after onset of chest pain, no incremental reduction in mortality rate is seen with beta blockers, but recurrent ischemia and reinfarction are reduced.*

**2009. STEMI patients with excellent long-term prognosis are?**
*Harrison's 20th Ed. Chapter 269 Page 1880*

A. Patients <55 years
B. Patients with no previous MI
C. Patients with normal ventricular function
D. All of the above

STEMI patients with excellent long-term prognosis are those with an expected mortality rate of <1% per year, patients <55 years, no previous MI, with normal ventricular function, no complex ventricular ectopy, and no angina.

**2010. High-risk STEMI patients are?**
*Harrison's 20th Ed. Chapter 269 Page 1880*

A. Those who are elderly
B. Those who have an anterior infarction
C. Those who have had a prior infarction
D. All of the above

**2011. ACE inhibitors should be continued indefinitely in patients who have?**
*Harrison's 20th Ed. Chapter 269 Page 1881*

A. Clinically evident CHF
B. In patients with reduction in global LV function
C. In patients with a large regional wall motion abnormality
D. All of the above

ACE inhibitors should be continued indefinitely in patients who have clinically evident CHF, in patients with a reduction in global LV function (LV ejection fraction ≤40%) or a large regional wall motion abnormality, or in hypertensive individuals.

**2012. Which of the following medication is least useful during the first 24–48 hours after the onset of myocardial infarction?**
*Harrison's 20th Ed. Chapter 269 Page 1881*

A. Intravenous nitroglycerin
B. Angiotensin-converting enzyme (ACE) inhibitors
C. Beta blockers
D. Unfractionated heparin (UFH)

Benefits of routine use of intravenous nitroglycerin are less in contemporary era where beta-adrenoceptor blockers & ACE inhibitors are routinely prescribed for patients with STEMI.

**2013. In STEMI, serum levels of which of the following should be corrected to minimize the risk of arrhythmias?**
*Harrison's 20th Ed. Chapter 269 Page 1881*

A. Calcium
B. Potassium
C. Magnesium
D. All of the above

Serum magnesium should be measured in all patients of STEMI on admission, and any deficits should be corrected to minimize the risk of arrhythmias.

**2014. After STEMI, left ventricle undergoes changes in which of the following in noninfarcted segments?**
*Harrison's 20th Ed. Chapter 269 Page 1881*

A. Shape
B. Size
C. Thickness
D. All of the above

After STEMI, left ventricle undergoes a series of changes in shape, size & thickness in both, infarcted and noninfarcted segments, a process referred to as ventricular remodeling.

**2015. Overall cardiac chamber enlargement is more following infarction of?**
*Harrison's 20th Ed. Chapter 269 Page 1881*

A. Inferior wall
B. Posterior wall
C. Anterior wall
D. Any of the above

Overall cardiac chamber enlargement is more following infarction of anterior wall & apex of left ventricle.

**2016. Which of the following is the primary cause of in-hospital death from STEMI?**
*Harrison's 20th Ed. Chapter 269 Page 1881*

A. Pump failure
B. Arrhythmia
C. Thromboembolism
D. Sepsis

Presently, pump failure is the primary cause of in-hospital death from STEMI.

**2017. Early mortality in STEMI refers to death within how many days of infarction?**
*Harrison's 20th Ed. Chapter 269 Page 1881*

A. 3 days
B. 7 days
C. 10 days
D. 14 days

Early mortality in STEMI refers to death within 10 days of infarction.

**2018. The most common clinical signs of pump failure is?**
*Harrison's 20th Ed. Chapter 269 Page 1881*

A. Tachycardia
B. Hypotension
C. Pulmonary rales
D. Raised JVP

The most common clinical signs of pump failure are pulmonary rales and S3 / S4 gallop sounds.

**2019. Which of the following is the characteristic hemodynamic finding of pump failure?**
*Harrison's 20th Ed. Chapter 269 Page 1881*

A. Elevated LV filling volume
B. Elevated RV filling volume
C. Elevated RA pressure
D. Elevated pulmonary artery pressure

Elevated LV filling pressure & elevated pulmonary artery pressure are the characteristic hemodynamic findings of pump failure.

**2020. Patients with rales at lung bases, S3 gallop, tachypnea, or signs of right heart failure belong to which Killip class?**
*Harrison's 20th Ed. Chapter 269 Page 1881*

A. Killip class I
B. Killip class II
C. Killip class III
D. Killip class IV

Killip classification divides patients into four groups. Class I–no signs of pulmonary or venous congestion, class II–rales at lung bases, S3 gallop, tachypnea, or signs of right heart failure, class III–severe heart failure, pulmonary edema and class IV–shock with systolic pressure <90 mm Hg, peripheral vasoconstriction, peripheral cyanosis, mental confusion, and oliguria.

**2021. Infarction of what percentage of left ventricle results in cardiogenic shock?**
*Harrison's 20th Ed. Chapter 269 Page 1881*

A. About 20%
B. About 30%
C. About 35%
D. About 40%

*Hemodynamic evidence of abnormal LV function appears when contraction is seriously impaired in 20 to 25% of the left ventricle. Infarction of ≥40% of left ventricle results in cardiogenic shock.*

**2022. After STEMI, which of the following is an ideal class of drugs for the long-term management of ventricular dysfunction?**
*Harrison's 20th Ed. Chapter 269 Page 1881*

A. Diuretics
B. Digitalis
C. Nitrates
D. ACE inhibitors

*ACE inhibitors are an ideal class of drugs for the long term management of ventricular dysfunction after STEMI.*

**2023. Incidence of cardiogenic shock is?**
*Harrison's 20th Ed. Chapter 269 Page 1882*

A. ~ 1%
B. ~ 3%
C. ~ 5%
D. ~ 7%

*The incidence of cardiogenic shock is ~7%. In recent years, practice of prompt reperfusion, efforts to reduce infarct size and treatment of ongoing ischemia and other complications of MI contributed to the reduction.*

**2024. In STEMI, what proportion of patients present with cardiogenic shock on admission?**
*Harrison's 20th Ed. Chapter 269 Page 1882*

A. 1%
B. 5%
C. 10%
D. 20%

*Only 10% of patients with STEMI present with cardiogenic shock on admission. 90% develop it during hospitalization.*

**2025. Which of the following is not true for cardiogenic shock?**
*Harrison's 20th Ed. Chapter 269 Page 1882*

A. Sustained systolic arterial pressure of <60 mm Hg
B. Cardiac index < 2.2 L/(min/m$_2$)
C. Elevated pulmonary capillary wedge pressure (>18 mm Hg)
D. Generally associated with mortality rate of >50%

*Cardiogenic shock (CS) is characterized by systemic hypoperfusion due to severe depression of cardiac index [<2.2 (L/min)/m2] & sustained systolic arterial hypotension (<90 mm Hg), despite an elevated filling pressure (PCWP > 18 mm Hg). In-hospital mortality rate is >50%.*

**2026. Clinically significant RV infarction can cause?**
*Harrison's 20th Ed. Chapter 269 Page 1882*

A. Jugular venous distention
B. Kussmaul's sign
C. Hepatomegaly
D. All of the above

*Approximately one-third of patients with inferior infarction demonstrate at least a minor degree of RV necrosis. Clinically significant RV infarction causes signs of severe RV failure i.e. jugular venous distention, Kussmaul's sign, hepatomegaly with or without hypotension.*

**2027. Which of the following ECG lead is most helpful in diagnosing right ventricular myocardial infarction?**
*Harrison's 20th Ed. Chapter 269 Page 1882*

A. $V_1R$
B. $V_2R$
C. $V_3R$
D. $V_4R$

*ST-segment elevations of right-sided precordial ECG leads, particularly lead $V_4R$, are frequently present in the first 24 hours in patients with RV infarction.*

**2028. What is true for right ventricular myocardial infarction?**
*Harrison's 20th Ed. Chapter 269 Page 1882*

A. Associated with occlusion of proximal RCA
B. ST-segment elevation of >1 mm in lead $V_4R$
C. Upright T wave in lead $V_4R$ during initial hours
D. All of the above

**2029. Catheterization study in a patient with right ventricular myocardial infarction resembles?**
*Harrison's 20th Ed. Chapter 269 Page 1882*

A. Constrictive pericarditis
B. Pericardial effusion
C. Cardiac tamponade
D. Any of the above

*In RV infarction, catheterization study of the right side of heart resembles constrictive pericarditis i.e. steep right atrial "y" descent and an early diastolic dip & plateau in RV waveforms.*

**2030. Objective of therapy for RV infarction is?**
*Harrison's 20th Ed. Chapter 269 Page 1882*

A. To maintain adequate RV preload
B. To reduce pulmonary capillary wedge
C. To reduce pulmonary arterial pressures
D. All of the above

*Therapy for RV infarction consists of volume expansion to maintain adequate RV preload, efforts to improve LV performance with attendant reduction in pulmonary capillary wedge & pulmonary arterial pressures.*

**2031. Mechanisms responsible for infarction-related arrhythmias is?**
*Harrison's 20th Ed. Chapter 269 Page 1882*

A. Autonomic nervous system imbalance
B. Electrolyte disturbances
C. Slowed conduction in zones of ischemic myocardium
D. All of the above

*The mechanisms responsible for infarction-related arrhythmias include autonomic nervous system imbalance, electrolyte disturbances, ischemia and slowed conduction in zones of ischemic myocardium.*

**2032. Warning arrhythmia refers to?**
*Harrison's 20th Ed. Chapter 269 Page 1882*

A. Early systolic ventricular extrasystoles
B. Early diastolic ventricular extrasystoles
C. Late systolic ventricular extrasystoles
D. Late diastolic ventricular extrasystoles

**2033. Which of the following is effective in abolishing ventricular ectopic activity in patients with STEMI?**
*Harrison's 20th Ed. Chapter 269 Page 1882*

A. Nitrates
B. Beta-adrenoceptor blocking agents
C. Inhibitors of the P2Y$_{12}$ ADP receptor
D. Digitalis

*Beta-adrenoceptor blocking agents are effective in abolishing ventricular ectopic activity in patients with STEMI and in the prevention of ventricular fibrillation.*

**2034. In patients with STEMI, serum magnesium should be adjusted to?**
*Harrison's 20th Ed. Chapter 269 Page 1882*

A. ~ 1.0 mmol / L
B. ~ 2.0 mmol / L
C. ~ 3.0 mmol / L
D. ~ 4.0 mmol / L

*Hypokalemia and hypomagnesemia are risk factors for ventricular fibrillation in patients with STEMI. To reduce the risk, serum potassium concentration should be adjusted to ~4.5 mmol/L and magnesium to ~2.0 mmol/L.*

**2035. Prophylactic use of lidocaine in STEMI increases?**
*Harrison's 20th Ed. Chapter 269 Page 1882*

A. Overall mortality
B. Risk of bradycardia
C. Risk of asystole
D. All of the above

**2036. Ventricular tachycardia or fibrillation refractory to electroshock is more responsive after patient is treated with?**
*Harrison's 20th Ed. Chapter 269 Page 1882*

A. Epinephrine
B. Bretylium
C. Amiodarone
D. All of the above

*Ventricular tachycardia or fibrillation that is refractory to electroshock may be more responsive after patient is treated with epinephrine (1 mg intravenously or 10 mL of a 1:10,000 solution via the intracardiac route), bretylium (5 mg/kg bolus) or amiodarone (75 to 150 mg bolus).*

**2037. Torsades des pointes may occur in patients with STEMI with the use of?**
*Harrison's 20th Ed. Chapter 269 Page 1882*

A. Amiodarone
B. Lidocaine
C. Quinidine
D. All of the above

*Torsades des pointes may occur in patients with STEMI as a consequence of hypoxia, hypokalemia, or co-administration of digoxin or quinidine.*

**2038. Which of the following about accelerated idioventricular rhythm (AIVR) is false?**
*Harrison's 20th Ed. Chapter 269 Page 1882*

A. Benign
B. Occurs transiently during fibrinolytic therapy
C. Ventricular rate is 60-100 beats/minute
D. None of the above

*Accelerated idioventricular rhythm (AIVR) or "slow ventricular tachycardia" is a ventricular rhythm with a rate of 60- 100 beats/minute. It often occurs transiently during fibrinolytic therapy at the time of reperfusion. AIVR is benign and does not presage the development of classic ventricular tachycardia. Most episodes of AIVR do not require treatment.*

**2039. Synchronized electroshock is recommended if supraventricular abnormal rhythm persists for?**
*Harrison's 20th Ed. Chapter 269 Page 1882*

A. > 2 hours
B. > 6 hours
C. > 12 hours
D. > 24 hours

*If supraventricular abnormal rhythm persists for >2 hours with a ventricular rate > 120 beats/minute, or if tachycardia induces heart failure, shock, or ischemia, a synchronized electroshock (100-200 J monophasic waveform) should be used.*

**2040. Which of the following about accelerated junctional rhythms is false?**
*Harrison's 20th Ed. Chapter 269 Page 1882*

A. Occur in patients with inferoposterior infarction
B. Occur in patients with digitalis excess
C. Right atrial or coronary sinus pacing is indicated
D. None of the above

**2041. Heart block in inferior infarction results from the release of?**
*Harrison's 20th Ed. Chapter 269 Page 1882*

A. Adenosine
B. Bradykinin
C. Natriuretic peptide
D. All of the above

*Heart block in inferior infarction results from increased vagal tone and/or the release of adenosine and therefore is transient.*

**2042. Implantable cardioverter/defibrillator (ICD) is recommended for which of the following?**
*Harrison's 19th Ed. 1609, Figure 295-5*

A. LVEF is <30-40% and NYHA class II
B. LVEF is <30-40% and NYHA class III
C. LVEF is <30-35% and NYHA class I
D. All of the above

*Patients with depressed left ventricular function at least 40 days post-STEMI are referred for insertion of an implantable cardioverter/defibrillator (ICD) if the LVEF is <30–40% with NYHA class II-III or if LVEF is <30–35% with NYHA class I functional status. Patients with preserved left ventricular function (LVEF >40%) do not receive an ICD regardless of NYHA functional class.*

**2043. Which of the following is false about recurrent post STEMI angina?**
*Harrison's 20th Ed. Chapter 269 Page 1884*

A. Develops in ~25% of patients hospitalized for STEMI
B. More frequent in those who have successful fibrinolysis
C. Repeat fibrinolysis is an alternative
D. None of the above

*Recurrent angina develops in ~25% of patients hospitalized for STEMI. It is even higher in patients who undergo successful fibrinolysis. Repeat administration of a fibrinolytic agent is an alternative to early mechanical revascularization.*

**2044. Pain of pericarditis radiates to?**
*Harrison's 20th Ed. Chapter 269 Page 1884*

A. Right trapezius muscle
B. Left trapezius muscle
C. Both trapezius muscles
D. Any of the above

*Pain radiating to either trapezius muscle is typical of pericarditis.*

**2045. Complication of LV aneurysm is?**
*Harrison's 20th Ed. Chapter 269 Page 1882*

A. CHF
B. Arterial embolism
C. Ventricular arrhythmias
D. All of the above

*Complications of LV aneurysm do not usually occur for weeks to months after STEMI. They include CHF, arterial embolism and ventricular arrhythmias. Apical aneurysms are the most common.*

**2046. Maximal (symptom limited) exercise stress test may be carried out how many weeks after myocardial infarction?**
*Harrison's 20th Ed. Chapter 269 Page 1882*

A. 2-4 weeks
B. 4-6 weeks
C. 6-10 weeks
D. 10-12 weeks

*Maximal (symptom limited) exercise stress test may be carried out 4-6 weeks after myocardial infarction to detect residual ischemia and ventricular ectopy.*

**2047. Usual duration of hospitalization for an uncomplicated STEMI is about?**
*Harrison's 20th Ed. Chapter 269 Page 1882*

A. 3 days
B. 5 days
C. 7 days
D. 10 days

*Usual duration of hospitalization for an uncomplicated STEMI is about 5 days.*

**2048. Intravenous antiplatelet drugs include?**
*Journal of Blood Medicine 2012:3:33-42*

A. Abciximab
B. Eptifibatide
C. Tirofiban
D. All of the above

*Three potent parenteral GpIIb/IIIa inhibitors are Abciximab (chimeric monoclonal Fab fragment of human & murine protein that binds to GpIIb/IIIa), Eptifibatide (synthetic cyclic heptapeptide with a KGD sequence) and Tirofiban (synthetic peptidomimetic based on the RGD sequence).*

**2049. ATP in "National Cholesterol Education Project ATP III" stands for?**
*N Engl J Med. 2014; 370:1422-1431*

A. Adult Treatment Panel
B. Advanced Treatment Panel
C. Aggressive Treatment Panel
D. Angina Treatment Panel

*Adult Treatment Panel III (ATP III).*

**2050. The technique "Percutaneous transluminal coronary angioplasty" (PTCA) was first introduced by?**
*N Engl J Med. 2001; 344:144-145*

A. Andreas Gruentzig
B. Denton Cooley
C. Michael DeBakey
D. Christian Bernard

*In 1977, Andreas Gruentzig introduced percutaneous transluminal coronary angioplasty (PTCA).*

**2051. During percutaneous coronary intervention (PCI), steerable guidewire put into coronary artery lumen has a diameter of?**
*BMJ. 2003;326(7399):1137-1140*

A. < 0.4 mm
B. < 0.6 mm
C. < 0.8 mm
D. < 1 mm

*During PCI, steerable guidewire put into coronary artery lumen has a diameter of < 0.4 mm.*

**2052. What suggests involvement of right coronary artery rather than left circumflex artery as the culprit vessel in inferior MI?**
*N Engl J Med. 2003;348:933-40*

A. Greater ST-segment elevation in lead II than in lead III & ST-segment depression of >1 mm in leads I & aVL
B. Greater ST-segment elevation in lead III than in lead II & ST-segment depression of >1 mm in leads I & aVL
C. Greater ST-segment elevation in lead aVF than in lead II or III & ST-segment depression of >1 mm in leads I & aVL
D. Greater ST-segment elevation in lead II & III than in lead aVF & ST-segment depression of >1 mm in leads I & aVL

**2053. In inferior MI, ST-segment depression in leads V1 and V2 suggest concomitant infarction of?**
*N Engl J Med. 2003;348:933-40*

A. Lateral wall of left ventricle
B. Posterior wall of left ventricle
C. Anterior wall of left ventricle
D. Atrial infarction

**2054. Most sensitive electrocardiographic sign of right ventricular infarction is?**
*N Engl J Med. 2003;348:933-40*

A. ST-segment elevation of >1 mm in $V_4R$ with upright T wave during first 12 hours
B. ST-segment elevation of >1 mm in $V_4R$ with inverted T wave during first 12 hours
C. ST-segment elevation of >1 mm in $V_4R$ with upright T wave after first 12 hours
D. ST-segment elevation of >1 mm in $V_4R$ with inverted T wave after first 12 hours

**2055. Proximal occlusion of the left anterior descending artery is indicated by?**
*N Engl J Med. 2003;348:933-40*

A. Anterior wall MI, ST elevation in $V_1$, $V_2$, and $V_3$
B. Anterior wall MI, ST elevation in $V_1$, $V_2$, and $V_3$ & aVL
C. Anterior wall MI, ST elevation in $V_1$, $V_2$, $V_3$ & aVL with ST depression of >1 mm in lead aVF
D. Anterior wall MI, ST elevation in $V_1$, $V_2$, $V_3$ & aVL with ST depression of >1 mm in lead II, III and aVF

2056. Which of the following statements about blood supply of sinus node is true?
   *N Engl J Med. 2003;348:933-40*

   A. Supplied by RCA in 60% of people and by the left circumflex artery in 40%
   B. Supplied by RCA in 40% of people and by left circumflex artery in 60%
   C. Supplied by RCA in 80% of people and by left circumflex artery in 20%
   D. Supplied by RCA in 60% of people and by left anterior descending artery in 40%

2057. Which of the following statements about blood supply of atrioventricular node is true?
   *N Engl J Med. 2003;348:933-40*

   A. Supplied by RCA in 50% of people and by left circumflex artery in 50%
   B. Supplied by RCA in 60% of people and by left circumflex artery in 40%
   C. Supplied by RCA in 75% of people and by left circumflex artery in 25%
   D. Supplied by RCA in 90% of people and by left circumflex artery in 10%

2058. Which of the following statements about blood supply of bundle of His is true?
   *N Engl J Med. 2003;348:933-40*

   A. Supplied by atrioventricular nodal branch of LAD
   B. Supplied by atrioventricular nodal branch of RCA + septal perforators of LAD
   C. Supplied by atrioventricular nodal branch of left circumflex artery + septal perforators of LAD
   D. Supplied by septal branch of left circumflex artery

2059. Which of the following statements about blood supply of right bundle branch is true?
   *N Engl J Med. 2003;348:933-40*

   A. Supplied by septal perforators of LAD
   B. Supplied by septal perforators of RCA
   C. Supplied by septal perforators of left circumflex artery
   D. None of the above

2060. Which of the following is an electrocardiographic predictor of myocardial reperfusion following thrombolysis?
   *N Engl J Med. 2003;348:933-40*

   A. T-wave inversion in < 4 hours after MI
   B. ST-segment resolution during first 90 minutes
   C. Accelerated idioventricular rhythm
   D. All of the above

## Hypertensive Vascular Disease

**2061.** According to JNC 7, stage 2 hypertension is?
*N Engl J Med. 2006;355:385-92*

 A. 120/80 mm Hg
 B. 140-159/90-99
 C. ≥ 160/100 mm Hg
 D. 180/110 mm Hg

**2062.** Isolated systolic hypertension is defined as a systolic pressure of >=140 mm Hg and a diastolic pressure below?
*N Engl J Med. 2006;355:385-92*

 A. 70 mm Hg
 B. 80 mm Hg
 C. 90 mm Hg
 D. 100 mm Hg

**2063.** Among adults, diastolic blood pressure increases progressively until what age, after which it tends to decrease?
*Harrison's 20th Ed. Chapter 271 Page 1891*

 A. ~ 45 years
 B. ~ 55 years
 C. ~ 65 years
 D. ~ 75 years

*Among adults, diastolic blood pressure increases progressively with age until ~55 years, after which it tends to decrease.*

**2064.** The probability that a middle-aged or elderly individual will develop hypertension in his or her lifetime is?
*Harrison's 20th Ed. Chapter 271 Page 1891*

 A. 10%
 B. 30%
 C. 60%
 D. 90%

*Probability that a middle-aged / elderly individual will develop hypertension in lifetime is 90%.*

**2065.** Which of the following statements about age-related increase of blood pressure is false?
*Harrison's 20th Ed. Chapter 271 Page 1891*

 A. Augmented by high NaCl intake
 B. Augmented by low dietary intakes of calcium
 C. Augmented by low dietary intakes of potassium
 D. None of the above

*Hypertension prevalence is related to dietary NaCl intake, & age-related increase of BP is augmented by high NaCl intake. Low dietary intakes of calcium & potassium contribute to risk of hypertension.*

**2066.** Which of the following is a stronger correlate of blood pressure?
*Harrison's 20th Ed. Chapter 271 Page 1891*

 A. Urine sodium
 B. Urine potassium
 C. Urine sodium-to-potassium ratio
 D. All of the above

*The urine sodium-to-potassium ratio is a stronger correlate of blood pressure than is either sodium or potassium alone.*

**2067.** High BP before age 55 occurs how many times more frequently among persons with a positive family history of hypertension?
*Harrison's 19th Ed. 1612*

 A. 1.8 times
 B. 2.8 times
 C. 3.8 times
 D. 4.8 times

*High blood pressure before age 55 occurs 3.8 times more frequently among persons with a positive family history of hypertension.*

**2068.** Which of the following is considered as a hypertension-related gene?
*Harrison's 20th Ed. Chapter 271 Page 1891*

 A. Alpha-adducin gene
 B. MDR1 gene
 C. NAT2 gene
 D. All of the above

*Alpha adducin gene encodes a cytoskeletal protein important for renal tubular sodium absorption. It is thought to be associated with increased renal tubular absorption of sodium, and variants of this gene may be associated with hypertension and salt sensitivity of blood pressure.*

**2069.** Which of the following best relate to the genetics of hypertension?
*Harrison's 20th Ed. Chapter 271 Page 1891*

 A. Epigenetic signature
 B. Epigenetic reset
 C. Epigenetic dysregulation
 D. Epigenetic imprint

**2070.** Hypertension-related genes relate to?
*Harrison's 20th Ed. Chapter 271 Page 1891*

 A. Renin-angiotensin aldosterone system
 B. Atrial natriuretic peptide
 C. Beta-2 adrenoreceptor
 D. All of the above

**2071.** Which of the following genes is possibly related to hypertension?
*Harrison's 20th Ed. Chapter 271 Page 1891*

 A. Gene encoding $AT_1$ receptor
 B. Gene encoding aldosterone synthase
 C. Gene encoding $\beta_2$ adrenoreceptor
 D. All of the above

*Genes possibly related to hypertension include genes encoding the AT1 receptor, aldosterone synthase, atrial natriuretic peptide and the b2 adrenoreceptor.*

**2072.** Which of the following statements about genesis of hypertension is false?
*Harrison's 20th Ed. Chapter 271 Page 1892*

A. Vascular volume is a primary determinant of arterial pressure over the long term
B. Nonchloride salts of sodium have little or no effect on blood pressure
C. Salt-wasting disorders are associated with low blood pressure levels
D. None of the above

**2073. Which of the following modulate blood pressure over the short term?**
*Harrison's 20th Ed. Chapter 271 Page 1892*

A. Adrenergic reflexes
B. Hormonal factors
C. Volume-related factors
D. All of the above

*Adrenergic reflexes modulate blood pressure over the short term. Adrenergic function, in concert with hormonal & volume-related factors contributes to long-term regulation of arterial pressure.*

**2074. Which of the following is an endogenous catecholamine?**
*Harrison's 20th Ed. Chapter 271 Page 1892, British J of Pharmacology. 2012;165:2015-2033*

A. Norepinephrine
B. Epinephrine
C. Dopamine
D. All of the above

*The three endogenous catecholamines are norepinephrine, epinephrine, and dopamine. They play important roles in tonic and phasic cardiovascular regulation.*

**2075. The activities of the adrenergic receptors are mediated by?**
*Harrison's 20th Ed. Chapter 271 Page 1892*

A. Receptor Tyrosine Kinase
B. Cytokine Receptor–Linked Kinase
C. Guanosine nucleotide-binding regulatory proteins
D. Serine Kinase

*The activities of adrenergic receptors are mediated by guanosine nucleotide-binding regulatory proteins (G proteins) & by intracellular concentrations of downstream second messengers.*

**2076. Physiologic responsiveness to catecholamines depends on?**
*Harrison's 20th Ed. Chapter 271 Page 1892*

A. Receptor affinity
B. Receptor density
C. Receptor-effector coupling efficiency
D. All of the above

**2077. When activated by catecholamines, which of the following receptors act as negative feedback controllers, inhibiting further norepinephrine release?**
*Harrison's 20th Ed. Chapter 271 Page 1892*

A. $\alpha_1$
B. $\alpha_2$
C. $\beta_1$
D. $\beta_2$

*When activated by catecholamines, $\alpha_2$ receptors act as negative feedback controllers, inhibiting further norepinephrine release.*

**2078. In the kidney, activation of which of the following increases renal tubular reabsorption of sodium?**
*Harrison's 20th Ed. Chapter 271 Page 1892*

A. $\alpha_1$-adrenergic receptors
B. $\alpha_2$-adrenergic receptors
C. $\beta_1$-adrenergic receptors
D. $\beta_2$-adrenergic receptors

*In kidney, activation of $a_1$-adrenergic receptors increases renal tubular reabsorption of sodium.*

**2079. Activation of which of the following receptors by epinephrine relaxes vascular smooth muscle leading to vasodilation?**
*Harrison's 20th Ed. Chapter 271 Page 1892*

A. $\alpha_1$
B. $\alpha_2$
C. $\beta_1$
D. $\beta_2$

*Activation of $b_2$ receptors by epinephrine relaxes vascular smooth muscle & results in vasodilation.*

**2080. Antihypertensive agents act as?**
*Harrison's 20th Ed. Chapter 271 Page 1892*

A. $\alpha_1$ receptor inhibitors
B. $\alpha_2$ receptor agonists
C. $\beta_1$ receptor inhibitors
D. Any of the above

**2081. Which of the following about clonidine is false?**
*Harrison's 20th Ed. Chapter 271 Page 1892*

A. Antihypertensive agent
B. Centrally acting $\alpha_1$ agonist
C. Inhibits sympathetic outflow
D. Abrupt cessation of therapy leads to rebound hypertension due to upregulation of $\alpha_1$ receptors

*Clonidine is a centrally acting α2 agonist.*

**2082. The autonomic nervous system maintains cardiovascular homeostasis via which of the following signals?**
*Harrison's 20th Ed. Chapter 271 Page 1892*

A. Pressure signals
B. Volume signals
C. Chemoreceptor signals
D. All of the above

*The autonomic nervous system maintains cardiovascular homeostasis via pressure, volume, and chemoreceptor signals.*

**2083. Which of the following is false about Renin?**
*Harrison's 20th Ed. Chapter 271 Page 1892*

A. Prorenin is an enzymatically inactive precursor
B. Synthesized in renal afferent renal arteriole
C. Plasma contains 2–5 times more prorenin than renin
D. None of the above

**2084. Which of the following is not a primary stimuli for renin secretion?**
*Harrison's 20th Ed. Chapter 271 Page 1892*

A. Decreased NaCl transport in thick ascending limb of loop of Henle
B. Increased NaCl transport in thick ascending limb of loop of Henle
C. Decreased pressure or stretch within renal afferent arteriole
D. Sympathetic nervous system stimulation of renin-secreting cells via beta$_1$ adrenoreceptors

Three primary stimuli for renin secretion are decreased NaCl transport in thick ascending limb of loop of Henle (macula densa mechanism), decreased pressure or stretch within renal afferent arteriole (baroreceptor mechanism), and sympathetic nervous system stimulation of renin-secreting cells via beta1 adrenoreceptors. Renin secretion is inhibited by increased NaCl transport in thick ascending limb of loop of Henle.

**2085. Renin is best related to which of the following?**
*Harrison's 20th Ed. Chapter 271 Page 1892*

A. Metallo-protease
B. Aspartyl protease
C. Cysteine protease
D. Serine protease

Renin is an aspartyl protease that is synthesized as an enzymatically inactive precursor called prorenin.

**2086. Most renin in the circulation is synthesized in?**
*Harrison's 20th Ed. Chapter 271 Page 1892*

A. Renal afferent renal arteriole
B. Renal efferent renal arteriole
C. Glomeruli
D. All of the above

Most renin in the circulation is synthesized in the renal afferent renal arteriole.

**2087. Which of the following directly inhibits renin secretion?**
*Harrison's 20th Ed. Chapter 271 Page 1892*

A. Angiotensin I
B. Angiotensin II
C. Angiotensinogen
D. Prorenin

Angiotensin II directly inhibits renin secretion due to angiotensin II type 1 receptors on juxtaglomerular cells. Renin secretion increases in response to pharmacologic blockade of ACE or angiotensin II receptors.

**2088. Which of the following statements is false?**
*Harrison's 20th Ed. Chapter 271 Page 1893*

A. Angiotensin I is an inactive decapeptide
B. Angiotensin II is an active octapeptide
C. ACE-kininase II is located in pulmonary circulation
D. ACE-kininase II activates bradykinin

In circulation, active renin cleaves angiotensinogen to form an inactive decapeptide, angiotensin I. ACE-kininase II is a converting enzyme, located primarily in pulmonary circulation, converts angiotensin I to active octapeptide, angiotensin II. It also inactivates vasodilator bradykinin.

**2089. Which of the following statements is false about angiotensin II?**
*Harrison's 20th Ed. Chapter 271 Page 1893*

A. Acts on angiotensin II type 1 receptors on cell membranes
B. Potent pressor substance
C. Stimulates secretion of aldosterone
D. None of the above

**2090. Which of the following is a functional effect of angiotensin II type 2 receptor (AT$_2$)?**
*Harrison's 20th Ed. Chapter 271 Page 1893*

A. Vasodilation
B. Sodium excretion
C. Inhibition of cell growth & matrix formation
D. All of the above

Angiotensin II type 2 (AT$_2$) receptor is widely distributed in kidneys and has the opposite functional effects of AT$_1$ receptor. AT$_2$ receptor induces vasodilation, sodium excretion and inhibition of cell growth and matrix formation.

**2091. Which of the following is a renin-secreting tumor?**
*Harrison's 20th Ed. Chapter 271 Page 1893*

A. Germinoma
B. Benign hemangiopericytoma
C. Choriocarcinoma
D. Osteoblastoma

Renin-secreting tumors include benign hemangiopericytomas of the juxtaglomerular apparatus, renal carcinomas & Wilms tumors.

**2092. Renin-producing carcinomas may be found in?**
*Harrison's 20th Ed. Chapter 271 Page 1893*

A. Lung
B. Liver
C. Pancreas
D. All of the above

Renin-producing carcinomas have been described in lung, liver, pancreas, colon and adrenals.

**2093. Angiotensinogen, renin, and angiotensin II are also synthesized locally in?**
*Harrison's 20th Ed. Chapter 271 Page 1893*

A. Uterus
B. Brain
C. Spleen
D. All of the above

Angiotensinogen, renin, and angiotensin II are also synthesized locally in brain, pituitary, aorta, arteries, heart, adrenal glands, kidneys, adipocytes, leukocytes, ovaries, testes, uterus, spleen, and skin.

**2094. Angiotensin II in tissues may be formed by the enzymatic activity of?**
*Harrison's 20th Ed. Chapter 271 Page 1893*

A. Tonin
B. Chymase
C. Cathepsins
D. All of the above

Angiotensin II in tissues may be formed by the enzymatic activity of renin or by other proteases like tonin, chymase, and cathepsins.

**2095. Which of the following is the primary trophic factor regulating synthesis & secretion of aldosterone by zona glomerulosa of adrenal cortex?**
*Harrison's 20th Ed. Chapter 271 Page 1893*

A. Potassium
B. Adrenocorticotropic hormone (ACTH)

C. Angiotensin II
D. All of the above

*Angiotensin II is the primary trophic factor regulating synthesis & secretion of aldosterone by zona glomerulosa of adrenal cortex. Aldosterone synthesis is also dependent on potassium and acute elevations of adrenocorticotropic hormone (ACTH).*

**2096. Excess tissue angiotensin II contributes to?**
*Harrison's 20th Ed. Chapter 271 Page 1893*

A. Atherosclerosis
B. Cardiac hypertrophy
C. Renal failure
D. All of the above

*Excess tissue angiotensin II contributes to atherosclerosis, cardiac hypertrophy & renal failure.*

**2097. Which of the following best relates to angiotensin II?**
*Harrison's 20th Ed. Chapter 271 Page 1893*

A. Anaphylactoid reaction
B. Mitogen
C. Thrombocytopenia
D. Hyperlipidemia

*Tissue angiotensin II is a mitogen that stimulates growth and contributes to modeling and repair.*

**2098. Which of the following influence the synthesis & secretion of aldosterone by zona glomerulosa of adrenal cortex?**
*Harrison's 20th Ed. Chapter 271 Page 1893*

A. Angiotensin II
B. Potassium
C. Adrenocorticotropic hormone (ACTH)
D. All of the above

**2099. Which of the following is the primary tropic factor regulating synthesis & secretion of aldosterone by zona glomerulosa?**
*Harrison's 20th Ed. Chapter 271 Page 1893*

A. Angiotensin II
B. Potassium
C. Adrenocorticotropic hormone (ACTH)
D. All of the above

*Angiotensin II is the primary tropic factor regulating synthesis & secretion of aldosterone by zona glomerulosa of adrenal cortex. Aldosterone secretion may be decreased in potassium-depleted individuals. Acute elevations of adrenocorticotropic hormone (ACTH) increase aldosterone secretion.*

**2100. Aldosterone increases sodium reabsorption by?**
*Harrison's 20th Ed. Chapter 271 Page 1893*

A. ATP-sensitive potassium channel
B. Voltage-sensitive sodium channel
C. Amiloride-sensitive Na+ channel
D. All of the above

**2101. Increased aldosterone secretion may result in?**
*Harrison's 20th Ed. Chapter 271 Page 1893*

A. Hypokalemia
B. Alkalosis
C. Endothelial dysfunction
D. All of the above

*Aldosterone is a potent mineralocorticoid that increases sodium reabsorption by amiloride-sensitive epithelial sodium channels (ENaC) on apical surface of principal cells of renal cortical collecting duct. Increased aldosterone secretion may result in hypokalemia, alkalosis, fibrosis, endothelial dysfunction, inflammation, and oxidative stress, as well as an overall increase in cardiovascular morbidity & mortality.*

**2102. Mineralocorticoid receptors are expressed in which of the following?**
*Harrison's 19th Ed. 1614*

A. Colon
B. Salivary glands
C. Sweat glands
D. All of the above

*Mineralocorticoid receptors also are expressed in the colon, salivary glands, and sweat glands.*

**2103. Which of the following has no affinity for the mineralocorticoid receptor?**
*Harrison's 20th Ed. Chapter 271 Page 1893*

A. Aldosterone
B. Cortisol
C. Cortisone
D. All of the above

*Cortisol binds to mineralocorticoid receptors but is a less potent mineralocorticoid than aldosterone because cortisol is converted to cortisone by enzyme 11 β-hydroxysteroid dehydrogenase type 2. Cortisone has no affinity for the mineralocorticoid receptor.*

**2104. Myocardial fibrosis, nephrosclerosis, vascular inflammation and remodeling are the effects of which of the following?**
*Harrison's 20th Ed. Chapter 271 Page 1893*

A. Aldosterone
B. Cortisol
C. Cortisone
D. All of the above

*Aldosterone and/or mineralocorticoid receptor activation induces structural & functional alterations in heart, kidney & blood vessels, leading to myocardial fibrosis, nephrosclerosis & vascular inflammation and remodeling, as a consequence of oxidative stress. These effects are amplified by a high salt intake.*

**2105. In CHF, low-dose spironolactone reduces the risk of progressive heart failure & sudden death from cardiac causes by?**
*Harrison's 20th Ed. Chapter 271 Page 1893*

A. 10%
B. 20%
C. 30%
D. 40%

*In CHF, low-dose spironolactone reduces the risk of progressive heart failure and sudden death from cardiac causes by 30%.*

**2106. Resistance to blood flow varies inversely with?**
*Harrison's 20th Ed. Chapter 271 Page 1893*

A. Second power of the radius
B. Third power of the radius
C. Fourth power of the radius
D. Fifth power of the radius

*Vascular radius & compliance of resistance arteries are important determinants of arterial pressure. Resistance to flow varies inversely with the fourth power of the radius.*

### 2107. Which of the following contribute to vascular remodeling?
*Harrison's 20th Ed. Chapter 271 Page 1893*

A. Apoptosis
B. Low-grade inflammation
C. Vascular fibrosis
D. All of the above

### 2108. Which of the following is related to the functional properties of large arteries?
*Harrison's 20th Ed. Chapter 271 Page 1893*

A. Cardiac output
B. Peripheral resistance
C. Pulse pressure
D. All of the above

*Pulse pressure is related to the functional properties of large arteries.*

### 2109. Aortic augmentation index is calculated as the ratio of?
*Harrison's 20th Ed. Chapter 271 Page 1894*

A. Central arterial pressure - to - pulse pressure
B. Pulse pressure - to - central arterial pressure
C. Central arterial pressure - to - mean blood pressure
D. Mean blood pressure - to - central arterial pressure

*The aortic augmentation index is a surrogate index of arterial stiffening. It is calculated as the ratio of central arterial pressure-to-pulse pressure. Central blood pressure and the aortic augmentation index are strong, independent predictors of cardiovascular disease and all-cause mortality.*

### 2110. Intracellular pH (pHi) is regulated by?
*Harrison's 20th Ed. Chapter 271 Page 1894*

A. $Na^+$ - $H^+$ exchange
B. $Na^+$ - dependent $HCO_3^-$ - $Cl^-$ exchange
C. Cation-independent $HCO_3^-$ - $Cl^-$ exchange
D. All of the above

*Intracellular pH (pHi) of vascular smooth muscle cells determine vascular tone and vascular growth. Ion transport mechanisms that regulate pHi include $Na^+$-$H^+$ exchange, $Na^+$-dependent $HCO_3^-$-$Cl^-$ exchange and cation-independent $HCO_3^-$-$Cl^-$ exchange.*

### 2111. Which of the following is increased in hypertension?
*Harrison's 20th Ed. Chapter 271 Page 1894*

A. Sympathetic outflow
B. Activity of the $Na^+$ - $H^+$ exchanger
C. Atrial natriuretic factor
D. All of the above

### 2112. Which of the following is a vasoconstrictor?
*Harrison's 20th Ed. Chapter 271 Page 1894*

A. Nitric oxide
B. Acetylcholine
C. Endothelin
D. All of the above

*Vascular endothelium synthesizes & releases nitric oxide, a potent vasodilator. Acetylcholine is an endothelium-dependent vasodilator. Endothelin is a vasoconstrictor peptide produced by endothelium.*

### 2113. Which of the following occurs in hypertension?
*Harrison's 20th Ed. Chapter 271 Page 1894*

A. Impaired endothelium-dependent vasodilation
B. Increased circulating levels of autoantibodies
C. Disruption of renal pressure-natriuresis curve
D. All of the above

### 2114. Which of the following is an early consequence of hypertension-related heart disease?
*Harrison's 20th Ed. Chapter 271 Page 1894*

A. Systolic dysfunction
B. Diastolic dysfunction
C. Left ventricular hypertrophy
D. All of the above

*Diastolic dysfunction is an early consequence of hypertension-related heart disease.*

### 2115. Cerebral blood flow remains unchanged when mean arterial pressure is between?
*Harrison's 20th Ed. Chapter 271 Page 1894*

A. 50–100 mm Hg
B. 50–150 mm Hg
C. 50–200 mm Hg
D. 50–250 mm Hg

*Cerebral blood flow remains unchanged over mean arterial pressure of 50–150 mm Hg.*

### 2116. Differential diagnosis of hypertensive encephalopathy includes?
*Harrison's 20th Ed. Chapter 271 Page 1895*

A. Pseudotumor cerebri
B. Acute intermittent porphyria
C. Uremic encephalopathy
D. All of the above

### 2117. Mechanisms of kidney-related hypertension is?
*Harrison's 20th Ed. Chapter 271 Page 1895*

A. Diminished capacity to excrete sodium
B. Excessive renin secretion in relation to volume status
C. Sympathetic nervous system overactivity
D. All of the above

### 2118. Which of the following is synthesized in adrenal medulla and released into circulation upon adrenal stimulation?
*Harrison's 19th Ed. 1615*

A. Epinephrine
B. Norepinephrine
C. Dopamine
D. All of the above

*Adrenergic neurons synthesize norepinephrine & dopamine, which are stored in vesicles within neuron. When neuron is stimulated, these neurotransmitters are released into synaptic cleft. Epinephrine is synthesized in adrenal medulla & released into circulation upon adrenal stimulation.*

### 2119. Atherosclerotic, hypertension-related vascular lesions in the kidney primarily affect?
*Harrison's 20th Ed. Chapter 271 Page 1895*

A. Preglomerular arterioles
B. Glomerular capillaries
C. Postglomerular arterioles
D. All of the above

*Atherosclerotic, hypertension-related vascular lesions in the kidney primarily affect preglomerular arterioles, resulting in ischemic changes in the glomeruli and postglomerular structures.*

**2120. Renal lesion associated with malignant hypertension is?**
*Harrison's 20th Ed. Chapter 271 Page 1895*

A. Fibrinoid necrosis of afferent arterioles
B. Fibrinoid necrosis of glomerular capillaries
C. Fibrinoid necrosis of efferent arterioles
D. All of the above

*Renal lesion associated with malignant hypertension consists of fibrinoid necrosis of the afferent arterioles.*

**2121. For every 20 mm Hg increase in SBP & 10 mm Hg increase in DBP, cardiovascular disease risk increases by?**
*Harrison's 20th Ed. Chapter 271 Page 1895*

A. 1.5 times
B. 2 times
C. 2.5 times
D. 3 times

*Cardiovascular disease risk doubles for every 20 mm Hg increase in systolic and 10 mm Hg increase in diastolic pressure.*

**2122. Among older individuals, which of the following is the least powerful predictor of cardiovascular disease?**
*Harrison's 20th Ed. Chapter 271 Page 1895*

A. Systolic blood pressure
B. Diastolic blood pressure
C. Pulse pressure
D. None of the above

*Among older individuals, systolic blood pressure & pulse pressure are more powerful predictors of cardiovascular disease than diastolic blood pressure.*

**2123. Blood pressure tends to be higher during which of the following times?**
*Harrison's 20th Ed. Chapter 271 Page 1895*

A. Early morning hours soon after waking
B. Following meals
C. Evenings
D. Night

*Blood pressure tends to be higher in the early morning hours, soon after waking, than at other times of day. Myocardial infarction and stroke are more frequent in the early morning hours.*

**2124. Generally, night time blood pressures are lower than day time blood pressures by?**
*Harrison's 20th Ed. Chapter 271 Page 1895*

A. 5–10%
B. 10–20%
C. 20–30%
D. 30–40%

*Nighttime blood pressures are generally 10–20% lower than daytime blood pressures.*

**2125. Which of the following about hypertension is false?**
*Harrison's 20th Ed. Chapter 271 Page 1895*

A. More severe in glomerular than in interstitial diseases
B. Low-renin patients have volume-dependent hypertension
C. White coat hypertension does not develop into sustained hypertension
D. ~80–95% of hypertensive patients have essential hypertension

*Individuals with white coat hypertension are at increased risk for developing sustained hypertension.*

**2126. Which of the following is a secondary cause of systolic & diastolic hypertension?**
*Harrison's 20th Ed. Chapter 271 Page 1896 Table 271-3*

A. 17α-hydroxylase deficiency
B. 11β-hydroxylase deficiency
C. 11-hydroxysteroid dehydrogenase deficiency
D. All of the above

**2127. Which of the following is a secondary cause of systolic & diastolic hypertension?**
*Harrison's 20th Ed. Chapter 271 Page 1896 Table 271-3*

A. Hypothyroidism
B. Hyperthyroidism
C. Hypercalcemia
D. All of the above

**2128. Which of the following is a secondary cause of systolic & diastolic hypertension?**
*Harrison's 20th Ed. Chapter 271 Page 1896 Table 271-3*

A. Cyclosporine
B. High-dose estrogens
C. Erythropoietin
D. All of the above

**2129. Which of the following about primary hypertension is false?**
*Harrison's 20th Ed. Chapter 271 Page 1896*

A. Tends to be familial
B. High-renin patients have vasoconstrictor form of hypertension
C. Low-renin patients have volume-dependent hypertension
D. None of the above

**2130. Association between aldosterone & blood pressure is striking in?**
*Harrison's 20th Ed. Chapter 271 Page 1896*

A. Native American
B. Polynesian
C. African Americans
D. Maori population

*Association between aldosterone & blood pressure is more striking in African Americans. Aldosterone antagonist Spironolactone may be an effective antihypertensive agent.*

**2131. Metabolic syndrome consists of all except?**
*Harrison's 20th Ed. Chapter 271 Page 1896*

A. Diabetes mellitus
B. Abdominal obesity
C. Hypertension
D. Dyslipidemia

*Constellation of insulin resistance, abdominal obesity, hypertension & dyslipidemia is called metabolic syndrome.*

**2132. Which of the following is the most common cause of secondary hypertension?**
*Harrison's 20th Ed. Chapter 271 Page 1896*

A. Obesity & metabolic syndrome
B. Renal disease
C. Obstructive sleep apnea
D. Psychogenic

*Virtually all disorders of kidney may cause hypertension and renal disease is the most common cause of secondary hypertension.*

**2133. Which of the following about patients with fibromuscular dysplasia is false?**
*Harrison's 20th Ed. Chapter 271 Page 1896*

A. Lesions are frequently bilateral
B. Strong predilection for young black women
C. Have more favorable outcomes with vascular repair
D. Potentially curable form of hypertension

*Fibromuscular dysplasia may occur at any age and it has a strong predilection for young white women.*

**2134. Which is the most common histologic variant of fibromuscular dysplasia?**
*Harrison's 19th Ed. 1617*

A. Medial fibroplasia
B. Perimedial fibroplasia
C. Medial hyperplasia
D. Intimal fibroplasia

*Histologic variants of fibromuscular dysplasia include medial fibroplasia, perimedial fibroplasia, medial hyperplasia & intimal fibroplasia. Medial fibroplasia is the most common variant (66%).*

**2135. Lesions of fibromuscular dysplasia mostly affect which portion of renal artery?**
*Harrison's 20th Ed. Chapter 271 Page 1897*

A. Proximal
B. Mid
C. Distal
D. Any of the above

*Lesions of fibromuscular dysplasia are frequently bilateral and in contrast to atherosclerotic renovascular disease tend to affect more distal portions of renal artery.*

**2136. Which of the following raises the possibility of renovascular hypertension?**
*Harrison's 20th Ed. Chapter 271 Page 1897*

A. Severe or refractory hypertension
B. Recent loss of hypertension control
C. Deterioration of renal function with ACE inhibitor use
D. All of the above

**2137. What percentage of patients with renovascular hypertension have an abdominal or flank bruit?**
*Harrison's 20th Ed. Chapter 271 Page 1897*

A. ~ 10%
B. ~ 25%
C. ~ 50%
D. ~ 75%

*~50% of patients with renovascular hypertension have an abdominal or flank bruit. Bruit is more likely to be hemodynamically significant if it lateralizes or extends throughout systole into diastole.*

**2138. Which of the following serves as "gold standard" for evaluation and identification of renal artery lesions?**
*Harrison's 20th Ed. Chapter 271 Page 1897*

A. DTPA scan
B. Gadolinium-contrast magnetic resonance angiography
C. Contrast arteriography
D. Doppler ultrasound of the renal arteries

*Contrast arteriography remains the "gold standard" for evaluation and identification of renal artery lesions.*

**2139. Renal blood flow may be evaluated with?**
*Harrison's 20th Ed. Chapter 271 Page 1897*

A. 2-[$^{18}$F]fluoro-2-deoxy-D-glucose (FDG) scan
B. [$^{131}$I]-orthoiodohippurate (OIH) scan
C. $^{99m}$Tc scan
D. $^{90}$Yttrium scan

*As a screening test, renal blood flow is evaluated with a radionuclide [$^{131}$I]-orthoiodohippurate (OIH) scan.*

**2140. [$^{99m}$Tc]-diethylenetriamine pentaacetic acid (DTPA) scan estimates which of the following?**
*Harrison's 20th Ed. Chapter 271 Page 1897*

A. Renal blood flow
B. Renal blood flow velocity
C. Glomerular filtration rate
D. All of the above

*Glomerular filtration rate (GFR) is evaluated with a [$^{99m}$Tc]-diethylenetriamine pentaacetic acid (DTPA) scan before and after a single dose of captopril.*

**2141. Which of the following test is sufficiently reliable for a causal relationship between a renal artery lesion & hypertension?**
*Harrison's 20th Ed. Chapter 271 Page 1897*

A. DTPA scan
B. Gadolinium-contrast magnetic resonance angiography
C. Doppler ultrasound of the renal arteries
D. None of the above

*No single test is sufficiently reliable to determine a causal relationship between a renal artery lesion and hypertension.*

**2142. In renal artery obstruction, functionally significant lesions occlude?**
*Harrison's 20th Ed. Chapter 271 Page 1897*

A. > 30% of the lumen
B. > 50% of the lumen
C. > 70% of the lumen
D. > 90% of the lumen

*Functionally significant renal artery lesions generally occlude more than 70% of the lumen of the affected renal artery.*

**2143. Which of the following predict a functionally significant renal artery and response to vascular repair?**
*Harrison's 20th Ed. Chapter 271 Page 1897*

A. Occlusion of >70% of lumen of the affected renal artery
B. Presence of collateral vessels to the ischemic kidney

C. Lateralizing renal vein renin ratio
D. All of the above

*Renin secretion is increased in the ischemic kidney but is suppressed in the contralateral kidney. The ratio of the measurement from ischemic kidney to the measurement from contralateral kidney is the renal vein renin ratio. A ratio higher than 1.5 constitutes a positive test result and is suggestive of functionally important renovascular disease.*

### 2144. Which of the following is false about primary aldosteronism?
*Harrison's 20th Ed. Chapter 271 Page 1897*

A. Potentially curable form of hypertension
B. Aldosterone production is independent of RAS
C. Patients rarely have edema
D. None of the above

### 2145. Which of the following is not a feature of primary aldosteronism?
*Harrison's 20th Ed. Chapter 271 Page 1897*

A. Sodium retention
B. Mild to moderate hypertension
C. Unprovoked hypokalemia
D. High PRA

*Excess aldosterone production in primary aldosteronism is independent of the renin-angiotensin system (RAS) and leads to sodium retention, hypertension, hypokalemia, and low PRA. In patients on diuretics, serum potassium <3.1 mEq/L also raises the possibility of primary aldosteronism.*

### 2146. Hypokalemic hypertension is seen in?
*Harrison's 20th Ed. Chapter 271 Page 1897*

A. Primary aldosteronism
B. Glucocorticoid-induced hypertension
C. Pheochromocytoma
D. All of the above

*Besides primary aldosteronism, hypokalemic hypertension may be a consequence of secondary aldosteronism, other mineralocorticoid- and glucocorticoid-induced hypertensive disorders, and pheochromocytoma.*

### 2147. Plasma aldosterone (adult) level in supine position with patient on normal sodium diet normally is?
*Harrison's 18th Ed., Appendix: Laboratory Values of Clinical Importance, Table 2*

A. < 16 ng/dL
B. < 32 ng/dL
C. < 48 ng/dL
D. < 72 ng/dL

### 2148. What ratio of plasma aldosterone to plasma renin activity is indicative of aldosterone-producing adenoma?
*Harrison's 20th Ed. Chapter 271 Page 1897*

A. > 10 : 1
B. > 20 : 1
C. > 30 : 1
D. > 40 : 1

*A ratio of >30 : 1 of plasma aldosterone to plasma renin activity (PA / PRA) is indicative of aldosterone-producing adenoma provided plasma aldosterone concentration is >555 pmol/L (>20 ng/dL). It can be confirmed by demonstrating failure to suppress plasma aldosterone to <277 pmol/L (<10 ng/dL) after IV infusion of 2 liters of isotonic saline over 4 hours.*

### 2149. Plasma aldosterone is suppressed by all except?
*Harrison's 20th Ed. Chapter 271 Page 1897*

A. Oral NaCl load
B. Fludrocortisone
C. Captopril
D. Spironolactone

*Aldosterone antagonists, angiotensin receptor antagonists, and ACE inhibitors may increase renin. Aldosterone antagonists may increase aldosterone. IV infusion of isotonic saline, oral NaCl load, fludrocortisone, or captopril suppress aldosterone.*

### 2150. Which of the following is the most common cause of sporadic primary aldosteronism?
*Harrison's 20th Ed. Chapter 271 Page 1898*

A. Glucocorticoid-remediable primary aldosteronism
B. Bilateral adrenal hyperplasia
C. Familial aldosteronism type II
D. Familial aldosteronism type III

*The two most common causes of sporadic primary aldosteronism are an aldosterone-producing adenoma and bilateral adrenal hyperplasia. Together, they account for >90% of all patients with primary aldosteronism.*

### 2151. Which of the following is false about aldosterone-producing adrenal adenoma?
*Harrison's 20th Ed. Chapter 271 Page 1898*

A. Tumor is almost always unilateral
B. Measures < 3 cm in diameter
C. Aldosterone biosynthesis more responsive to ACTH
D. None of the above

### 2152. Glucocorticoid-remediable hyperaldosteronism (GRA) best relates to?
*Harrison's 20th Ed. Chapter 271 Page 1898*

A. Mutations in KCNJ5 gene
B. Chimeric karyotype
C. Chimeric gene duplication
D. All of the above

*Glucocorticoid-remediable hyperaldosteronism is a monogenic autosomal dominant disorder characterized by moderate to severe early age hypertension. Hypokalemia is usually mild or absent. Normally, angiotensin II stimulates aldosterone production by adrenal zona glomerulosa, whereas ACTH stimulates cortisol production in zona fasciculata. Due to a chimeric gene on chromosome 8, ACTH also regulates aldosterone secretion by zona fasciculata in glucocorticoid-remediable hyperaldosteronism. Consequently, there is overproduction in zona fasciculata of both aldosterone & hybrid steroids (18-hydroxycortisol & 18-oxocortisol). Suppression of ACTH with low-dose glucocorticoids corrects hyperaldosteronism, hypertension & hypokalemia.*

### 2153. Glucocorticoid-remediable hyperaldosteronism is also called?
*Harrison's 20th Ed. Chapter 49 Page 305*

A. Familial hyperaldosteronism type I (FH-I)
B. Familial hyperaldosteronism type II (FH-II)
C. Familial hyperaldosteronism type III (FH-III)
D. Familial hyperaldosteronism type IV (FH-IV)

*Familial hyperaldosteronism type I (FH-I) is also known as glucocorticoid-remediable hyperaldosteronism. FH-I is caused by a chimeric gene duplication between the homologous 11β-hydroxylase (CYP11B1) and aldosterone synthase (CYP11B2) genes, fusing the adrenocorticotropic hormone (ACTH) responsive 11β-hydroxylase promoter to the coding region of aldosterone synthase. This chimeric gene is under the control of ACTH and thus repressible by glucocorticoids.*

### 2154. Which of the following is caused by mutations in the KCNJ5 gene?
*Harrison's 20th Ed. Chapter 49 Page 305*

A. Familial hyperaldosteronism type I (FH-I)
B. Familial hyperaldosteronism type II (FH-II)
C. Familial hyperaldosteronism type III (FH-III)
D. Familial hyperaldosteronism type IV (FH-IV)

*Familial hyperaldosteronism type III (FH-III) is caused by mutations in the KCNJ5 gene, which encodes G-protein-activated inward rectifier K⁺ channel 4 (GIRK4).*

**2155. Surgery is not indicated in which of the following?**
*Harrison's 20th Ed. Chapter 271 Page 1898*

A. Bilateral adrenal hyperplasia
B. Glucocorticoid-remediable primary aldosteronism
C. Familial aldosteronism type II
D. All of the above

**2156. Laboratory screening for Cushing's syndrome is done by?**
*Harrison's 20th Ed. Chapter 271 Page 1898*

A. 24-hour excretion rates of urine-free cortisol
B. Overnight dexamethasone-suppression test
C. Late night salivary cortisol
D. All of the above

**2157. In pheochromocytoma, hypotension rather than hypertension is the presentation, the hormone secreted is?**
*Harrison's 20th Ed. Chapter 271 Page 1898*

A. Epinephrine
B. Norepinephrine
C. Corticosterone
D. Cortisol

When epinephrine is the predominant catecholamine secreted in pheochromocytoma, the patients may present with hypotension rather than hypertension.

**2158. Inherited pheochromocytomas may be associated with?**
*Harrison's 20th Ed. Chapter 271 Page 1898*

A. Multiple endocrine neoplasia (MEN) type 2A & type 2B
B. von Hippel-Lindau disease
C. Neurofibromatosis
D. All of the above

~20% of pheochromocytomas are familial with autosomal dominant inheritance. Inherited pheochromocytomas may be associated with multiple endocrine neoplasia (MEN) type 2A and type 2B, von Hippel-Lindau disease and neurofibromatosis.

**2159. Mutations of which of the following genes are associated with paraganglioma syndromes?**
*Harrison's 20th Ed. Chapter 271 Page 1898*

A. Activin receptor–like kinase gene
B. Succinate dehydrogenase genes
C. Tyrosinase gene
D. Serine threonine kinase gene

Mutations of succinate dehydrogenase genes are associated with paraganglioma syndromes, characterized by head and neck paragangliomas.

**2160. Which of the following is the most common congenital cardiovascular cause of hypertension?**
*Harrison's 20th Ed. Chapter 271 Page 1899*

A. Patent ductus arteriosus
B. Venrticular septal defect
C. Coarctation of the aorta
D. Atrial septal defect

**2161. Coarctation of the aorta is associated with which of the following syndromes?**
*Harrison's 20th Ed. Chapter 271 Page 1899*

A. Klinefelter's syndrome
B. Parkes Weber syndrome
C. Hennekam's syndrome
D. Turner's syndrome

Coarctation of the aorta is the most common congenital cardiovascular cause of hypertension. The incidence is 1–8 per 1000 live births. It is usually sporadic but occurs in 35% of children with Turner's syndrome.

**2162. Which of the following is a complication of coarctation of the aorta?**
*Harrison's 20th Ed. Chapter 271 Page 1899*

A. Ischemic heart disease
B. Cerebral hemorrhage
C. Aortic aneurysm
D. All of the above

**2163. In which of the following conditions, males may present with pseudohermaphroditism and hypertension?**
*Harrison's 20th Ed. Chapter 271 Page 1899 Table 271-4*

A. Glucocorticoid-remediable hyperaldosteronism
B. 11β-hydroxylase deficiency
C. 17α-hydroxylase deficiency
D. 11β-hydroxysteroid dehydrogenase deficiency

With 17α-hydroxylase deficiency, synthesis of sex hormones & cortisol is decreased. Consequently, these individuals do not mature sexually. Males may present with pseudohermaphroditism and females with primary amenorrhea and absent secondary sexual characteristics. Because cortisol-induced negative feedback on pituitary ACTH production is diminished, ACTH-stimulated adrenal steroid synthesis proximal to the enzymatic block is increased. Hypertension and hypokalemia are consequences of increased synthesis of mineralocorticoids proximal to the enzymatic block, particularly desoxycorticosterone. Increased steroid production and, hence, hypertension may be treated with low-dose glucocorticoids.

**2164. Which of the following conditions may result in hypertension?**
*Harrison's 20th Ed. Chapter 271 Page 1899*

A. Hypercalcemia
B. Acromegaly
C. Hypothyroidism, hyperthyroidism
D. All of the above

**2165. Which of the following is a form of monogenic hypertension?**
*Harrison's 20th Ed. Chapter 271 Page 1899*

A. Liddle's syndrome
B. Hypertension exacerbated in pregnancy
C. Glucocorticoid-remediable primary aldosteronism
D. All of the above

**2166. Supplementation of which of the following may be associated with reduced stroke mortality?**
*Harrison's 20th Ed. Chapter 271 Page 1901*

A. Potassium
B. Calcium
C. Sodium
D. Alcohol

Potassium supplementation may be associated with reduced stroke mortality.

**2167.** "Hypertensive headache" occurs during?
*Harrison's 19th Ed. 1621*

A. Morning
B. Afternoon
C. Evening
D. Night

**2168.** "Hypertensive headache" is localized to?
*Harrison's 19th Ed. 1621*

A. Occipital region
B. Frontal region
C. Temporal region
D. Any of the above

*Characteristically, hypertensive headache occurs in morning & is localized to occipital region.*

**2169.** Width of the blood pressure bladder cuff should equal at least what percentage of the arm circumference?
*Harrison's 19th Ed. 1445*

A. 10%
B. 20%
C. 30%
D. 40%

**2170.** Length of blood pressure bladder cuff bladder should encircle at least what percentage of the arm circumference?
*Harrison's 19th Ed. 1445*

A. 20%
B. 40%
C. 60%
D. 80%

*Width of the blood pressure bladder cuff should equal at least 40% of the arm circumference; the length of the cuff bladder should encircle at least 80% of the arm circumference.*

**2171.** Optical funduscopic changes in hypertension include?
*Harrison's 19th Ed. 1622*

A. Increased arteriolar light reflex
B. Arteriovenous crossing defects
C. Hemorrhages and exudates
D. All of the above

*With increasing severity of hypertension and atherosclerotic disease, progressive funduscopic changes include increased arteriolar light reflex, arteriovenous crossing defects, hemorrhages and exudates and in patients with malignant hypertension — papilledema.*

**2172.** Blunting of the day-night blood pressure pattern occurs in?
*Harrison's 19th Ed. 1627*

A. Sleep apnea
B. Autonomic neuropathy
C. African Americans populations
D. All of the above

*Attenuated nighttime blood pressure "dip" is associated with increased cardiovascular disease risk. Blunting of day-night blood pressure pattern occurs in sleep apnea, autonomic neuropathy & in African Americans.*

**2173.** One standard drink contains how many grams of ethanol?
*Harrison's 20th Ed. Chapter 271 Page 1901*

A. ~ 10 grams
B. ~ 14 grams
C. ~ 18 grams
D. ~ 24 grams

*One standard drink contains ~14 grams of ethanol.*

**2174.** DASH trial stands for?
*Harrison's 20th Ed. Chapter 271 Page 1901*

A. Death and survival in hypertension
B. Diastolic and systolic hypertension
C. Dietary approaches to stop hypertension
D. Duration and severity of hypertension

*DASH stands for Dietary Approaches to Stop Hypertension.*

**2175.** Which of the following about lowering of SBP & DBP is false?
*Harrison's 20th Ed. Chapter 271 Page 1901*

A. Risk reductions of 35–40% for stroke
B. Risk reductions of 12–16% for CHD
C. Risk reductions of > 50% for heart failure
D. Risk reductions of > 75% for renal failure

*Lowering SBP by 10-12 mm Hg & DBP by 5-6 mm Hg reduces relative risk by 35-40% for stroke, 12-16% for CHD within 5 years of initiation of treatment and >50% risk reduction of heart failure. Benefit of BP lowering on progression of renal failure is less apparent.*

**2176.** Additive blood pressure lowering effect of thiazide diuretics is least when combined with?
*Harrison's 20th Ed. Chapter 271 Page 1901*

A. Beta blockers
B. Calcium channel blocker
C. Angiotensin-converting enzyme inhibitors (ACEIs)
D. Angiotensin receptor blockers (ARBs)

**2177.** Which of the following is a side effect of thiazide diuretic?
*Harrison's 20th Ed. Chapter 271 Page 1901*

A. Hypokalemia
B. Insulin resistance
C. Increased cholesterol
D. All of the above

**2178.** Which of the following act by inhibiting epithelial sodium channels in the distal nephron?
*Harrison's 20th Ed. Chapter 271 Page 1901*

A. Thiazides
B. Furosemide
C. Eplerenone
D. Amiloride

*Potassium-sparing diuretics, amiloride and triamterene, act by inhibiting epithelial sodium channels in the distal nephron. Thiazides inhibit the $Na^+/Cl^-$ pump in the distal convoluted tubule and hence increase sodium excretion. Loop diuretics inhibit the $Na^+$-$K^+$-$2Cl^-$ cotransporter in the thick ascending limb of the loop of Henle. Eplerenone is an aldosterone antagonist.*

**2179. Angiotensin-converting enzyme inhibitors act by which of the following mechanism?**
*Harrison's 20th Ed. Chapter 271 Page 1901*

A. Decrease production of angiotensin II
B. Increase bradykinin levels
C. Reduce sympathetic nervous system activity
D. All of the above

*ACEIs decrease the production of angiotensin II, increase bradykinin levels, and reduce sympathetic nervous system activity.*

**2180. Angiotensin receptor blockers (ARB) provide selective blockade of?**
*Harrison's 20th Ed. Chapter 271 Page 1901*

A. $AT_1$ receptors
B. $AT_2$ receptors
C. $AT_3$ receptors
D. $AT_4$ receptors

*ARBs provide selective blockade of $AT_1$ receptors, and the effect of angiotensin II on unblocked $AT_2$ receptors may augment their hypotensive effect.*

**2181. Which of the following diminishes the adverse effects of diuretics on glucose metabolism?**
*Harrison's 20th Ed. Chapter 271 Page 1902*

A. ACEIs and ARBs
B. Beta blockers
C. Calcium antagonists
D. Alpha antagonists

*ACEIs & ARBs improve insulin action & ameliorate the adverse effects of diuretics on glucose metabolism.*

**2182. Which of the following reduces the risk of developing diabetes in high-risk hypertensive patients?**
*Harrison's 20th Ed. Chapter 271 Page 1902*

A. Valsartan
B. Lisinopril
C. Captopril
D. Ramipril

*Valsartan (an ARB) reduces the risk of developing diabetes in high-risk hypertensive patients.*

**2183. Combining angiotensin-converting enzyme inhibitors with which of the following is associated with more adverse events?**
*Harrison's 20th Ed. Chapter 271 Page 1902*

A. Angiotensin receptor blockers
B. Beta blockers
C. Calcium channel blocker
D. Alpha blocking agents

*ACEI/ARB combination therapy is associated with more adverse events like cardiovascular death, myocardial infarction, stroke, and hospitalization for heart failure, without increases in benefit.*

**2184. Which of the following predisposes to renal insufficiency induced by ACEIs and ARBs?**
*Harrison's 20th Ed. Chapter 271 Page 1902*

A. Dehydration
B. CHF
C. Use of nonsteroidal anti-inflammatory drugs
D. All of the above

**2185. Dry cough occurs in what percentage of patients taking ACEIs?**
*Harrison's 20th Ed. Chapter 271 Page 1902*

A. ~ 5%
B. ~ 10%
C. ~ 15%
D. ~ 20%

*Dry cough occurs in ~15% of patients, and angioedema occurs in <1% of patients taking ACEIs.*

**2186. Which of the following is a direct renin inhibitor?**
*Harrison's 20th Ed. Chapter 271 Page 1902*

A. Guanfacine
B. Doxazosin
C. Aliskiren
D. Terazosin

*Aliskiren is an oral, nonpeptide competitive inhibitors of the enzymatic activity of renin.*

**2187. Which of the following trials studied Aliskiren in Type 2 Diabetes?**
*N Engl J Med. 2012; 367:2204-2213*

A. ALTITUDE
B. ATMOSPHERE
C. CHARM-Added
D. Val-HeFT

*ALTITUDE Clinical Trial studied the addition of aliskiren to standard therapy with renin–angiotensin system blockade in patients with type 2 diabetes who are at high risk for cardiovascular & renal events. It concluded that addition may be harmful.*

**2188. Which of the following about spironolactone is false?**
*Harrison's 20th Ed. Chapter 271 Page 1903*

A. Nonselective aldosterone antagonist
B. Binds to progesterone
C. Binds to androgen receptors
D. None of the above

**2189. Spironolactone is effective in patients with?**
*Harrison's 20th Ed. Chapter 271 Page 1903*

A. Low-renin essential hypertension
B. Resistant hypertension
C. Primary aldosteronism
D. All of the above

*Spironolactone is a nonselective aldosterone antagonist that may be used alone or in combination with a thiazide diuretic. It is particularly effective agent in patients with low-renin essential hypertension, resistant hypertension, and primary aldosteronism. Because spironolactone binds to progesterone and androgen receptors, side effects may include gynecomastia, impotence, and menstrual abnormalities.*

**2190. Which of the following is a selective aldosterone antagonist?**
*Harrison's 20th Ed. Chapter 271 Page 1903*

A. Aliskiren
B. Eplerenone
C. Candesartan
D. Minoxidil

*Eplerenone is a selective aldosterone antagonist.*

**2191. Which of the following clinical trials evaluated eplerenone?**
*N Engl J Med. 2011; 364:11-21*

A. SHIFT trial
B. CHARM-Added trial
C. RALES trial
D. EPHESUS trial

*Eplerenone Post–Acute Myocardial Infarction Heart Failure Efficacy and Survival Study (EPHESUS).*

**2192. β-Adrenergic receptor blockers lower blood pressure by?**
*Harrison's 20th Ed. Chapter 271 Page 1903*

A. Decreasing cardiac output
B. Central nervous system effect
C. Inhibition of renin release
D. All of the above

*β-Adrenergic receptor blockers lower blood pressure by decreasing cardiac output (reduction of heart rate & contractility). Other mechanisms include a central nervous system effect & inhibition of renin release.*

**2193. Which of the following blocks both β receptors and peripheral α-adrenergic receptors?**
*Harrison's 20th Ed. Chapter 271 Page 1903*

A. Carvedilol
B. Aliskiren
C. Eplerenone
D. Minoxidil

*Carvedilol and labetalol block both β receptors and peripheral α-adrenergic receptors.*

**2194. Which of the following about Nebivolol is false?**
*Harrison's 20th Ed. Chapter 271 Page 1903*

A. Beta blocker
B. Cardioselective
C. Enhances nitric oxide activity
D. None of the above

*Nebivolol is a cardioselective β blocker with vasodilator action due to enhancement of nitric oxide activity.*

**2195. Selective alpha antagonists include all except?**
*Harrison's 20th Ed. Chapter 271 Page 1902 Table 271-8*

A. Prazosin
B. Doxazosin
C. Terazosin
D. Phenoxybenzamine

*Phenoxybenzamine is a nonselective alpha antagonist.*

**2196. Which of the following antihypertensive drugs is contraindicated in pregnancy?**
*Harrison's 20th Ed. Chapter 271 Page 1902 Table 271-8*

A. Aliskiren
B. Minoxidil
C. Clonidine
D. All of the above

**2197. Which of the following drug is contraindicated in pregnancy?**
*Harrison's 20th Ed. Chapter 271 Page 1902 Table 271-8*

A. Captopril
B. Losartan
C. Aliskiren
D. All of the above

**2198. Which of the following is false about α-Adrenergic Blockers?**
*Harrison's 20th Ed. Chapter 271 Page 1903*

A. Do not reduce cardiovascular morbidity / mortality & CHF
B. Effective in treating men with prostatic hypertrophy
C. Useful in management of patients with pheochromocytoma
D. None of the above

**2199. Peripheral sympatholytics act by depleting nerve terminal?**
*Harrison's 20th Ed. Chapter 271 Page 1903*

A. Epinephrine
B. Norepinephrine
C. Acethylcholine
D. All of the above

*Peripheral sympatholytics decrease peripheral resistance and venous constriction by depleting nerve terminal norepinephrine.*

**2200. Calcium antagonists reduce vascular resistance through?**
*Harrison's 20th Ed. Chapter 271 Page 1903*

A. K - channel blockade
B. L - channel blockade
C. M - channel blockade
D. N - channel blockade

*Calcium antagonists reduce vascular resistance through L-channel blockade, which reduces intracellular calcium and blunts vasoconstriction.*

**2201. Which of the following is not a class of calcium antagonists?**
*Harrison's 20th Ed. Chapter 271 Page 1903*

A. Phenylalkylamines
B. Phenylpyridines
C. Benzothiazepines
D. Dihydropyridines

*Calcium antagonists are of three classes — phenylalkylamines (verapamil), benzothiazepines (diltiazem), and 1,4-dihydropyridines (amlodipine, felodipine, isradipine, nicardipine, nifedipine and nisoldipine).*

**2202. Edema with dihydropyridine calcium channel blockers is due to?**
*Harrison's 20th Ed. Chapter 271 Page 1903*

A. Net salt retention
B. Net water retention
C. Increase in transcapillary pressure gradients
D. All of the above

*Edema with dihydropyridine use are related to their potencies as arteriolar dilators. Edema is due to an increase in transcapillary pressure gradients, not to net salt and water retention.*

**2203. Which of the following is a direct vasodilator?**
*Harrison's 20th Ed. Chapter 271 Page 1903*

A. Hydralazine
B. Minoxidil
C. Sodium nitroprusside
D. All of the above

**2204. Which of the following is true about Hydralazine?**
*Harrison's 20th Ed. Chapter 271 Page 1903*

A. Direct vasodilator
B. Antioxidant
C. Nitric-oxide enhancer
D. All of the above

*Hydralazine is a potent direct vasodilator that has antioxidant and nitric-oxide enhancing actions.*

**2205. Which of the following drug is used in patients with renal insufficiency who are refractory to all other drugs?**
*Harrison's 20th Ed. Chapter 271 Page 1903*

A. Minoxidil
B. Aliskiren
C. Hydralazine
D. Methyldopa

*Minoxidil is used most frequently in patients with renal insufficiency who are refractory to all other drugs.*

**2206. Patients with high-renin hypertension may be more responsive to which of the following?**
*Harrison's 20th Ed. Chapter 271 Page 1903*

A. ACE inhibitors
B. Beta blockers
C. Calcium antagonists
D. Diuretics

**2207. Patients with low-renin hypertension are more responsive to which of the following?**
*Harrison's 20th Ed. Chapter 271 Page 1903*

A. ACE inhibitors
B. Beta blockers
C. Calcium antagonists
D. Direct vasodilators

*Younger patients may be more responsive to beta blockers & ACE inhibitors, whereas patients over age 50 may be more responsive to diuretics & calcium antagonists. Patients with high-renin hypertension may be more responsive to ACE inhibitors & angiotensin receptor blockers, whereas patients with low-renin hypertension are more responsive to diuretics and calcium antagonists.*

**2208. Which of the following influences the selection of antihypertensive agents?**
*Harrison's 20th Ed. Chapter 271 Page 1903*

A. Age
B. Ethnicity
C. Comorbid conditions
D. All of the above

**2209. In HOPE (Heart Outcomes Prevention Evaluation) trial, which of the following ACE inhibitors was studied?**
*The American Journal of Medicine 2005;118, 695-705*

A. Lisinopril
B. Ramipril
C. Enalapril
D. Perindopril

**2210. In ALLHAT (Antihypertensive and Lipid-Lowering Treatment to Prevent Heart Attack Trial), which of the following ACE inhibitors was studied?**
*The American Journal of Medicine 2005;118, 695-705*

A. Lisinopril
B. Ramipril
C. Enalapril
D. Perindopril

**2211. Which of the following antihypertensives is inferior to other agents in reducing all-cause mortality?**
*Harrison's 20th Ed. Chapter 271 Page 1904*

A. ACE Inhibitors
B. Diuretics
C. Calcium antagonists
D. Beta blockers

*Antihypertensive and Lipid-Lowering Treatment to Prevent Heart Attack Trial (ALLHAT) concluded that occurrence of CHD, nonfatal MI & overall mortality was virtually identical in hypertensive patients treated with either ACEI (lisinopril), a diuretic (chlorthalidone), or a calcium antagonist (amlodipine). However, Beta blockers are inferior to other classes of agents for prevention of cardiovascular events, stroke, renal failure, and all-cause mortality.*

**2212. Which of the following drug has renal protective effects?**
*Harrison's 20th Ed. Chapter 271 Page 1904*

A. Aliskiren
B. ACE Inhibitors
C. ARBs
D. All of the above

*In hypertension & diabetes, renal protection with aliskiren is comparable to that with ACEIs & ARBs.*

**2213. Better stroke protection is provided by?**
*Harrison's 20th Ed. Chapter 271 Page 1904*

A. ACE inhibitors
B. Beta blockers
C. Calcium channel blockers
D. All of the above

*ACE inhibitors provide better coronary protection than calcium channel blockers, whereas calcium channel blockers provide more stroke protection than either ACE inhibitors or beta blockers.*

**2214. Resistant hypertension refers to BP persistently above what level despite taking 3 or more antihypertensives, including a diuretic, in reasonable combination and at full doses?**
*Harrison's 20th Ed. Chapter 271 Page 1905*

A. >130/90 mm Hg
B. >140/90 mm Hg
C. >150/90 mm Hg
D. >160/90 mm Hg

*Resistant hypertension refers to patients with BP persistently >140/90 mm Hg despite taking three or more antihypertensive agents, including a diuretic, in reasonable combination & at full doses.*

**2215. "Pseudoresistance" refers to?**
*Harrison's 20th Ed. Chapter 271 Page 1905*

A. Lower office and high home blood pressures
B. High office and lower home blood pressures
C. Higher office and high home blood pressures
D. Lower office and low home blood pressures

*"Pseudoresistance" refers to high office blood pressures & lower home blood pressures.*

**2216. If the radial pulse remains palpable despite occlusion of the brachial artery by the cuff, the maneuver is called?**
*Harrison's 20th Ed. Chapter 271 Page 1905*

A. Roger maneuver
B. Osler maneuver
C. Happit maneuver
D. Weber maneuver

*Osler maneuver refers to the radial pulse that remains palpable despite occlusion of brachial artery by cuff.*

**2217. Which of the following is most important in malignant hypertension?**

*Harrison's 20th Ed. Chapter 271 Page 1905*

A. Underlying hypertension
B. Absolute level of blood pressure
C. Rate of rise of blood pressure
D. Response to treatment

*In malignant hypertension, absolute level of blood pressure is not as important as its rate of rise.*

**2218. Which of the following occurs pathologically in malignant hypertension?**

*Harrison's 20th Ed. Chapter 271 Page 1905*

A. Diffuse necrotizing vasculitis
B. Arteriolar thrombi
C. Fibrin deposition in arteriolar walls
D. All of the above

*Pathologically, malignant hypertension is associated with diffuse necrotizing vasculitis, arteriolar thrombi, and fibrin deposition in arteriolar walls.*

**2219. Malignant hypertension is associated with?**

*Harrison's 20th Ed. Chapter 271 Page 1905*

A. Progressive retinopathy
B. Microangiopathic hemolytic anemia
C. Encephalopathy
D. All of the above

*Clinically, in malignant hypertension, there occurs progressive retinopathy (arteriolar spasm, hemorrhages, exudates, and papilledema), deteriorating renal function with proteinuria, microangiopathic hemolytic anemia, and encephalopathy.*

**2220. Which of the following can contribute to the development of malignant hypertension?**

*Harrison's 20th Ed. Chapter 271 Page 1905*

A. Monoamine oxidase inhibitors
B. Cocaine
C. Amphetamines
D. All of the above

**2221. In malignant hypertension, the initial goal of therapy is to reduce mean arterial blood pressure by no more than?**

*Harrison's 20th Ed. Chapter 271 Page 1905*

A. 10%
B. 25%
C. 40%
D. 60%

*In malignant hypertension, the initial goal of therapy is to reduce mean arterial blood pressure by no more than 25% within minutes to 2 hours or to a blood pressure in the range of 160/100 - 110 mm Hg.*

**2222. Which of the following drugs is used in the treatment of hypertensive encephalopathy?**

*Harrison's 20th Ed. Chapter 271 Page 1905*

A. Nitroprusside
B. Labetalol
C. Nicardipine
D. All of the above

**2223. Which of the following is a short-acting oral antihypertensive useful in the management of malignant hypertension without encephalopathy?**

*Harrison's 20th Ed. Chapter 271 Page 1905*

A. Captopril
B. Clonidine
C. Labetalol
D. All of the above

**2224. SBP above what level should be lowered in patients with cerebral infarction who are not candidates for thrombolytic therapy?**

*Harrison's 20th Ed. Chapter 271 Page 1905*

A. > 180 mm Hg
B. > 200 mm Hg
C. > 220 mm Hg
D. > 240 mm Hg

**2225. DBP above what level should be lowered in patients with cerebral infarction who are not candidates for thrombolytic therapy?**

*Harrison's 20th Ed. Chapter 271 Page 1905*

A. > 100 mm Hg
B. > 110 mm Hg
C. > 120 mm Hg
D. > 130 mm Hg

*For patients with cerebral infarction who are not candidates for thrombolytic therapy, antihypertensive therapy is given only for those with a systolic blood pressure >220 mm Hg or a diastolic blood pressure >130 mm Hg.*

**2226. Recommended BP goal for patients with cerebral infarction who are undergoing thrombolytic therapy is?**

*Harrison's 20th Ed. Chapter 271 Page 1905*

A. SBP < 200 mm Hg and DBP < 110 mm Hg
B. SBP < 185 mm Hg and DBP < 110 mm Hg
C. SBP < 200 mm Hg and DBP < 100 mm Hg
D. SBP < 185 mm Hg and DBP < 100 mm Hg

*If thrombolytic therapy is to be used in patients with cerebral infarction, the recommended goal blood pressure is <185 mm Hg systolic pressure and <110 mm Hg diastolic pressure.*

**2227. Adrenergic crisis due to catecholamine excess is due to?**

*Harrison's 20th Ed. Chapter 271 Page 1905*

A. Cocaine or amphetamine overdose
B. Acute spinal cord injuries
C. Interaction of tyramine-containing compounds with monoamine oxidase inhibitors
D. All of the above

**2228. Adrenergic crisis is treated with?**

*Harrison's 20th Ed. Chapter 271 Page 1905*

A. Labetalol
B. Esmolol
C. Phentolamine
D. Hydralazine

*Besides pheochromocytoma, adrenergic crisis due to catecholamine excess may be due to cocaine or amphetamine overdose, clonidine withdrawal, acute spinal cord injuries and an interaction of tyramine-containing compounds with monoamine oxidase inhibitors. These patients may be treated with phentolamine or nitroprusside.*

**2229. Esmolol is the preferred parenteral drug for?**
*Harrison's 20th Ed. Chapter 271 Page 1905 Table 271-9*

A. Aortic dissection
B. Preeclampsia/eclampsia of pregnancy
C. Stroke
D. Adrenergic crisis

**2230. Preferred parenteral drug for hypertensive emergency during preeclampsia / eclampsia of pregnancy is?**
*Harrison's 20th Ed. Chapter 271 Page 1905 Table 271-9*

A. Hydralazine
B. Labetalol
C. Nicardipine
D. All of the above

**2231. Which of the following antihypertensive agents is given as "IV bolus" in hypertensive emergencies?**
*Harrison's 20th Ed. Chapter 271 Page 1905 Table 271-10*

A. Hydralazine
B. Esmolol
C. Phentolamine
D. Labetalol

**2232. Risk factors for preeclampsia include all except?**
*Harrison's 20th Ed. Chapter 466 Page 3440*

A. Nulliparity
B. Diabetes mellitus
C. Anemia
D. Obesity

Risk factors for the development of preeclampsia include nulliparity, diabetes mellitus, a history of renal disease or chronic hypertension, a prior history of preeclampsia, extremes of maternal age (>35 years or <15 years), obesity, antiphospholipid antibody syndrome and multiple gestation.

**2233. Risk factors for preeclampsia include all except?**
*Harrison's 20th Ed. Chapter 466 Page 3440*

A. Factor V Leiden mutation
B. Angiotensinogen gene T235
C. Antiphospholipid antibody syndrome
D. Smoking

**2234. Medications or substances that can raise blood pressure or antagonize effects of antihypertensive drugs include all except?**
*N Engl J Med. 2006;355:385-92*

A. Ginseng
B. Anabolic steroids
C. Erythropoietin
D. Chloroquine

**2235. Medications or substances that can raise blood pressure or antagonize effects of antihypertensive drugs include all except?**
*N Engl J Med. 2006;355:385-92*

A. Nonsteroidal antiinflammatory drugs
B. Excessive alcohol use
C. High sodium intake
D. Appetite stimulants

**2236. High sodium intake is defined by?**
*N Engl J Med. 2006;355:385-92*

A. Urinary sodium excretion of >50 mmol per day
B. Urinary sodium excretion of >100 mmol per day
C. Urinary sodium excretion of >150 mmol per day
D. None of the above

**2237. Frequency of salt sensitivity is increased among?**
*N Engl J Med. 2006;355:385-92*

A. > 60 years of age
B. Black or obese
C. Renal impairment
D. All of the above

**2238. Which of the following suggest a diagnosis of atherosclerotic renovascular disease?**
*N Engl J Med. 2006;355:385-92*

A. Abdominal bruit
B. Hypokalemia
C. Recent increase in severity of hypertension
D. All of the above

**2239. Which of the following suggest aldosteronism as cause of secondary hypertension?**
*N Engl J Med. 2006;355:385-92*

A. Abnormal ratio of aldosterone to renin
B. Abnormal response to sodium loading
C. Adrenal adenoma on CT or MRI
D. All of the above

**2240. Which of the following suggest pheochromocytoma as cause of secondary hypertension?**
*N Engl J Med. 2006;355:385-92*

A. Norepinephrine >80 µg/24 hours
B. VMA >5 mg/24 hours
C. Elevated plasma metanephrines
D. All of the above

**2241. To prevent hypertensive crisis, patients taking MAOIs must avoid?**
*N Engl J Med. 2005;353:1819-34*

A. Phenylalanine diet
B. Tryptophan diet
C. Tyramine diet
D. All of the above

**2242. Which of the following is amino acid derived hormone?**
*N Engl J Med. 2005;353:1819-34*

A. Dopamine
B. Catecholamines
C. Thyroid hormone
D. All of the above

**2243. In hypertension during pregnancy, which of the following drugs would be safest?**
*N Engl J Med. 1998;338:1131*

A. Labetalol
B. Beta-adrenergic–receptor antagonists
C. Prazosin
D. Calcium channel blocker

**2244. If ACE inhibitors are given during pregnancy, what teratogenic effects can happen?**
*N Engl J Med. 1998;338:1131*

A. Prolonged renal failure in neonates
B. Decreased skull ossification
C. Renal tubular dysgenesis
D. All of the above

**2245. If Warfarin is given during pregnancy, what teratogenic effect can happen?**
*N Engl J Med. 1998;338:1131*

A. Neonatal meconium ileus
B. Anomalies of teeth and bone
C. Ebstein's anomaly
D. Dandy–Walker syndrome

**2246. Mothers who took warfarin during 1st trimester could have all of the following congenital malformations in infants except?**
*Harrison's 20th Ed. Chapter 114 Page 854, N Engl J Med. 2002;347:110*

A. Severe nasal hypoplasia
B. Stippled epiphyseal calcifications
C. Chondrodysplasia punctata
D. Chiari type I malformation

*Warfarin crosses the placenta and can cause fetal abnormalities that include a characteristic embryopathy, which consists of nasal hypoplasia and stippled epiphyses. The risk of embryopathy is highest if warfarin is given in the first trimester of pregnancy.*

**2247. Which of the following anticoagulants does not cross placenta?**
*Harrison's 20th Ed. Chapter 114 Page 854*

A. Warfarin
B. Anisindione
C. Heparin
D. None of the above

*Heparin, LMWH, or fondaparinux can be given during pregnancy for prevention or treatment of thrombosis.*

**2248. Which of the following is a vasoconstrictor?**
*Lancet 2005;365:417-430*

A. Norepinephrine
B. Endothelin
C. Angiotensin II
D. All of the above

**2249. Hypertensive retinopathy was first described by?**
*N Engl J Med. 2004;351:2310-7*

A. Marcus Gunn
B. William Osler
C. Keith Wegener
D. Alexender Fleming

**2250. Which of the following is called "Age pigment"?**
*Heart Lung and Circulation 2005;14:107-114*

A. Calpains
B. Melanin
C. Lipofuscin
D. Bilirubin

## Renovascular Disease

**2251.** Which of the following regions of kidney have blood circulation excess of its metabolic requirements?
*Harrison's 20th Ed. Chapter 272 Page 1906*

- A. Renal cortex
- B. Superficial medullary segments
- C. Deeper medullary segments
- D. Renal papilla

*Renal vasculature is complex with rich arteriolar flow to cortex in excess of metabolic requirements, consistent with its primary function as a filtering organ.*

**2252.** Vascular disorders that commonly threaten the blood supply of the kidney include?
*Harrison's 20th Ed. Chapter 272 Page 1906*

- A. Large vessel atherosclerosis
- B. Fibromuscular diseases
- C. Embolic disorders
- D. All of the above

**2253.** Which of the following is predictive of systemic atherosclerotic disease events?
*Harrison's 20th Ed. Chapter 272 Page 1906*

- A. Microalbuminuria
- B. Urinary albumin excretion (UAE)
- C. Urine albumin / creatinine ratio
- D. All of the above

**2254.** Large-vessel renal artery occlusive disease most commonly results from?
*Harrison's 20th Ed. Chapter 272 Page 1906*

- A. Intimal dissection
- B. Fibromuscular dysplasia (FMD)
- C. Atherosclerotic disease
- D. Extrinsic compression of the vessel

*Large-vessel renal artery occlusive disease results most commonly from atherosclerotic disease. Also from extrinsic compression of the vessel, intimal dissection & fibromuscular dysplasia (FMD).*

**2255.** Which of the following about systemic hypertension due to renal artery stenosis is false?
*Harrison's 20th Ed. Chapter 272 Page 1906*

- A. Angiotensin dependence in the early stages
- B. Loss of circadian blood pressure (BP) rhythms
- C. Accelerated target organ injury
- D. Revascularization lowers BP to normal

*Revascularization (endovascular or surgical) alone rarely lowers BP to normal in renal artery stenosis.*

**2256.** Minimum renal artery velocity that predicts hemodynamically significant lesion is?
*Harrison's 20th Ed. Chapter 272 Page 1906*

- A. > 100 cm per second
- B. > 200 cm per second
- C. > 300 cm per second
- D. > 400 cm per second

*Minimum renal artery velocity (by Doppler ultrasound) that predicts hemodynamically significant (>60% vessel lumen occlusion) lesion is >200 cm per second.*

**2257.** Normal study of which of the following investigations excludes renovascular hypertension?
*Harrison's 20th Ed. Chapter 272 Page 1907 Table 272-1*

- A. Captopril renography with $^{99m}$Tc MAG3
- B. Duplex ultrasonography
- C. Computed tomographic angiography
- D. Magnetic resonance angiography

*Captopril-enhanced renography has a strong negative predictive value when normal.*

**2258.** Which of the following is considered as "gold standard" for diagnosis of large-vessel renal disease?
*Harrison's 20th Ed. Chapter 272 Page 1907 Table 272-1*

- A. Intraarterial angiography
- B. Duplex ultrasonography
- C. Computed tomographic angiography
- D. Magnetic resonance angiography

**2259.** Vascular lesions in malignant hypertension best relate to?
*Harrison's 20th Ed. Chapter 272 Page 1909*

- A. Avascular necrosis
- B. Cystic medial necrosis
- C. Fibrinoid necrosis
- D. Subintimal foam cells

*The hemodynamic stress of malignant hypertension leads to fibrinoid necrosis of small blood vessels, thrombotic microangiography, a nephritic urinalysis, and acute renal failure. The renal lesion associated with malignant hypertension consists of fibrinoid necrosis of the afferent arterioles, extending into glomerulus, and may result in focal necrosis of glomerular tuft.*

**2260.** Which of the following predispose to subtle focal sclerosing glomerular disease, with severe hypertension?
*Harrison's 20th Ed. Chapter 272 Page 1909*

- A. SERPINA1
- B. APOL1
- C. TCR-α
- D. DRB1

**2261.** Vascular lesions of hypertensive nephrosclerosis are also seen in?
*Harrison's 20th Ed. Chapter 272 Page 1909*

- A. Aging
- B. Dyslipidemia
- C. Glucose intolerance
- D. All of the above

# Deep Venous Thrombosis and Pulmonary Thromboembolism

**2262.** Which is the most common preventable cause of death among hospitalized patients?
*Harrison's 20th Ed. Chapter 273 Page 1910*

A. Deep venous thrombosis (DVT)
B. Pulmonary embolism (PE)
C. Postthrombotic syndrome
D. All of the above

*PE is the most common preventable cause of death among hospitalized patients.*

**2263.** Postthrombotic syndrome is also known as?
*Harrison's 20th Ed. Chapter 273 Page 1910*

A. Chronic thromboembolic pulmonary hypertension
B. Chronic venous insufficiency
C. Deep venous thrombosis
D. Pulmonary embolism

*Postthrombotic syndrome is also known as chronic venous insufficiency.*

**2264.** Virchow's triad consists of all except?
*Harrison's 20th Ed. Chapter 273 Page 1910*

A. Inflammation
B. Venous stasis
C. Hypercoagulability
D. Endothelial injury

*Virchow's triad of venous stasis, hypercoagulability and endothelial injury leads to recruitment of activated platelets, which release microparticles.*

**2265.** Wells Clinical Prediction Rule is used for?
*Harrison's 20th Ed. Chapter 3 Page 19*

A. ILD
B. COPD
C. Pulmonary embolism
D. Cystic fibrosis

*Wells Clinical Prediction Rule is a semi-quantitative clinical scoring system for suspected pulmonary embolism (PE). The Wells Scoring System has a maximum of 12.5 points. If the score is <= 4 points, the likelihood of PE is only 8%.*

**2266.** Microparticles contain proinflammatory mediators that bind?
*Harrison's 20th Ed. Chapter 273 Page 1910*

A. Platelets
B. Neutrophils
C. Eosinophils
D. Basophils

**2267.** Which of the following about neutrophil extracellular traps is false?
*Harrison's 20th Ed. Chapter 273 Page 1910*

A. Nuclear material of neutrophils
B. Web-like extracellular networks
C. Prothrombotic
D. None of the above

*Microparticles contain proinflammatory mediators that bind neutrophils, stimulating them to release their nuclear material and form web-like extracellular prothrombotic networks called neutrophil extracellular traps which contain histones that stimulate platelet aggregation and promote platelet-dependent thrombin generation.*

**2268.** Which of the following intracellular components has antimicrobial properties?
*Harrison's 20th Ed. Chapter 116 Page 871*

A. Histones
B. Myeloperoxidase
C. Elastase
D. All of the above

*Neutrophil extracellular traps (NETs) are composed of DNA and other intracellular components with antimicrobial properties, such as histones, myeloperoxidase, and elastase.*

**2269.** Venous thrombi form and flourish in an environment of?
*Harrison's 20th Ed. Chapter 273 Page 1910*

A. Stasis
B. Low oxygen tension
C. Upregulation of proinflammatory genes
D. All of the above

*Venous thrombi form and flourish in an environment of stasis, low oxygen tension and upregulation of proinflammatory genes.*

**2270.** Which of the following is the most common autosomal dominant genetic mutation that leads to a prothrombotic state?
*Harrison's 20th Ed. Chapter 273 Page 1910*

A. Prothrombin gene mutation
B. Thrombin gene mutation
C. Fibrinogen gene mutation
D. Fibrin gene mutation

*Factor V Leiden and prothrombin gene mutation are the two most common autosomal dominant genetic mutation that lead to a prothrombotic state. Presence of genetic mutations such as heterozygous factor V Leiden and prothrombin gene mutation does not appear to increase the risk of recurrent VTE.*

**2271.** Leiden is the name of a city in?
*Cleveland Clinic J of Medicine 2000;67(11):825*

A. Austria
B. Netherland
C. France
D. Germany

**2272.** Factor V Leiden best relates to which of the following?
*Cleveland Clinic J of Medicine 2000;67(11):825*

A. G1691A
B. G1691B
C. G1691C
D. G1691D

*Factor V Leiden is a single point mutation. A G-to-A substitution at nucleotide 1691 (G1691A) of the gene that codes for factor V occurs. Inherited in an autosomal-dominant fashion, it has the effect of rendering factors V and Va resistant to degradation by activated protein C.*

**2273.** Factor V Leiden results in a condition known as?
*Circulation. 2003;107:e94-e97*

A. Activated protein S resistance
B. Activated antithrombin resistance

C. Activated protein C resistance
D. All of the above

*Activated protein C, a natural anticoagulant, breaks down factor Va and factor VIIIa, resulting in less thrombin generation and less fibrin. Activated protein C resistance was first described in 1993. >90% of cases are due to factor V Leiden mutation. Remaining 10% being due to pregnancy, OCP use, select antiphospholipid antibodies, and other factor V point mutations such as factor V Hong Kong and factor V Cambridge.*

**2274. Heterozygous Factor V Leiden increases the lifetime risk of having a venous thromboembolic event by?**
*Cleveland Clinic J of Medicine 2000;67(11):825*

A. ~ 3 fold
B. ~ 5 fold
C. ~ 7 fold
D. ~ 9 fold

*Factor V Leiden increases the risk of developing a DVT during pregnancy by about 7-fold. Persons homozygous for the mutation (who have two abnormal copies) have an astounding 80-fold increased risk.*

**2275. A woman who has factor V Leiden and takes oral contraceptive pills (OCP) has an increased risk of developing a DVT by?**
*Circulation. 2003;107:e94-e97*

A. ~ 15 fold
B. ~ 25 fold
C. ~ 35 fold
D. ~ 45 fold

*A woman who has factor V Leiden and takes oral contraceptive pills (OCP) has a 35-fold increased risk of developing a DVT.*

**2276. Factor V Leiden causes resistance to?**
*Harrison's 20th Ed. Chapter 273 Page 1910*

A. Antithrombin
B. Protein C
C. Protein S
D. All of the above

*Factor V Leiden causes resistance to the endogenous anticoagulant - activated protein C. Activated protein C inactivates clotting factors V and VIII.*

**2277. Which of the following is a naturally occurring coagulation inhibitor?**
*Harrison's 20th Ed. Chapter 273 Page 1910*

A. Antithrombin
B. Protein C
C. Protein S
D. All of the above

*Antithrombin, protein C and protein S are naturally occurring coagulation inhibitors.*

**2278. Which of the following is the most common acquired cause of thrombophilia?**
*Harrison's 20th Ed. Chapter 273 Page 1910*

A. Antiphospholipid antibody syndrome
B. Cigarette smoking
C. Chronic obstructive pulmonary disease
D. Oral contraceptives

*Antiphospholipid antibody syndrome is the most common acquired cause of thrombophilia and is associated with venous or arterial thrombosis.*

**2279. Which of the following is a predisposing factor of thrombophilia?**
*Harrison's 20th Ed. Chapter 273 Page 1910*

A. Air pollution
B. Systemic arterial hypertension
C. Obesity
D. All of the above

*Common predisposing factors of thrombophilia include cancer, obesity, cigarette smoking, systemic arterial hypertension, chronic obstructive pulmonary disease, chronic kidney disease, blood transfusion, long-haul air travel, air pollution, oral contraceptives, pregnancy, postmenopausal hormone replacement, surgery and trauma.*

**2280. Which of the following medical conditions contribute to the likelihood of VTE?**
*Harrison's 20th Ed. Chapter 273 Page 1910*

A. Antiphospholipid antibody syndrome
B. Systemic arterial hypertension
C. Chronic obstructive pulmonary disease
D. All of the above

*Acquired predispositions to VTE include long-haul air travel, obesity, cigarette smoking, oral contraceptives, pregnancy, postmenopausal hormone replacement, surgery, trauma. Medical conditions include APLA syndrome, cancer, systemic arterial hypertension & COPD.*

**2281. Increased pulmonary vascular resistance leads to increase in?**
*Harrison's 20th Ed. Chapter 273 Page 1910*

A. Serotonin
B. Brain natriuretic peptide
C. Cardiac troponin
D. All of the above

**2282. Which of the following is not a pathophysiologic abnormality in pulmonary embolism?**
*Harrison's 20th Ed. Chapter 273 Page 1911*

A. Impaired gas exchange
B. Alveolar hypoventilation
C. Increased airway resistance
D. Decreased pulmonary compliance

**2283. Massive pulmonary embolism is characterized by extensive thrombosis affecting how much of the pulmonary vasculature?**
*Harrison's 20th Ed. Chapter 273 Page 1911*

A. At least 10%
B. At least 25%
C. At least 33%
D. At least 50%

*Massive pulmonary embolism is characterized by extensive thrombosis affecting at least half of the pulmonary vasculature.*

**2284. Which of the following is the hallmark of massive PE?**
*Harrison's 20th Ed. Chapter 273 Page 1911*

A. Dyspnea
B. Cyanosis
C. Hypotension
D. All of the above

*Dyspnea, syncope, hypotension and cyanosis are hallmarks of massive PE.*

**2285. Which of the following is normal in submassive PE?**
*Harrison's 20th Ed. Chapter 273 Page 1911*

A. Pulmonary artery pressure
B. Right ventricular diastolic function
C. Right ventricular systolic function
D. Systemic arterial pressure

Submassive PE is characterized by RV dysfunction despite normal systemic arterial pressure. The combination of right heart failure & release of cardiac biomarkers indicates a high risk of clinical deterioration.

**2286. Lower extremity DVT usually begins in?**
*Harrison's 20th Ed. Chapter 273 Page 1911*

A. Calf
B. Thigh
C. Pelvis
D. Any of the above

Lower extremity DVT usually begins in the calf and propagates proximally to the popliteal vein, femoral vein and iliac veins.

**2287. Which of the following signs is related to DVT?**
*N Engl J Med. 1946; 234:288-291, J Am Med Assoc. 1949;140(5):476*

A. Peabody's sign
B. Pratt's test
C. Lisker's sign
D. All of the above

**2288. "LEFT" rule used in the diagnosis of deep-vein thrombosis in pregnancy consists of all except?**
*N Engl J Med. 2015;373:540-7*

A. Left calf circumference ≥2 cm more than right calf
B. Edema
C. First-trimester presentation
D. Tachycardia

The "LEFT" rule is used to assess three variables to predict the likelihood of a diagnosis of deep-vein thrombosis in pregnancy: left (L) calf circumference (a difference of ≥2 cm or more from the right calf is positive), edema (E), and first-trimester presentation (FT).

**2289. Which of the following is false for gestational deep-vein thrombosis?**
*N Engl J Med. 2015;373:540-7*

A. Usually occurs in the left leg
B. Proximal rather than distal
C. Associated with increased risk of embolic complications
D. None of the above

**2290. Which of the following signs is related to DVT?**
*JAPI. 2007;55:5-30*

A. Louvel's sign
B. Lowenberg's sign
C. Bancroft's sign
D. All of the above

Peabody's sign - calf muscle spasm occurs on raising the affected leg with the foot extended. Pratt's test - pain elicited by compression on the popliteal vein in the proximal calf. Lisker's sign - tenderness when anteromedial part of tibia is percussed. Louvel's sign - pain in the distribution of affected vein which occurs during coughing or sneezing (Valsalva maneuver), and which disappears when the vein is compressed proximally. Lowenberg's sign - pain is elicited rapidly when a blood pressure cuff is placed around calf and inflated to ~80mm Hg. Bancroft's sign (Also known as Moses' sign) - pain is elicited when calf muscle is compressed forwards against tibia, but not when the calf muscle is compressed from side to side.

**2291. Which of the following is also called dorsiflexion sign of DVT?**
*JAPI. 2007;55:5-30*

A. Louvel's sign
B. Lowenberg's sign
C. Bancroft's sign
D. Homans' sign

Homans' sign or the dorsiflexion sign refers to discomfort behind the knee on forced dorsiflexion of the foot.

**2292. Which of the following is a part of the classification of pulmonary embolism?**
*Harrison's 20th Ed. Chapter 273 Page 1911*

A. Massive PE
B. Submassive PE
C. Low-risk PE
D. All of the above

**2293. Eponym "The Great Masquerader" is used for?**
*Harrison's 20th Ed. Chapter 273 Page 1911*

A. Deep venous thrombosis (DVT)
B. Pulmonary embolism (PE)
C. Venous thromboembolism (VTE)
D. All of the above

**2294. "The Great Masquerader" eponym applies to?**
*Harrison's 20th Ed. Chapter 273 Page 1911 (2616, 2740)*

A. Fibromyalgia
B. Pulmonary embolism (PE)
C. Pheochromocytoma
D. All of the above

Apart from PE, term masquerader has been used for fibromyalgia & pheochromocytoma. Historically, syphilis and tuberculosis were labeled as the "great masqueraders"

**2295. The most common symptom of pulmonary embolism is?**
*Harrison's 20th Ed. Chapter 273 Page 1911*

A. Unexplained breathlessness
B. Unexplained syncope
C. Unexplained hypotension
D. Unexplained cyanosis

The most common symptom of pulmonary embolism is unexplained breathlessness.

**2296. Clinical improvement often fails to occur in which of the following when occult PE occurs concomitantly?**
*Harrison's 20th Ed. Chapter 273 Page 1911*

A. Asthma
B. Pneumonia
C. Sarcoidosis
D. All of the above

When occult PE occurs concomitantly with overt congestive heart failure or pneumonia, clinical improvement often fails to occur despite standard medical treatment of the concomitant illness. This scenario presents a clinical clue to the possible coexistence of PE.

**2297. Which of the following eponyms is used to describe presentation of DVT?**
*Harrison's 20th Ed. Chapter 273 Page 1911*

A. Creepy ant
B. Blueberry muffin
C. Charley horse
D. Goose bump

With DVT, the most common symptom is a cramp or "charley horse" in the lower calf that persists and intensifies over several days.

**2298. DVT is likely if?**
*Harrison's 20th Ed. Chapter 273 Page 1911*

A. Sudden, severe calf discomfort
B. Fever and chills
C. Marked thigh swelling, tenderness and erythema
D. Leg is diffusely edematous

**2299. Which of the following is likely in massive DVT?**
*Harrison's 20th Ed. Chapter 273 Page 1911*

A. Sudden, severe calf discomfort
B. Severe thigh swelling
C. Diffusely edematous leg
D. Any of the above

Sudden, severe calf discomfort suggests a ruptured Baker's cyst. Severe thigh swelling & marked tenderness in inguinal area & common femoral vein occurs in massive DVT. If leg is diffusely edematous, DVT is unlikely, rather acute exacerbation of venous insufficiency due to postphlebitic syndrome is likely.

**2300. Upper extremity venous thrombosis may present with?**
*Harrison's 20th Ed. Chapter 273 Page 1911*

A. Numbness in fingers
B. Asymmetry in supraclavicular fossa
C. Pain in nail beds of fingers
D. All of the above

Upper extremity venous thrombosis may present with asymmetry in the supraclavicular fossa or in the circumference of the upper arms.

**2301. May-Thurner Syndrome best relates to?**
*Proc (Bayl Univ Med Cent) 2012;25(3):231-233*

A. Right Iliofemoral deep venous thrombosis
B. Left Iliofemoral deep venous thrombosis
C. Bilateral Iliofemoral deep venous thrombosis
D. Any of the above

First described in 1957, May-Thurner syndrome (MTS) is also known as the iliac vein compression syndrome. In this anatomical variant an overriding right common iliac artery causes compression of the left common iliac vein against the lumbar spine (L5). The anatomical defect occurs high in the pelvis, an area that is not easily visualized by ultrasound.

**2302. Which of the following suggests a small pulmonary embolism?**
*Harrison's 20th Ed. Chapter 273 Page 1912*

A. Dyspnea
B. Pleuritic pain
C. Syncope
D. Hypotension

**2303. Which of the following suggests a massive pulmonary embolism?**
*Harrison's 19th Ed. 1632*

A. Cough
B. Pleuritic pain
C. Dyspnea
D. Hemoptysis

Dyspnea is the most frequent symptom of PE, and tachypnea is its most frequent sign. Dyspnea, syncope, hypotension or cyanosis indicates a massive PE. Pleuritic pain, cough or hemoptysis suggests a small embolism located distally near the pleura. This condition is exquisitely painful because the thrombus lodges peripherally, near the innervation of pleural nerves.

**2304. Which of the following nonthrombotic PE can occur after total hip or knee replacement?**
*Harrison's 20th Ed. Chapter 273 Page 1912*

A. Fat
B. Bone marrow
C. Cotton
D. Bony fragment

Nonthrombotic PE etiologies include fat embolism after pelvic or long bone fracture, tumor embolism, bone marrow and air embolism. Cement embolism and bony fragment embolism can occur after total hip or knee replacement. Intravenous drug users may inject themselves with substances that can embolize such as hair, talc and cotton. Amniotic fluid embolism occurs when fetal membranes leak or tear at placental margin.

**2305. The sensitivity of the D-dimer for DVT is?**
*Harrison's 20th Ed. Chapter 273 Page 1912*

A. > 60%
B. > 70%
C. > 80%
D. > 90%

**2306. The sensitivity of the D-dimer for PE is?**
*Harrison's 20th Ed. Chapter 273 Page 1912*

A. > 65%
B. > 75%
C. > 85%
D. > 95%

The sensitivity of the D-dimer is >80% for DVT (including isolated calf DVT) and >95% for PE.

**2307. Levels of D-dimer increase in?**
*Harrison's 20th Ed. Chapter 273 Page 1912*

A. Myocardial infarction
B. Sepsis
C. Second or third trimester of pregnancy
D. All of the above

Levels of D-dimer increase in myocardial infarction, pneumonia, sepsis, cancer, postoperative state, and second or third trimester of pregnancy.

**2308. All are true for pulmonary embolism except?**
*Harrison's 20th Ed. Chapter 273 Page 1912*

A. Plasma D-dimer ELISA assay has high (-) predictive value
B. ABG lacks diagnostic utility
C. Westermark's sign in chest X-ray is focal oligemia
D. Palla's sign is enlarged (L) descending pulmonary artery

Quantitative ELISA plasma D-dimer level is elevated (>500 ng/mL) in more than 90% of patients with PE, reflecting plasmin's breakdown of fibrin and indicating endogenous thrombolysis. D-dimer assay is not specific and levels increase in patients with MI, sepsis etc. Plasma D-dimer ELISA has a high negative predictive value (99.6%) and can be used to help exclude PE. It has a sensitivity of 96.4%. Arterial blood gases lack diagnostic utility for PE.

**2309. Which of the following biomarkers increase in PE?**
*Harrison's 20th Ed. Chapter 273 Page 1912*

A. Serum troponin
B. Plasma heart-type fatty acid-binding protein
C. NT-pro-brain natriuretic peptide
D. All of the above

Serum troponin and plasma heart-type fatty acid-binding protein levels increase because of RV microinfarction. Myocardial stretch causes release of brain natriuretic peptide or NT-pro-brain natriuretic peptide.

**2310. ECG change in pulmonary embolism include?**
*Harrison's 20th Ed. Chapter 273 Page 1912*

A. T wave inversion in $V_{1-4}$
B. Sinus tachycardia
C. $S_1Q_3T_3$ pattern
D. All of the above

ECG abnormalities in PE include sinus tachycardia and $S_1Q_3T_3$ sign (S wave in lead I, Q wave in lead III & an inverted T wave in lead III).

**2311. Most frequent ECG finding in pulmonary embolism is?**
*Harrison's 20th Ed. Chapter 273 Page 1912*

A. New-onset atrial fibrillation
B. $S_1Q_3T_3$ pattern
C. QRS axis greater than 90°
D. T-wave inversion in leads $V_1$ to $V_4$

In PE, T-wave inversion in leads $V_1$ to $V_4$ is the most frequent change (right ventricular strain).

**2312. Which of the following parameter is looked at in venous ultrasonography for DVT?**
*Harrison's 20th Ed. Chapter 273 Page 1912*

A. Intima-media thickness
B. Diameter of the vein
C. Vein compressibility
D. All of the above

Venous ultrasonography of deep-venous system relies on loss of vein compressibility as the primary diagnostic criterion for DVT.

**2313. Which of the following is found in venous ultrasonography for the diagnosis of acute DVT?**
*Harrison's 20th Ed. Chapter 273 Page 1912*

A. Homogeneous and low echogenicity thrombus
B. Hetrogeneous and low echogenicity thrombus
C. Homogeneous and high echogenicity thrombus
D. Hetrogeneous and high echogenicity thrombus

The diagnosis of acute DVT is more reliable when thrombus is directly visualized which is homogeneous & with low echogenicity.

**2314. Which of the following is found in venous ultrasonography for the diagnosis of acute DVT?**
*Harrison's 20th Ed. Chapter 273 Page 1912*

A. Dilated vein
B. Loss of vein compressibility
C. Absent collateral channels
D. All of the above

Venous flow dynamics can be examined with Doppler imaging.

**2315. Augmentation of Doppler flow pattern in venous Doppler imaging is done by?**
*Harrison's 20th Ed. Chapter 273 Page 1912*

A. Valsalva maneuver
B. Passive leg raising
C. Manual calf compression
D. All of the above

Loss of normal respiratory variation is caused by an obstructing DVT in venous flow dynamics study with Doppler imaging. Normally, manual calf compression causes augmentation of the Doppler flow pattern.

**2316. Which of the following is a feature of pulmonary embolism on chest X-ray?**
*Harrison's 20th Ed. Chapter 273 Page 1912*

A. Westermark's sign
B. Hampton's hump
C. Palla's sign
D. All of the above

**2317. Palla's sign refers to?**
*Harrison's 20th Ed. Chapter 273 Page 1912*

A. Focal oligemia
B. Peripheral wedged-shaped density above diaphragm
C. Enlarged right descending pulmonary artery
D. Enlarged left descending pulmonary artery

**2318. Westermark's sign refers to?**
*Harrison's 20th Ed. Chapter 273 Page 1912*

A. Focal oligemia
B. Peripheral wedged-shaped density above diaphragm
C. Enlarged right descending pulmonary artery
D. Enlarged left descending pulmonary artery

**2319. Hampton's hump refers to?**
*Harrison's 20th Ed. Chapter 273 Page 1912*

A. Focal oligemia
B. Peripheral wedged-shaped density above diaphragm
C. Enlarged right descending pulmonary artery
D. Enlarged left descending pulmonary artery

In a dyspneic patient, a normal or near-normal chest X-ray suggests PE. Other abnormalities include focal oligemia (Westermark's sign), a peripheral wedged-shaped density above the diaphragm (Hampton's hump), or an enlarged right descending pulmonary artery (Palla's sign).

**2320. Which of the following is the principal imaging test for the diagnosis of PE?**
*Harrison's 20th Ed. Chapter 273 Page 1912*

A. Lung Scanning
B. Chest X-ray
C. Chest CT with intravenous contrast
D. Echocardiography

Computed tomography of chest with intravenous contrast is the principal imaging test for diagnosis of PE. Multidetector-row spiral CT scanners can image small peripheral emboli. Sixth-order branches can be visualized with resolution superior to that of conventional invasive contrast pulmonary angiography.

**2321. "Triple rule-out CT" helps in the diagnosis of?**
*Harrison's 20th Ed. Chapter 273 Page 1912*

A. Pulmonary embolism
B. Acute aortic syndrome
C. Acute coronary syndrome
D. All of the above

**2322. "Triple rule-out CT" best relates to?**
*Harrison's 20th Ed. Chapter 273 Page 1912*

A. Ultrasonography
B. ECG
C. Echocardiography
D. All of the above

"Triple rule-out CT" utilizes ECG synchronized acquisition, adjusts contrast material timing & opacifies both thoracic aorta & pulmonary artery circulation to exclude PE, acute aortic & acute coronary syndrome.

**2323. Which of the following is false?**
*Harrison's 20th Ed. Chapter 273 Page 1913*

A. Normal or nearly normal chest X-ray often occurs in PE
B. Normal venous ultrasound does not exclude PE
C. Lung scanning is the second-line diagnostic test for PE
D. None of the above

PE is unlikely in normal/nearly normal lung scan. Echocardiography is not a reliable diagnostic tool for acute PE.

**2324. Pulmonary perfusion scan that has a high probability for PE should have how many segmental perfusion defects in the presence of normal ventilation scan?**
*Harrison's 20th Ed. Chapter 273 Page 1913*

A. One or more
B. Two or more
C. Three or more
D. Four or more

A high probability pulmonary perfusion scan for PE is defined as having two or more segmental perfusion defects in the presence of normal ventilation scan.

**2325. Which of the following radiolabeled inhaled gas is used in ventilation scan?**
*Harrison's 20th Ed. Chapter 273 Page 1912*

A. Helium (He)
B. Neon (Ne)
C. Krypton (Kr)
D. Argon (Ar)

Xenon-133, Krypton-81m, or Technetium-99m DTPA are the radiolabeled inhaled gases used in ventilation scan which improves the specificity of the perfusion scan.

**2326. Which of the following about perfusion scan is false?**
*Harrison's 20th Ed. Chapter 273 Page 1912*

A. Agent used is macro aggregated albumin labeled with a gamma-emitting radionuclide like technetium$^{99}$m ($^{99m}$Tc-MAA).
B. Injected intravenously
C. Gamma camera acquires the images
D. None of the above

**2327. Echocardiography is the least useful diagnostic tool for?**
*Harrison's 20th Ed. Chapter 273 Page 1913*

A. Acute myocardial infarction
B. Pulmonary embolism
C. Pericardial tamponade
D. Aortic dissection

Echocardiography is not a reliable diagnostic imaging tool for acute PE because most patients with PE have normal echocardiograms.

**2328. In echocadiography, McConnell's sign is specific for which of the following?**
*Harrison's 20th Ed. Chapter 273 Page 1913*

A. HOCM
B. Pulmonary embolism
C. Acute rheumatic fever
D. Infective endocarditis

Echocardiographic McConnell's sign refers to right ventricular free wall hypokinesis with normal or hyperkinetic right ventricular apical motion and is specific for PE.

**2329. Transesophageal echocardiography can identify which of the following?**
*Harrison's 20th Ed. Chapter 273 Page 1913*

A. Saddle PE
B. Right main PE
C. Left main PE
D. All of the above

Transesophageal echocardiography can identify saddle, right main or left main PE.

**2330. Definitive diagnostic test for pulmonary embolism is?**
*Harrison's 20th Ed. Chapter 273 Page 1913*

A. V/Q scan
B. MR Angiography
C. CT Chest
D. Selective pulmonary angiography

Selective pulmonary angiography demonstrating intraluminal filling defect in more than one projection is the most specific examination available for establishing the definitive diagnosis of PE. Although chest CT with contrast has replaced invasive pulmonary angiography as a diagnostic test, invasive catheter-based diagnostic testing is reserved for patients with technically unsatisfactory chest CTs and those in whom an interventional procedure such as catheter-directed thrombolysis or embolectomy is planned.

**2331. Secondary signs of PE on pulmonary angiography include?**
*Harrison's 20th Ed. Chapter 273 Page 1913*

A. Prolonged arterial phase with slow filling
B. Tortuous, tapering peripheral vessels
C. Segmental oligemia or avascularity
D. All of the above

Secondary signs of PE on pulmonary angiography include abrupt occlusion ("cutoff") of vessels, segmental oligemia or avascularity, prolonged arterial phase with slow filling & tortuous, tapering peripheral vessels.

**2332. In pulmonary embolism, which of the following identify high-risk patients?**
*Harrison's 20th Ed. Chapter 273 Page 1914*

A. Hemodynamic instability
B. Right ventricular dysfunction on echocardiography

C. Elevation of troponin level
D. All of the above

*Hemodynamic instability, right ventricular dysfunction on echocardiography, or elevation of the troponin level due to right ventricular microinfarction identify high-risk PE. RV enlargement on chest CT indicates a 5x increased likelihood of death within next 30 days compared with PE patients with normal RV size on chest CT.*

### 2333. In PE, which of the following is the most widely used approach to risk stratification?
*Harrison's 20th Ed. Chapter 273 Page 1914*

A. Elevation of troponin level
B. $S_1Q_3T_3$ pattern in ECG
C. Detection of RV hypokinesis by echocardiography
D. Increased levels of D-dimer

*In PE, detection of RV hypokinesis on echocardiography is most widely used for risk stratification.*

### 2334. Which of the following is a heparin-based parenteral anticoagulant?
*Harrison's 20th Ed. Chapter 273 Page 1914*

A. Argatroban
B. Rivaroxaban
C. Fondaparinux
D. Bivalirudin

*The three heparin-based parenteral anticoagulants are unfractionated heparin (UFH), low-molecular-weight heparin (LMWH) and fondaparinux.*

### 2335. Which of the following is a direct thrombin inhibitor?
*Harrison's 20th Ed. Chapter 273 Page 1914*

A. Argatroban
B. Dabigatran
C. Bivalirudin
D. All of the above

*Direct thrombin inhibitors are argatroban, dabigatran, or bivalirudin and should be used in patients with proven or suspected heparin-induced thrombocytopenia.*

### 2336. Primary therapy of PE is?
*Harrison's 20th Ed. Chapter 273 Page 1914*

A. Anticoagulation with heparin
B. Anticoagulation with warfarin
C. Thrombolysis
D. Placement of inferior vena cava filter

*Primary therapy consists of clot dissolution with thrombolysis or removal of PE by embolectomy. Anticoagulation with heparin and warfarin or placement of an inferior vena cava filter constitutes secondary prevention of recurrent PE.*

### 2337. Which of the following prevents postphlebitic syndrome?
*Harrison's 20th Ed. Chapter 273 Page 1914*

A. Vascular compression stockings
B. Aspirin
C. Warfarin
D. Clopidogrel

*Only therapy to prevent postphlebitic syndrome is daily use of below-knee 30 - 40 mm Hg vascular compression stockings.*

### 2338. In massive pulmonary embolism, immediately effective anticoagulation is initiated with?
*Harrison's 20th Ed. Chapter 273 Page 1914*

A. Unfractionated heparin (UFH)
B. Low molecular weight heparin (LMWH)
C. Fondaparinux
D. Any of the above

*In massive PE, immediately effective anticoagulation is initiated with a parenteral drug - UFH, LMWH (Enoxaparin, Tinzaparin), fondaparinux, argatroban, bivalirudin, rivaroxaban or apixaban.*

### 2339. A typical initial intravenous bolus of unfractionated heparin in PE is?
*Harrison's 20th Ed. Chapter 273 Page 1914*

A. 60 U / kg
B. 80 U / kg
C. 100 U / kg
D. 120 U / kg

*UFH is dosed to achieve a target activated partial thromboplastin time (aPTT) that is 2 - 3 times the upper limit of laboratory normal. This is usually equivalent to an aPTT of 60 - 80 seconds. For UFH, a typical initial intravenous bolus is 80 U/kg, followed by an initial infusion rate of 18/kg per hour.*

### 2340. What is the dose of Fondaparinux in patients weighing between 50 - 100 kg?
*Harrison's 20th Ed. Chapter 114 Page 851*

A. 2.5 mg
B. 5 mg
C. 7.5 mg
D. 10 mg

*Fondaparinux is an anti-Xa pentasaccharide. It is administered by once-daily subcutaneous injection. Patients weighing <50 kg receive 5 mg, 50-100 kg patients receive 7.5 mg, and patients weighing >100 kg receive 10 mg. 2.5 mg of Fondaparinux is used to prevent VTE.*

### 2341. Warfarin inhibits which of the following?
*Harrison's 20th Ed. Chapter 114 Page 853*

A. Vitamin K epoxide reductase
B. Vitamin K epoxide oxidase
C. Vitamin K epoxide hydrolase
D. All of the above

*Warfarin inhibits vitamin K epoxide reductase (VKOR) thereby blocking the γ-carboxylation process. This results in the synthesis of vitamin K-dependent clotting proteins (factors II, VII, IX and X) that are only partially γ-carboxylated. Warfarin acts as an anticoagulant because these partially γ-carboxylated proteins have reduced or absent biologic activity.*

### 2342. Which of the following about warfarin is false?
*Harrison's 20th Ed. Chapter 114 Page 853*

A. Initially developed as a rodenticide
B. Warfarin is a racemic mixture of R and S isomers
C. S-warfarin is most active
D. None of the above

### 2343. Warfarin acts by preventing carboxylation activation of which coagulation factor?
*Harrison's 20th Ed. Chapter 273 Page 1914*

A. II
B. VII
C. X
D. All of the above

*Warfarin is a vitamin K antagonist that prevents carboxylation activation of coagulation factors II, VII, IX, and X.*

**2344. Heparin should be overlapped with oral anticoagulation for at least how many days?**
*Harrison's 20th Ed. Chapter 273 Page 1914*

A. 2 to 3 days
B. 3 to 4 days
C. 4 to 5 days
D. 5 to 6 days

Warfarin requires 5-7 days to achieve a therapeutic effect. During that period, the parenteral and oral agents are overlapped. If warfarin is initiated as monotherapy during an acute thrombotic illness, a paradoxical exacerbation of hypercoagulability increases the likelihood of thrombosis. Overlapping UFH, LMWH, fondaparinux or parenteral direct thrombin inhibitors with warfarin for at least 5 days will nullify the early procoagulant effect of warfarin.

**2345. Which of the following affect warfarin metabolism?**
*Harrison's 20th Ed. Chapter 273 Page 1914*

A. Drug-drug and drug-food interactions
B. Age, sex, weight
C. Concomitant drugs
D. All of the above

**2346. Antidote for bleeding from fondaparinux is?**
*Harrison's 20th Ed. Chapter 273 Page 1914*

A. Protamine sulfate
B. Vitamin K
C. Recombinant factor VIIa
D. None of the above

There is no specific antidote for bleeding from fondaparinux, direct thrombin inhibitors or factor Xa inhibitors.

**2347. Which of the following is an oral anticoagulant?**
*Harrison's 20th Ed. Chapter 114 Page 848*

A. Dabigatran etexilate
B. Rivaroxaban
C. Apixaban
D. All of the above

**2348. Which of the following is an oral anticoagulant?**
*Harrison's 20th Ed. Chapter 114 Page 848*

A. Lepirudin
B. Bivalirudin
C. Argatroban
D. None of the above

Currently available oral anticoagulants include warfarin; dabigatran etexilate, an oral thrombin inhibitor; and rivaroxaban, apixaban, and edoxaban, which are oral factor Xa inhibitors. Parenteral anticoagulants include heparin, low molecular-weight heparin (LMWH), fondaparinux (a synthetic pentasaccharide), lepirudin, desirudin, bivalirudin, and argatroban.

**2349. Catastrophic bleeding associated with warfarin administration is best treated by?**
*Harrison's 20th Ed. Chapter 112 Page 837*

A. Fresh-frozen plasma
B. Recombinant factor VIIa therapy (rFVIIa)
C. Vitamin K
D. All of the above

For life-threatening or intracranial hemorrhage due to heparin or LMWH, protamine sulfate can be administered. Major bleeding from warfarin is best managed with prothrombin complex concentrate. With non-life threatening bleeding, fresh-frozen plasma can be used. Recombinant human coagulation factor VIIa (rFVIIa) is used to manage catastrophic bleeding from warfarin. For minor bleeding or to manage an excessively high INR in the absence of bleeding, oral vitamin K may be administered.

**2350. Individuals with loss-of-function alleles in which of the following are at increased risk for bleeding with warfarin?**
*Harrison's 20th Ed. Chapter 63 Page 423*

A. CYP2C8
B. CYP2C9
C. CYP2C19
D. CYP2C21

CYP2C9 mediates elimination of warfarin. Individuals with loss-of-function alleles in CYP2C9, responsible for metabolism of the active S-enantiomer of warfarin are at increased risk for bleeding.

**2351. Risk of upper gastrointestinal bleeding is increased by how much in those taking warfarin and an NSAID?**
*Harrison's 20th Ed. Chapter 63 Page 426*

A. Twice
B. Thrice
C. Four times
D. Five times

In patients treated with warfarin, risk of upper gastrointestinal bleeding is increased almost threefold by concomitant use of an NSAID.

**2352. Most common nonbleeding side effect of warfarin is?**
*Harrison's 19th Ed. 354*

A. Alopecia
B. Skin necrosis
C. Seizure
D. Osteoporosis

Most common nonbleeding side effect of warfarin is alopecia. Warfarin-induced skin necrosis is rare.

**2353. Warfarin embryopathy occurs with warfarin exposure during?**
*Harrison's 20th Ed. Chapter 114 Page 854*

A. Second to sixth weeks of gestation
B. Sixth to twelfth weeks of gestation
C. Twelfth to sixteen weeks of gestation
D. Twenty to twenty four weeks of gestation

Warfarin is teratogenic. Warfarin embryopathy is most common with exposure during 6th to 12th weeks of gestation. Warfarin therapy is contraindicated in first trimester due to its association with fetal chondrodysplasia punctata. In the second and third trimesters, warfarin may cause fetal optic atrophy and mental retardation.

**2354. Warfarin can be administered safely during?**
*Harrison's 20th Ed. Chapter 114 Page 854*

A. Second trimester of pregnancy
B. Postpartum period
C. Breast feeding
D. All of the above

Warfarin is safe during second trimester, postpartum and breast feeding period.

**2355. Warfarin use during pregnancy can cause?**
*N Engl J Med. 2015;373:540-7*

A. Central nervous system abnormalities
B. Pregnancy loss
C. Fetal anticoagulation
D. All of the above

Warfarin is contraindicated in pregnancy as it crosses placenta and is associated with embryopathy, central nervous system abnormalities, pregnancy loss, and fetal anticoagulation with possible bleeding.

### 2356. Which of the following about Novel oral anticoagulants (NOACs) is false?
*Harrison's 20th Ed. Chapter 273 Page 1915*

A. Administered in a fixed dose
B. Establish effective anticoagulation within hours of ingestion
C. Require no laboratory coagulation monitoring
D. None of the above

Novel oral anticoagulants (NOACs) are administered in a fixed dose, result in effective anticoagulation within hours of ingestion, require no laboratory coagulation monitoring, and have few drug-drug or drug-food interactions.

### 2357. "Bridging" with a parenteral anticoagulant is required when which of the following is used?
*Harrison's 20th Ed. Chapter 273 Page 1915*

A. Betrixaban
B. Warfarin
C. Rivaroxaban
D. All of the above

Rivaroxaban is a factor Xa inhibitor, and dabigatran is a direct thrombin inhibitor. Because of these drugs' rapid onset of action & relatively short half-life compared with warfarin, "bridging" with a parenteral anticoagulant is not required.

### 2358. "Bridging" with a parenteral anticoagulant is required when which of the following is used?
*Harrison's 20th Ed. Chapter 273 Page 1915*

A. Betrixaban
B. Rivaroxaban
C. Apixaban
D. None of the above

Betrixaban, rivaroxaban and apixaban are direct factor Xa inhibitors, and are approved as monotherapy for acute and extended treatment of DVT and PE, without a parenteral "bridging" anticoagulant.

### 2359. Which of the following is a dabigatran antibody?
*Harrison's 20th Ed. Chapter 273 Page 1915*

A. Mepolizumab
B. Reslizumab
C. Idarucizumab
D. Benralizumab

The dabigatran antibody, idarucizumab, is an effective & rapidly acting antidote for dabigatran.

### 2360. Andexanet is an antidote for?
*Harrison's 20th Ed. Chapter 273 Page 1915*

A. Betrixaban
B. Rivaroxaban
C. Apixaban
D. All of the above

Andexanet is a universal anti-Xa antidote for betrixaban, rivaroxaban, apixaban & edoxaban.

### 2361. Bleeding from warfarin is managed with?
*Harrison's 20th Ed. Chapter 273 Page 1915*

A. Prothrombin complex concentrate
B. Fresh-frozen plasma
C. Intravenous vitamin K
D. All of the above

Major bleeding from warfarin is best managed with prothrombin complex concentrate. With less serious bleeding, fresh-frozen plasma or IV vitamin K can be used. Oral vitamin K is effective for managing minor bleeding or an excessively high INR in the absence of bleeding.

### 2362. Duration of anticoagulation for PE following surgery or trauma is?
*Harrison's 20th Ed. Chapter 273 Page 1915*

A. 3 - 6 months
B. 6 - 12 months
C. 12 - 18 months
D. Indefinite

Duration of anticoagulation for PE following surgery or trauma is 3 - 6 months.

### 2363. Duration of anticoagulation for PE with moderate or high levels of anticardiolipin antibodies is?
*Harrison's 20th Ed. Chapter 273 Page 1915*

A. 3 - 6 months
B. 6 - 12 months
C. 12 - 18 months
D. Indefinite

Duration of anticoagulation for PE with moderate or high levels of anticardiolipin antibodies is indefinite, even if initial VTE was provoked by trauma or surgery.

### 2364. Indefinite-duration anticoagulation is recommended for?
*Harrison's 20th Ed. Chapter 273 Page 1915*

A. Patients with high levels of anticardiolipin antibodies
B. Patients with idiopathic VTE
C. Patients with cancer and VTE
D. All of the above

### 2365. Which of the following is considered unprovoked VTE?
*Harrison's 20th Ed. Chapter 273 Page 1915*

A. That occurs following surgery, trauma
B. That occurs during long-haul air travel
C. That occurs following estrogen therapy
D. That occurs following indwelling central venous catheter

VTE that occurs during long-haul air travel is considered unprovoked. Among patients with idiopathic, unprovoked VTE, recurrence rate is high after cessation of anticoagulation.

### 2366. First-line inotropic agent for treatment of PE-related shock is?
*Harrison's 20th Ed. Chapter 273 Page 1915*

A. Dopamine / dobutamine
B. Phenylephrine
C. Vasopressin
D. Norepinephrine

Dopamine and dobutamine are first-line inotropic agents for treatment of PE-related shock. Other agents that may be effective include norepinephrine, vasopressin or phenylephrine.

### 2367. Successful fibrinolytic therapy in PE leads to?
*Harrison's 20th Ed. Chapter 273 Page 1915*

A. Rapidly reversal of right heart failure
B. Lowers rate of death
C. Prevention of recurrent PE
D. All of the above

The only FDA approved indication for PE fibrinolysis is massive PE. Successful fibrinolytic therapy in PE rapidly reverses right heart failure and leads to a lower rate of death and recurrent PE.

**2368. The preferred fibrinolytic regimen in PE is?**
*Harrison's 20th Ed. Chapter 273 Page 1915*

A. Recombinant tissue plasminogen activator (tPA)
B. Streptokinase
C. Urokinase
D. Alteplase

*Preferred fibrinolytic regimen is 100 mg of tPA administered as a continuous peripheral intravenous infusion over 2 hours. Lower dose i.e. 50 mg of TPA is associated with fewer bleeding complications.*

**2369. PE patients respond to fibrinolysis for up to how many days after the PE has occurred?**
*Harrison's 20th Ed. Chapter 273 Page 1915*

A. 1 day
B. 3 days
C. 7 days
D. 14 days

*PE patients respond to fibrinolysis for up to 14 days after the PE has occurred.*

**2370. What is the risk of intracranial hemorrhage following fibrinolysis in PE?**
*Harrison's 20th Ed. Chapter 273 Page 1915*

A. 0.1 - 0.3%
B. 0.3 - 0.9%
C. 0.9 - 1.9%
D. 2 - 3%

*The overall major bleeding rate is about 10%, including a 2 - 3% risk of intracranial hemorrhage.*

# Diseases of the Aorta

**2371.** In adults, aortic diameter at the origin is approximately?
*Harrison's 20th Ed. Chapter 274 Page 1917*

A. 2 cm
B. 3 cm
C. 4 cm
D. 5 cm

*In adults, aortic diameter at the origin is ~3 cm, 2.5 cm in descending portion in thorax, and 1.8 to 2 cm in abdomen.*

**2372.** Aortic wall intima is composed of all except?
*Harrison's 20th Ed. Chapter 274 Page 1917*

A. Endothelium
B. Subendothelial connective tissue
C. Internal elastic lamina
D. Smooth muscle cells

*Aortic wall thin intima is composed of endothelium, subendothelial connective tissue, and an internal elastic lamina.*

**2373.** Vasa vasorum and nervi vascularis are located in which of the following structures of aorta?
*Harrison's 20th Ed. Chapter 274 Page 1917*

A. Endothelium
B. Tunica media
C. Adventitia
D. All of the above

*Vasa vasorum & nervi vascularis are located in adventitia composed of connective tissue.*

**2374.** Kommerell's diverticulum is an anatomic remnant of?
*Harrison's 20th Ed. Chapter 274 Page 1917*

A. Left umbilical artery
B. Right aortic arch
C. Ductus arteriosus
D. Left atrial appendage

*Kommerell's diverticulum is an anatomic remnant of a right aortic arch.*

**2375.** Coarctation of the aorta may be associated with?
*Harrison's 20th Ed. Chapter 274 Page 1917*

A. Bicuspid aortic valve
B. Aortic arch hypoplasia
C. Intracranial aneurysms
D. All of the above

**2376.** Which of the following about coarctation of the aorta is false?
*Harrison's 20th Ed. Chapter 274 Page 1917*

A. Occurs near the insertion of ligamentum arteriosum
B. Occurs adjacent to the right subclavian artery
C. Associated with congenital heart defects
D. None of the above

**2377.** In a pseudoaneurysm, which of the following layers is not disrupted?
*Harrison's 20th Ed. Chapter 274 Page 1917*

A. Intima
B. Media
C. Adventitia
D. None of the above

*In pseudoaneurysm, intimal & medial layers are disrupted & dilatation is lined by adventitia only. A true aneurysm involves all three layers of the vessel wall.*

**2378.** A fusiform aneurysm affects what proportion of the circumference of a segment of the vessel?
*Harrison's 20th Ed. Chapter 274 Page 1917*

A. 25%
B. 50%
C. 75%
D. 100%

*A fusiform aneurysm affects the entire circumference of a segment of the vessel, resulting in a diffusely dilated artery. A saccular aneurysm involves only a portion of circumference, resulting in an outpouching of the vessel wall.*

**2379.** Which of the following factors is not associated with degenerative aortic aneurysms?
*Harrison's 20th Ed. Chapter 274 Page 1917*

A. Aging
B. Alcohol
C. Cigarette smoking
D. Hypercholesterolemia

*Factors associated with degenerative aortic aneurysms include aging, cigarette smoking, hypercholesterolemia, male sex, and a family history of aortic aneurysms.*

**2380.** The most common pathologic condition associated with degenerative aortic aneurysms is?
*Harrison's 20th Ed. Chapter 274 Page 1917*

A. Atherosclerosis
B. Genetic or developmental
C. Vasculitis
D. Infection

*Most common pathologic condition associated with degenerative aortic aneurysms is atherosclerosis.*

**2381.** Cystic medial necrosis affects which component of the aortic wall?
*Harrison's 20th Ed. Chapter 274 Page 1918*

A. Intima
B. Media
C. Adventitia
D. All of the above

*Cystic medial necrosis is a histopathologic term used to describe degeneration of collagen & elastic fibers in tunica media of aorta.*

**2382. Most common pathological condition for ascending aortic aneurysm is?**
*Harrison's 20th Ed. Chapter 274 Page 1918*

A. Hypertension
B. Atherosclerosis
C. Cystic medial necrosis
D. Tuberculosis

*Cystic medial necrosis characteristically affects the proximal aorta, leading to circumferential weakness, dilatation and development of fusiform aneurysm.*

**2383. Cystic medial necrosis is prevalent in patients with?**
*Harrison's 20th Ed. Chapter 274 Page 1918*

A. Marfan syndrome
B. Ehlers-Danlos syndrome type IV
C. Loeys-Dietz syndrome
D. All of the above

*Cystic medial necrosis is particularly prevalent in patients with Marfan syndrome, Loeys-Dietz syndrome, Ehlers-Danlos syndrome type IV, hypertension, congenital bicuspid aortic valves, and familial thoracic aortic aneurysm syndromes.*

**2384. Mutations of the gene that encodes fibrillin-1 are present in patients with?**
*Harrison's 20th Ed. Chapter 274 Page 1918*

A. Marfan syndrome
B. Ehlers-Danlos syndrome type IV
C. Loeys-Dietz syndrome
D. Osteogenesis Imperfecta (OI)

*Mutations of the gene that encodes fibrillin-1 are present in patients with Marfan syndrome.*

**2385. Loeys-Dietz syndrome is caused by mutations in the genes that encode?**
*Harrison's 20th Ed. Chapter 274 Page 1918*

A. COL5A1
B. TNXB
C. TGF-β receptors 1 (TGFBR1)
D. PLOD1

*Loeys-Dietz syndrome is due to mutations in genes that encode TGF-β 1 (TGFBR1) & 2 (TGFBR2).*

**2386. Loeys-Dietz syndrome (LDS) is characterized by all except?**
*Harrison's 20th Ed. Chapter 274 Page 1918*

A. Aortic aneurysms
B. Hearing loss
C. Cleft palate
D. Hypertelorism

*Loeys-Dietz syndrome (LDS) is characterized by aortic aneurysms, cleft palate & hypertelorism. LDS is related to Marfan Syndrome.*

**2387. Mutations of type III procollagen results in?**
*Harrison's 20th Ed. Chapter 274 Page 1918*

A. Ehlers-Danlos type I syndrome
B. Ehlers-Danlos type II syndrome
C. Ehlers-Danlos type III syndrome
D. Ehlers-Danlos type IV syndrome

*Mutations of type III procollagen have been implicated in Ehlers-Danlos type IV syndrome.*

**2388. Syphilitic aneurysms are mostly located in?**
*Harrison's 20th Ed. Chapter 274 Page 1918*

A. Ascending aorta
B. Thoracic aorta
C. Abdominal aorta
D. All of the above

*Approximately 90% of syphilitic aneurysms are located in ascending aorta or aortic arch. Syphilis is a relatively uncommon cause of aortic aneurysm.*

**2389. Tuberculous aneurysms are mostly located in?**
*Harrison's 20th Ed. Chapter 274 Page 1918*

A. Ascending aorta
B. Thoracic aorta
C. Abdominal aorta
D. All of the above

*Tuberculous aneurysms typically affect thoracic aorta. Direct extension of tubercular infection from hilar lymph nodes or contiguous abscesses or from bacterial seeding resulting granulomatous destruction of medial layer is the pathogenetic mechanism.*

**2390. All of the following conditions can lead to dilatation of the ascending aorta except?**
*Harrison's 20th Ed. Chapter 274 Page 1918*

A. Ankylosing spondylitis
B. Rheumatoid arthritis
C. Reiter's syndrome
D. Behcet's disease

*Spondyloarthropathies like ankylosing spondylitis, rheumatoid arthritis, psoriatic arthritis, relapsing polychondritis and Reiter's syndrome are associated with dilatation of the ascending aorta while Behcet's disease, IgG4-related systemic disease and Cogan's syndrome cause thoracic & abdominal aortic aneurysms.*

**2391. Most common pathological condition associated with aneurysms of aortic arch & descending thoracic aorta is?**
*Harrison's 20th Ed. Chapter 274 Page 1918*

A. Hypertension
B. Atherosclerosis
C. Cystic medial necrosis
D. Tuberculosis

*Atherosclerosis is the most frequent cause of aneurysms of aortic arch & descending thoracic aorta.*

**2392. Most common pathological condition for distal abdominal aortic aneurysm below renal arteries is?**
*Harrison's 20th Ed. Chapter 274 Page 1919*

A. Hypertension
B. Atherosclerosis
C. Cystic medial necrosis
D. Tuberculosis

*At least 90% of all abdominal aortic aneurysms >4.0 cm are affected by atherosclerosis, and most of these aneurysms are below the level of the renal arteries.*

**2393. What percentage of atherosclerotic aneurysms are located in distal abdominal aorta, below the renal arteries?**
*Harrison's 20th Ed. Chapter 274 Page 1919*

A. 25%
B. 33%
C. 50%
D. 75%

*75% of atherosclerotic aneurysms are located in distal abdominal aorta, below the renal arteries.*

**2394. For descending thoracic aneurysms, risk of rupture increases substantially beyond?**
*Harrison's 20th Ed. Chapter 274 Page 1918*

A. > 4 cm
B. > 5 cm
C. > 6 cm
D. > 7 cm

The average growth rate of thoracic aneurysms is 0.1 - 0.2 cm per year. Risk of rupture increases substantially for ascending aortic aneurysms >6 cm and descending thoracic aneurysms >7 cm.

**2395. The annual risk of aneurysmal rupture of thoracic aortic aneurysms that are > 6 cm in diameter is?**
*Harrison's 20th Ed. Chapter 274 Page 1918*

A. 3%
B. 5%
C. 7%
D. 9%

The risk of aneurysmal rupture is ~2 - 3% per year for thoracic aortic aneurysms <4.0 cm in diameter to 7% per year for those >6 cm in diameter.

**2396. Aneurysmal dilation of ascending aorta causes congestive heart failure as a consequence of?**
*Harrison's 20th Ed. Chapter 274 Page 1918*

A. Aortic stenosis
B. Aortic regurgitation
C. Hypertension
D. All of the above

Aneurysmal dilation of ascending aorta causes CHF as a consequence of aortic regurgitation.

**2397. Chest X-ray finding that suggests thoracic aortic aneurysm is?**
*Harrison's 20th Ed. Chapter 274 Page 1918*

A. Widening of the mediastinal shadow
B. Displacement or compression of trachea
C. Displacement or compression of left main stem bronchus
D. All of the above

**2398. Which of the following reduce rate of aortic dilation in Marfan's syndrome by blocking TGF-β signaling?**
*Harrison's 20th Ed. Chapter 274 Page 1918*

A. β-Adrenergic blockers
B. Angiotensin receptor antagonists
C. Diuretics
D. All of the above

Angiotensin receptor antagonists reduce the rate of aortic dilation in patients with Marfan's syndrome by blocking TGF-β signaling.

**2399. Operative repair is indicated in asymptomatic aneurysms when aortic root or ascending aortic diameter is?**
*Harrison's 20th Ed. Chapter 274 Page 1919*

A. ≥ 3.5 cm
B. ≥ 4.5 cm
C. ≥ 5.5 cm
D. ≥ 6.5 cm

**2400. Operative repair is indicated in asymptomatic aneurysms when growth rate is?**
*Harrison's 20th Ed. Chapter 274 Page 1919*

A. > 0.1 cm per year
B. > 0.3 cm per year
C. > 0.5 cm per year
D. > 0.7 cm per year

Operative repair with placement of a prosthetic graft is indicated in patients with symptomatic ascending thoracic aortic aneurysms and for most asymptomatic aneurysms, including those associated with bicuspid aortic valves, when aortic root or ascending aortic diameter is ≥5.5 cm, or when the growth rate is >0.5 cm per year.

**2401. As abdominal aortic aneurysms expand, patients complain of pain in?**
*Harrison's 20th Ed. Chapter 274 Page 1919*

A. Chest
B. Lower back
C. Scrotum
D. Any of the above

**2402. Which of the following is effective in managing abdominal aortic aneurysm?**
*Harrison's 20th Ed. Chapter 274 Page 1919*

A. Statins
B. β-adrenergic blockers
C. Renin-angiotensin inhibitors
D. All of the above

**2403. Which of the following is an acute aortic syndrome?**
*Harrison's 20th Ed. Chapter 274 Page 1919*

A. Aortic dissection
B. Intramural hematoma
C. Penetrating atherosclerotic ulcer
D. All of the above

The four major acute aortic syndromes are aortic rupture, aortic dissection, intramural hematoma and penetrating atherosclerotic ulcer.

**2404. Which of the following acute aortic syndromes is least aggressive?**
*Harrison's 20th Ed. Chapter 274 Page 1919*

A. Aortic dissection
B. Intramural hematoma
C. Penetrating atherosclerotic ulcer
D. Aortic rupture

Penetrating atherosclerotic ulcers are caused by erosion of a plaque into aortic media. They are usually localized and are not associated with extensive propagation.

**2405. Aortic dissection commonly occurs at?**
*Harrison's 20th Ed. Chapter 274 Page 1919*

A. Right lateral wall of ascending aorta
B. Left lateral wall of ascending aorta
C. Right lateral wall of thoracic descending aorta
D. Right lateral wall of thoracic descending aorta

Aortic dissection is caused by a circumferential or, less frequently, transverse tear of the intima. It often occurs along the right lateral wall of the ascending aorta where the hydraulic shear stress is high. Another common site is the descending thoracic aorta just below the ligamentum arteriosum.

### 2406. Acute intramural hematoma result from rupture of?
*Harrison's 20th Ed. Chapter 274 Page 1920*

A. Intima
B. Vasa vasorum
C. Collateral artery
D. Any of the above

*Acute intramural hematoma results from rupture of vasa vasorum with hemorrhage into wall of the aorta.*

### 2407. Acute intramural hematoma most commonly occurs in?
*Harrison's 20th Ed. Chapter 274 Page 1920*

A. Ascending aorta
B. Arch of aorta
C. Descending thoracic aorta
D. Descending abdominal aorta

*Most of acute intramural hematomas occur in descending thoracic aorta.*

### 2408. Stanford & DeBakey classifications are used to classify?
*Harrison's 20th Ed. Chapter 274 Page 1920*

A. Peripheral vascular disease
B. Aortic dissection
C. Renal artery stenosis
D. Internal carotid artery lesions

### 2409. Aortic dissection is the major cause of morbidity and mortality in patients with?
*Harrison's 20th Ed. Chapter 274 Page 1920*

A. Marfan's syndrome
B. Loeys-Dietz syndrome
C. Ehlers-Danlos syndrome
D. All of the above

### 2410. Incidence of aortic dissection is increased in patients with?
*Harrison's 20th Ed. Chapter 274 Page 1920*

A. Takayasu's arteritis
B. Bicuspid aortic valve
C. Coarctation of aorta
D. All of the above

### 2411. Incidence of aortic dissection is increased during which of the following period of pregnancy?
*Harrison's 20th Ed. Chapter 274 Page 1920*

A. Second trimester of pregnancy
B. Third trimester of pregnancy
C. Intrapartum period
D. Post partum period

*Incidence of aortic dissection is increased in normal women during 3rd trimester of pregnancy.*

### 2412. Which of the following about aortic dissection is false?
*Harrison's 20th Ed. Chapter 274 Page 1921*

A. Peak incidence is in sixth & seventh decades
B. Men are more affected than women (2:1)
C. Acute aortic regurgitation is common
D. None of the above

### 2413. Which of the following drugs should be avoided while managing hypertension in acute aortic dissection?
*Harrison's 20th Ed. Chapter 274 Page 1921*

A. Beta adrenergic blockers
B. Sodium nitroprusside
C. Diazoxide
D. Diltiazem

### 2414. Which of the following drugs should be avoided while managing hypertension in acute aortic dissection?
*Harrison's 20th Ed. Chapter 274 Page 1921*

A. Labetalol
B. Sodium nitroprusside
C. Hydralazine
D. Verapamil

*For acute dissection, parenteral beta-adrenergic blockers (IV propranolol, metoprolol, labetalol or esmolol) should be administered to achieve a heart rate of ~60 beats/min. Sodium nitroprusside infusion is used to lower SBP to <120 mm Hg. Verapamil, diltiazem or enalaprilat may be used parenterally. Isolated use of direct vasodilators like diazoxide and hydralazine is contraindicated because these agents can increase hydraulic shear and may propagate dissection.*

### 2415. Acute occlusion in distal abdominal aorta usually results from?
*Harrison's 20th Ed. Chapter 274 Page 1922*

A. Saddle embolus from the heart
B. In situ thrombosis
C. Extramural compression
D. Accidently during pelvic surgery

### 2416. Aortitis may be caused by?
*Harrison's 20th Ed. Chapter 274 Page 1922*

A. Cogan's syndrome
B. Erdheim-Chester disease
C. IgG4-related systemic disease
D. All of the above

### 2417. Infection that may cause aortitis is?
*Harrison's 20th Ed. Chapter 274 Page 1922*

A. Syphilis
B. Tuberculosis
C. Salmonella
D. All of the above

### 2418. Which of the following is termed pulseless disease?
*Harrison's 20th Ed. Chapter 274 Page 1922*

A. Infective aortitis
B. Giant cell arteritis
C. Takayasu's arteritis
D. Syphilitic aortitis

*Takayasu's arteritis is also termed pulseless disease because of the frequent occlusion of the large arteries originating from the aorta.*

### 2419. Takayasu's arteritis predominantly involves which of the following?
*Harrison's 20th Ed. Chapter 274 Page 1922*

A. Ascending aorta
B. Descending thoracic aorta
C. Descending abdominal aorta
D. All of the above

*Takayasu's arteritis is an inflammatory disease that involves the ascending aorta and aortic arch causing obstruction of the aorta and its major arteries.*

**2420. Which of the following about Takayasu's arteritis is false?**
*Harrison's 20th Ed. Chapter 274 Page 1922*

A. Panarteritis
B. Affects young females of Asian descent
C. Progressive course with no definitive therapy
D. None of the above

**2421. Which of the following may be associated with polymyalgia rheumatica?**
*Harrison's 20th Ed. Chapter 274 Page 1922*

A. Infective aortitis
B. Giant cell arteritis
C. Takayasu's arteritis
D. Syphilitic aortitis

*Giant cell arteritis is a disease of the old with focal granulomatous lesions involving the entire arterial wall. It may be associated with polymyalgia rheumatica.*

**2422. Which of the following disorders associated with aortitis involve the ascending aorta?**
*Harrison's 20th Ed. Chapter 274 Page 1922*

A. Rheumatoid arthritis
B. Ankylosing spondylitis
C. Psoriatic arthritis
D. All of the above

*Rheumatoid arthritis, ankylosing spondylitis, psoriatic arthritis, reactive arthritis (Reiter's syndrome), relapsing polychondritis and inflammatory bowel disorders may all be associated with aortitis involve the ascending aorta.*

**2423. Which of the following bacteria cause aortitis by infecting the aorta at sites of atherosclerotic plaque?**
*Harrison's 20th Ed. Chapter 274 Page 1922*

A. Staphylococcus
B. Streptococcus
C. Salmonella
D. All of the above

**2424. The initial lesion in syphilitic aortitis is in?**
*Harrison's 20th Ed. Chapter 274 Page 1922*

A. Intima
B. Media
C. Adventitia
D. All of the above

*The initial lesion in syphilitic aortitis is an obliterative endarteritis of the vasa vasorum, especially in the adventitia.*

**2425. Linear calcification of the ascending aorta is a feature of?**
*Harrison's 20th Ed. Chapter 274 Page 1922*

A. Infective aortitis
B. Giant cell arteritis
C. Takayasu's arteritis
D. Syphilitic aortitis

## Arterial Diseases of the Extremities

**2426. Which of the following is a cause of peripheral artery disease (PAD)?**
*Harrison's 20th Ed. Chapter 275 Page 1923*

A. Vasculitis
B. Entrapment
C. Cystic adventitial disease
D. All of the above

*Atherosclerosis is the leading cause of PAD in patients >40 years old. Other causes include thrombosis, embolism, vasculitis, fibromuscular dysplasia, entrapment, cystic adventitial disease and trauma.*

**2427. Out of the following vessels, which is the most often involved in PAD?**
*Harrison's 20th Ed. Chapter 275 Page 1923*

A. Abdominal aorta
B. Iliac arteries
C. Femoral and popliteal arteries
D. Tibial and peroneal arteries

*The primary sites of involvement are the abdominal aorta and iliac arteries (30% of symptomatic patients), the femoral and popliteal arteries (80-90% of patients) and the more distal vessels including the tibial and peroneal arteries (40-50% of patients).*

**2428. Which of the following about intermittent claudication is false?**
*Harrison's 20th Ed. Chapter 275 Page 1923*

A. Occurs during exercise & is relieved by rest
B. More common in lower than in upper extremities
C. Worse at night
D. None of the above

**2429. Which of the following is a physical finding of PAD?**
*Harrison's 20th Ed. Chapter 275 Page 1923*

A. Hair loss
B. Thickened nails
C. Smooth and shiny skin
D. All of the above

*Important physical findings of PAD include decreased or absent pulses distal to the obstruction, the presence of bruits over the narrowed artery and muscle atrophy. With more severe disease, hair loss, thickened nails, smooth and shiny skin, reduced skin temperature and pallor or cyanosis are common physical signs. In patients with critical limb ischemia, ulcers or gangrene may occur.*

**2430. In patients with peripheral arterial disease, the ankle:brachial index (ABI) is?**
*Harrison's 20th Ed. Chapter 275 Page 1923*

A. < 0.4
B. < 0.6
C. < 0.8
D. < 1

*In hemodynamically significant arterial stenoses, systolic blood pressure in leg is decreased. Ratio of ankle and brachial artery pressures (ankle:brachial index or ABI) is 1.00 to 1.40 in normal individuals. ABI <0.90 is abnormal and diagnostic of PAD. A ratio of <0.5 is consistent with severe ischemia.*

**2431. ABI > 1.40 indicates?**
*Harrison's 20th Ed. Chapter 275 Page 1923*

A. Hyperplastic artery
B. Noncompressible artery secondary to vascular calcification
C. Arteriovenous communication
D. None of the above

*ABIs > 1.40 indicates noncompressible arteries secondary to vascular calcification.*

**2432. Which of the following is false about PAD?**
*Harrison's 20th Ed. Chapter 275 Page 1923*

A. Decline of the ABI immediately after exercise
B. Blunting of amplitude of pulse volume contour
C. ABI values of 0.91 - 0.99 are considered borderline
D. None of the above

**2433. Which of the following drugs is effective in patients with PAD?**
*Harrison's 20th Ed. Chapter 275 Page 1924*

A. Cilostazol
B. Pentoxifylline
C. Angiotensin converting enzyme inhibitors
D. All of the above

*Cilostazol is a phosphodiesterase inhibitor with vasodilator and antiplatelet properties. Pentoxifylline is a substituted xanthine derivative and increases blood flow to the microcirculation and enhances tissue oxygenation.*

**2434. Which of the following about fibromuscular dysplasia is false?**
*Harrison's 20th Ed. Chapter 275 Page 1925*

A. Affects medium size and small arteries
B. Occurs predominantly in females
C. Usually involves renal and carotid arteries
D. None of the above

**2435. In fibromuscular dysplasia, which of the following is the most common histologic type?**
*Harrison's 20th Ed. Chapter 275 Page 1925*

A. Medial fibroplasia
B. Perimedial fibroplasia
C. Medial hyperplasia
D. Intimal fibroplasia

*The histologic classification of fibromuscular dysplasia includes intimal fibroplasia, medial dysplasia and adventitial hyperplasia. Medial dysplasia is subdivided into medial fibroplasia, perimedial fibroplasia and medial hyperplasia. Medial fibroplasia is the most common type and is characterized by alternating areas of thinned media and fibromuscular ridges. The internal elastic lamina usually is preserved.*

**2436. "String of beads" appearance on angiography is typical of?**
*Harrison's 20th Ed. Chapter 275 Page 1925*

A. Fibromuscular dysplasia
B. Thromboangiitis obliterans
C. Takayasu's arteritis
D. Giant cell (temporal) arteritis

*"String of beads" appearance on angiography is characteristic of fibromuscular dysplasia caused by thickened fibromuscular ridges contiguous with thin, less-involved portions of the arterial wall.*

**2437. Clinical features of thromboangiitis obliterans include?**
*Harrison's 20th Ed. Chapter 275 Page 1925*

A. Claudication of affected extremity
B. Raynaud's phenomenon
C. Migratory superficial vein thrombophlebitis
D. All of the above

Clinical features of thromboangiitis obliterans include a triad of claudication of the affected extremity, Raynaud's phenomenon, and migratory superficial vein thrombophlebitis.

**2438. Which out of the following is false about thromboangiitis obliterans?**
*Harrison's 20th Ed. Chapter 275 Page 1925*

A. Most frequently in men < 40 years of age
B. Definite relationship to cigarette smoking
C. Involves small & medium-size arteries & veins of extremities
D. None of the above

**2439. Which out of the following is false about thromboangiitis obliterans?**
*Harrison's 20th Ed. Chapter 275 Page 1925*

A. Smooth tapering segmental lesions in distal vessels
B. Collateral vessels at sites of vascular occlusion
C. Proximal atherosclerotic disease is usually absent
D. None of the above

**2440. Which of the following is a cause of acute arterial occlusion?**
*Harrison's 20th Ed. Chapter 275 Page 1926*

A. Embolism
B. Thrombus in situ
C. Arterial dissection
D. All of the above

Principal causes of acute arterial occlusion include embolism, thrombus in situ, arterial dissection and trauma.

**2441. In lower extremities, emboli lodge most frequently in?**
*Harrison's 20th Ed. Chapter 275 Page 1926*

A. Femoral artery
B. Iliac artery
C. Popliteal artery
D. Tibioperoneal arteries

In lower extremities, emboli lodge most frequently in femoral artery, followed by iliac artery, aorta, and popliteal and tibioperoneal arteries.

**2442. "Blue toe" syndrome is best related to?**
*Harrison's 20th Ed. Chapter 275 Page 1927 Figure 275-2*

A. Frostbite
B. Raynaud's phenomenon
C. Atheroembolism
D. Arteriovenous Fistula

Atheroembolism causes cyanotic discoloration & impending necrosis of the toes termed as "blue toe syndrome".

**2443. Paget-Schroetter syndrome is best related to?**
*Harrison's 20th Ed. Chapter 275 Page 1927*

A. Frostbite
B. Thoracic Outlet Compression Syndrome
C. Atheroembolism
D. Arteriovenous Fistula

Thoracic outlet compression syndrome may be divided into arterial, venous & neurogenic forms. Patients with neurogenic thoracic outlet compression may develop shoulder & arm pain, weakness, & paresthesias. Patients with arterial compression experience claudication, Raynaud's phenomenon, ischemic tissue loss & gangrene. Venous compression causes thrombosis of subclavian & axillary veins, often associated with effort & is referred to as Paget-Schroetter syndrome.

**2444. Which of the following maneuvers is useful in diagnosis of thoracic outlet compression syndrome?**
*Harrison's 20th Ed. Chapter 275 Page 1927*

A. Hyperabduction maneuver
B. Scalene maneuver
C. Costoclavicular maneuver
D. All of the above

Maneuvers used for diagnosis of thoracic outlet compression syndrome include abduction & external rotation test, in which affected arm is abducted by 90° & shoulder is externally rotated. Scalene maneuver (extension of neck & rotation of head to side of symptoms). Costoclavicular maneuver (posterior rotation of shoulders) & hyperabduction maneuver (raising arm to 180°).

**2445. Which of the following is the most common peripheral artery aneurysm?**
*Harrison's 20th Ed. Chapter 275 Page 1927*

A. Femoral artery
B. Popliteal artery
C. Tibial artery
D. Dorsalis pedis artery

Popliteal artery aneurysms are the most common peripheral artery aneurysms.

**2446. Nicoladoni-Branham sign refers to?**
*Harrison's 20th Ed. Chapter 275 Page 1927*

A. Tenderness in supraclavicular fossa
B. Compression of large arteriovenous fistula causing reflex slowing of heart rate
C. Hyperabduction maneuver causing subclavian bruits
D. Hyperabduction maneuver causing loss of pulses in arm

Compression of a large arteriovenous fistula may cause reflex slowing of the heart rate. This is called Nicoladoni-Branham sign.

**2447. On cold exposure, which of the following is the first to occur in Raynaud's phenomenon?**
*Harrison's 20th Ed. Chapter 275 Page 1928*

A. Pallor
B. Cyanosis
C. Rubor
D. None of the above

Raynaud's phenomenon is characterized by episodic digital ischemia, manifested clinically by sequential development of digital blanching or pallor, cyanosis, & rubor of fingers or toes following cold exposure & subsequent rewarming.

**2448. In Raynaud's phenomenon, patients experience throbbing pain during which phase?**
*Harrison's 20th Ed. Chapter 275 Page 1928*

A. Pallor
B. Cyanosis
C. Rubor
D. None of the above

Blanching or pallor represents the ischemic phase of Raynaud's phenomenon and results from vasospasm of digital arteries. During ischemic phase, capillaries & venules dilate and cyanosis results from deoxygenated blood that is present in these vessels. A sensation of cold or numbness or paresthesia of the digits often accompanies the phases of pallor and cyanosis. With rewarming, the digital vasospasm resolves, and blood flow into the dilated arterioles and capillaries increases dramatically. This "reactive hyperemia" imparts a bright red color to the digits. In addition to rubor and warmth, patients often experience a throbbing, painful sensation during the hyperemic phase.

2449. Which of the following about Raynaud's disease is false?

*Harrison's 20th Ed. Chapter 275 Page 1928*

A. 50% with Raynaud's phenomenon have Raynaud's disease
B. Women are affected 5 times more than men
C. Age of presentation is between 20 and 40 years
D. Toes are involved more frequently than fingers

Over 50% of patients with Raynaud's phenomenon have Raynaud's disease. Women are affected about five times more often than men, and the age of presentation is usually between 20 and 40 years. Fingers are involved more frequently than the toes.

2450. Which of the following may be involved in Raynaud's phenomenon?

*Harrison's 20th Ed. Chapter 275 Page 1929*

A. Earlobes
B. Tip of the nose
C. Penis
D. All of the above

Rarely, the earlobes, the tip of the nose and the penis are involved in Raynaud's phenomenon.

2451. Which of the following about Raynaud's phenomenon is false?

*Harrison's 20th Ed. Chapter 275 Page 1929*

A. Occurs frequently in patients who also have migraine
B. Occurs frequently in patients who also have variant angina
C. Radial, ulnar and pedal pulses are abnormal
D. Fingers and toes perspire excessively between attacks

Raynaud's phenomenon occurs frequently in patients who also have migraine headaches or variant angina. Radial, ulnar, and pedal pulses are normal. The fingers and toes may be cool between attacks and may perspire excessively.

2452. Which of the following drugs does not cause Raynaud's phenomenon?

*Harrison's 20th Ed. Chapter 275 Page 1929*

A. Methysergide
B. α-adrenergic receptor antagonists
C. β-adrenergic receptor antagonists
D. None of the above

2453. Which of the following drugs cause Raynaud's phenomenon?

*Harrison's 20th Ed. Chapter 275 Page 1928 Table 275–1*

A. Bleomycin
B. Vinblastine
C. Cisplatin
D. All of the above

Drugs that can cause Raynaud's phenomenon include ergot derivatives, methysergide, beta-adrenergic receptor blockers, bleomycin, vinblastine and cisplatin.

2454. Which of the following diseases can present as Raynaud's phenomenon?

*Harrison's 20th Ed. Chapter 275 Page 1929*

A. Scleroderma
B. Systemic lupus erythematosus
C. Dermatomyositis or polymyositis
D. All of the above

Raynaud's phenomenon occurs in patients with systemic sclerosis (scleroderma), systemic lupus erythematosus (SLE), dermatomyositis or polymyositis, rheumatoid arthritis, atherosclerosis of extremities, thromboangiitis obliterans, acute occlusion of large and medium-sized arteries by a thrombus or embolus, thoracic outlet compression syndrome, primary pulmonary hypertension, blood dyscrasias, use of vibrating hand tools, pianists and keyboard operators. Electric shock injury to the hands or frostbite may lead to the later development of Raynaud's phenomenon.

2455. Which of the following drug is useful in Raynaud's phenomenon?

*Harrison's 20th Ed. Chapter 275 Page 1929*

A. Nifedipine
B. Prazosin
C. Methyldopa
D. All of the above

2456. Which of the following drug is useful in Raynaud's phenomenon?

*Harrison's 20th Ed. Chapter 275 Page 1929*

A. Amlodipine
B. Terazosin
C. Phenoxybenzamine
D. All of the above

Dihydropyridine calcium channel antagonists (nifedipine, isradipine, felodipine & amlodipine) are useful. Postsynaptic alpha 1-adrenergic antagonist prazosin, doxazosin & terazosin may be effective. Sympatholytic agents methyldopa, guanethidine & phenoxybenzamine may be useful. Digital sympathectomy is helpful in those who are unresponsive to medical therapy.

2457. Which of the following is false about acrocyanosis?

*Harrison's 20th Ed. Chapter 275 Page 1929*

A. Persistent cyanosis of the hands
B. Normal pulses
C. Trophic skin changes and ulcerations do not occur
D. None of the above

In acrocyanosis, there is arterial vasoconstriction & secondary dilation of capillaries & venules with resulting persistent cyanosis of hands & feet. Pain, ulcers & gangrene do not occur. Pulses are normal & blanching does not occur.

2458. Secondary acrocyanosis is associated with?

*Harrison's 20th Ed. Chapter 275 Page 1929*

A. Brain tumour
B. Lung cancer
C. Infective hepatitis
D. Anorexia nervosa

Secondary acrocyanosis may result from hypoxemia, connective tissue diseases, atheroembolism, antiphospholipid antibodies, cold agglutinins, or cryoglobulins, and is associated with anorexia nervosa and orthostatic tachycardia syndrome.

2459. "Atrophie blanche en plaque" is the term given to?

*Harrison's 20th Ed. Chapter 275 Page 1929*

A. Myxoedema dermopathy
B. Thyroid acropachy
C. Primary livedo reticularis with ulceration
D. Secondary livedo reticularis

*Primary livedo reticularis with ulceration is called atrophie blanche en plaque.*

**2460. Secondary livedo reticularis can occur with?**
*Harrison's 20th Ed. Chapter 275 Page 1929*

A. Atheroembolism
B. SLE
C. Anticardiolipin antibodies
D. All of the above

*Secondary livedo reticularis can occur with atheroembolism, SLE, anticardiolipin antibodies, hyperviscosity, cryoglobulinemia & Sneddon's syndrome (ischemic stroke & livedo reticularis).*

**2461. The other name of 'Pernio' is?**
*Harrison's 20th Ed. Chapter 275 Page 1930*

A. Acrocyanosis
B. Erythromelalgia
C. Chilblains
D. Frostbite

**2462. Which of the following best relates to Pernio (Chilblains)?**
*Harrison's 20th Ed. Chapter 275 Page 1930*

A. Atheroembolism
B. Mechanical trauma
C. Vasculitic disorder
D. All of the above

*Pernio (Chilblains) is a vasculitic disorder associated with exposure to cold. Raised erythematous lesions develop on lower part of legs & feet in cold weather. These are associated with pruritus and a burning sensation, and they may blister and ulcerate.*

**2463. Which of the following is false about erythromelalgia?**
*Harrison's 20th Ed. Chapter 275 Page 1930*

A. Characterized by burning pain and erythema of extremities
B. Feet involved more frequently than hands
C. Males affected more frequently than females
D. None of the above

*Erythromelalgia is characterized by burning pain and erythema of the extremities. The feet are involved more frequently than hands, and males are affected more frequently than females.*

**2464. Which of the following is false about erythromelalgia?**
*Harrison's 20th Ed. Chapter 275 Page 1930*

A. May be secondary to myeloproliferative disorders
B. May occur as an adverse effect of nifedipine
C. May occur as an adverse effect of bromocriptine
D. Burning sensation is precipitated by exposure to cold environment

*Secondary erythromelalgia occurs with myeloproliferative disorders such as polycythemia vera and essential thrombocytosis. Less-common causes include drugs, such as calcium channel blockers, bromocriptine, and pergolide; neuropathies; connective tissue diseases, such as SLE and paraneoplastic syndromes. Patients complain of burning in the extremities that is precipitated by exposure to a warm environment and aggravated by a dependent position. The symptoms are relieved by exposing the affected area to cool air or water or by elevation.*

**2465. Frostbite usually affects which of the following?**
*Harrison's 20th Ed. Chapter 275 Page 1930*

A. Nose
B. Chin
C. Cheeks
D. All of the above

*Frostbite affects distal aspects of extremities or exposed parts of face like ears, nose, chin & cheeks.*

**2466. In superficial frostbite, after rewarming, which of the following occurs?**
*Harrison's 20th Ed. Chapter 275 Page 1930*

A. Cyanosis and erythema
B. Wheal-and-flare formation
C. Edema and superficial blisters
D. All of the above

**2467. In frostbite, the temperature of the water bath used for rewarming should be?**
*Harrison's 20th Ed. Chapter 275 Page 1930*

A. 32° – 36°C
B. 36° – 40°C
C. 40° – 44°C
D. 44° – 48°C

*Initial treatment is rewarming, which is accomplished by immersion of the affected part in a water bath at temperatures of 40°–44°C (104°–111°F).*

# Chronic Venous Disease and Lymphedema

**2468. Chronic venous diseases include?**
*Harrison's 20th Ed. Chapter 276 Page 1930*

- A. Telangiectasias & reticular veins
- B. Varicose veins
- C. Chronic venous insufficiency
- D. All of the above

Chronic venous diseases include telangiectasias & reticular veins, varicose veins, chronic venous insufficiency with edema, skin changes, and ulceration.

**2469. Which of the following is the longest vein in the body?**
*Harrison's 20th Ed. Chapter 276 Page 1930*

- A. Popliteal vein
- B. Common iliac vein
- C. Great saphenous vein
- D. Common femoral vein

**2470. Which of the following about varicose veins is false?**
*Harrison's 20th Ed. Chapter 276 Page 1930*

- A. Deep veins
- B. Dilated, bulging, tortuous veins
- C. Measure at least 3 mm in diameter
- D. Due to defective structure & function of the valves

Varicose veins are dilated, bulging, tortuous superficial veins, measuring at least 3 mm in diameter.

**2471. Primary varicose veins result from?**
*Harrison's 20th Ed. Chapter 276 Page 1931*

- A. Defective structure & function of valves of saphenous veins
- B. Intrinsic weakness of the vein wall
- C. High intraluminal pressure
- D. All of the above

**2472. Secondary varicose veins result from?**
*Harrison's 20th Ed. Chapter 276 Page 1931*

- A. Deep-venous insufficiency
- B. Deep venous obstruction
- C. Incompetent perforating veins
- D. All of the above

Secondary varicose veins result from venous hypertension.

**2473. The Klippel-Trenaunay syndrome is characterized by?**
*J Cardiovasc Ultrasound. 2015;23(4):266-270*

- A. Vascular nevus
- B. Varicose veins
- C. Soft tissue and bony hypertrophy of limb
- D. All of the above

The Klippel-Trenaunay syndrome is characterized by a triad of vascular nevus, varicose veins, and soft tissue and bony hypertrophy of limb. The venous stasis in vascular malformations of lower limbs increases the chance of thrombus formation and PTE.

**2474. Venulitis is a feature of?**
*Harrison's 20th Ed. Chapter 276 Page 1930*

- A. Thromboangiitis obliterans
- B. Behçet's syndrome
- C. Homocystinuria
- D. All of the above

Venulitis occurring in thromboangiitis obliterans, Behçet's syndrome and homocystinuria may cause venous thrombosis.

**2475. 'Phlegmasia cerulea dolens' refers to?**
*N Engl J Med. 2007; 356:e3*

- A. Deoxygenated hemoglobin in stagnant veins giving cyanotic hue to limb
- B. Pain on antigravity movement of DVT affected limb
- C. DVT affected veins that are likely to embolize
- D. Chronic venous insufficiency

Phlegmasia cerulea dolens or blue, painful leg, is an uncommon manifestation of deep-vein thrombosis and results from massive thrombosis compromising venous outflow, which causes ischemia.

**2476. 'Phlegmasia alba dolens' refers to?**
*Damar Cer Derg 2017;26(3):111-115*

- A. Deoxygenated hemoglobin in stagnant veins giving cyanotic hue to limb
- B. Pain on antigravity movement of DVT affected limb
- C. DVT affected veins that are likely to embolize
- D. Pallor in markedly edematous DVT affected legs

Phlegmasia alba dolens is a condition characterized by limb swelling (edema), tenderness, pain, lividity, and bullous lesions followed by whitening of the limb due to venous stasis caused by femoral vein thrombosis. The collateral vessels are either not affected or affected less extensively than phlegmasia cerulea dolens.

**2477. Dermatologic findings associated with venous stasis include?**
*Harrison's 20th Ed. Chapter 276 Page 1931*

- A. Lipodermatosclerosis
- B. Atrophie blanche
- C. Phlebectasia corona
- D. All of the above

Dermatologic findings associated with venous stasis include hyperpigmentation, erythema, eczema, lipodermatosclerosis, atrophie blanche, and a phlebectasia corona.

**2478. Lipodermatosclerosis is best related to?**
*Harrison's 20th Ed. Chapter 276 Page 1931*

- A. Fat deposition
- B. Thrombin deposition
- C. Collagen deposition
- D. Hemosiderin deposition

Lipodermatosclerosis is the combination of induration, hemosiderin deposition, and inflammation, and typically occurs in the lower part of the leg just above the ankle.

**2479. Lipodermatosclerosis is a form of?**
*Harrison's 20th Ed. Chapter 54 Page 352*

A. Dermatitis
B. Vasculitis
C. Panniculitis
D. Cellulitis

Panniculitis, an inflammation of the fat. Various forms of panniculitis, are erythema nodosum, erythema induratum/nodular vasculitis, lupus panniculitis, lipodermatosclerosis, α1-antitrypsin deficiency, factitial, and fat necrosis secondary to pancreatic disease.

**2480. Which of the following is a feature of Atrophie blanche?**
*Harrison's 20th Ed. Chapter 276 Page 1931*

A. White patch of scar tissue
B. Focal telangiectasias and hyperpigmented border
C. Develops near medial malleolus
D. All of the above

Atrophie blanche is a white patch of scar tissue, often with focal telangiectasias and a hyperpigmented border that usually develops near medial malleolus.

**2481. Which of the following is the characteristic pattern of phlebectasia corona?**
*Harrison's 20th Ed. Chapter 276 Page 1931*

A. Crown-shaped
B. Fan-shaped
C. Tear drop-shaped
D. Dome-shaped

Phlebectasia corona is a fan-shaped pattern of intradermal veins near the ankle or on the foot.

**2482. Which of the following tests is used to diagnose varicose veins?**
*Harrison's 20th Ed. Chapter 276 Page 1932, Ann R Coll Surg Engl. 2006;88(3):309-312*

A. Brodie–Trendelenburg test
B. Perthes test
C. Schwarts test
D. All of the above

Brodie–Trendelenburg test is used to determine whether varicose veins are secondary to deep-venous insufficiency. As the patient is lying supine, the leg is elevated and the veins allowed to empty. Then, a tourniquet is placed on the proximal part of the thigh and the patient is asked to stand. Filling of the varicose veins within 30 s indicates that the varicose veins are caused by deep-venous insufficiency and incompetent perforating veins. Primary varicose veins with superficial venous insufficiency are the likely diagnosis if venous refilling occurs promptly after tourniquet removal. The Perthes test assesses the possibility of deep venous obstruction. A tourniquet is placed on the mid thigh after the patient has stood, and the varicose veins are filled. The patient is then instructed to walk for 5 min. A patent deep-venous system and competent perforating veins enable the superficial veins below the tourniquet to collapse. Deep venous obstruction is likely to be present if the superficial veins distend further with walking.
Brodie-Trendelenburg (tourniquet) test, cough impulse and tap test (Ann R Coll Surg Engl. 2006;88(3):309-312).
Brodie-Trendeleburg test, Schwarts test, Morrissey's cough impulse test, Parthe's test, multiple tourniquet test

**2483. Persistent lymphedema leads to infiltration of?**
*Harrison's 20th Ed. Chapter 276 Page 1933*

A. Mononuclear cells
B. Fibroblasts
C. Adipocytes
D. All of the above

Persistent lymphedema leads to inflammatory & immune responses characterized by infiltration of mononuclear cells, fibroblasts & adipocytes, leading to adipose & collagen deposition in skin & subcutaneous tissues.

**2484. Smooth muscle cells first appear in which of the following?**
*Harrison's 20th Ed. Chapter 276 Page 1933*

A. Lymphatic capillaries
B. Microlymphatic precollector vessels
C. Collecting lymphatic vessels
D. Larger lymphatic conduits

**2485. Bileaflet valves first appear in which of the following?**
*Harrison's 20th Ed. Chapter 276 Page 1933*

A. Lymphatic capillaries
B. Microlymphatic precollector vessels
C. Collecting lymphatic vessels
D. Larger lymphatic conduits

**2486. Superficial & deep lymphatic vessels in legs communicate at?**
*Harrison's 20th Ed. Chapter 276 Page 1933*

A. Popliteal lymph nodes
B. Pelvic lymph nodes
C. Para aortic lymph nodes
D. All of the above

Superficial & deep lymphatic vessels in legs communicate at the popliteal & inguinal lymph nodes.

**2487. Thoracic duct connects with?**
*Harrison's 20th Ed. Chapter 276 Page 1933*

A. Right brachiocephalic vein
B. Left brachiocephalic vein
C. Inferior vena cava
D. Superior vena cava

Pelvic lymphatic vessels drain into the thoracic duct, which connects with the left brachiocephalic vein.

**2488. Which of the following is a clinical subtype of primary lymphedema?**
*Harrison's 20th Ed. Chapter 276 Page 1933*

A. Congenital lymphedema
B. Lymphedema praecox
C. Lymphedema tarda
D. All of the above

**2489. Lymphedema tarda usually begins after the age of?**
*Harrison's 20th Ed. Chapter 276 Page 1933*

A. 1 year
B. 14 years
C. 25 years
D. 35 years

Congenital lymphedema appears shortly after birth, lymphedema praecox has its onset at the time of puberty and lymphedema tarda usually begins after age 35.

**2490. Which of the following genes is involved in the development of lymphatic valves?**
*Harrison's 20th Ed. Chapter 276 Page 1933*

A. KIF11
B. GATA2
C. CCBE1
D. FOXC2

Mutations of the GATA2 gene, which is involved in the development of lymphatic valves, cause lymphedema and predisposes to acute myeloid leukemia.

**2491. Milroy's disease is best described as?**
*Harrison's 20th Ed. Chapter 276 Page 1933*

A. Congenital lymphedema
B. Lymphedema praecox
C. Lymphedema tarda
D. Bacterial lymphangitis

*Familial forms of congenital lymphedema (Milroy's disease) and lymphedema praecox (Meige's disease) may be inherited in an autosomal dominant manner with variable penetrance.*

**2492. Mutations in which of the following genes causes Milroy's disease?**
*Harrison's 20th Ed. Chapter 276 Page 1933*

A. LSC1
B. VEGFR3
C. CCBE1
D. FOXC2

*Milroy's disease is caused by mutations in genes expressing vascular endothelial growth factor receptor 3 (VEGFR3) which determines lymphangiogenesis.*

**2493. Mutations in which of the following genes causes cholestasis-lymphedema syndrome?**
*Harrison's 20th Ed. Chapter 276 Page 1933*

A. LSC1
B. VEGFR3
C. CCBE1
D. FOXC2

**2494. Mutations in which of the following genes causes lymphedema-distichiasis syndrome?**
*Harrison's 20th Ed. Chapter 276 Page 1933*

A. LSC1
B. VEGFR3
C. CCBE1
D. FOXC2

**2495. Mutations in which of the following genes causes hypotrichosis, lymphedema, telangiectasia syndrome?**
*Harrison's 20th Ed. Chapter 276 Page 1933*

A. LSC1
B. VEGFR3
C. SOX18
D. FOXC2

**2496. Double row of eyelashes relates to which of the following genes?**
*Harrison's 20th Ed. Chapter 276 Page 1933*

A. LSC1
B. VEGFR3
C. SOX18
D. FOXC2

**2497. Mutations in which of the following genes causes microcephaly-lymphedema syndrome?**
*Harrison's 20th Ed. Chapter 276 Page 1933*

A. KIF11
B. GATA2
C. CCBE1
D. FOXC2

**2498. Primary lymphedema may be associated with?**
*Harrison's 20th Ed. Chapter 276 Page 1934*

A. Turner syndrome
B. Klinefelter syndrome
C. Noonan syndrome
D. All of the above

**2499. Primary lymphedema may be associated with?**
*Harrison's 20th Ed. Chapter 276 Page 1934*

A. Yellow nail syndrome
B. Intestinal lymphangiectasia syndrome
C. Lymphangiomyomatosis
D. All of the above

*Primary lymphedema may be associated with Turner's syndrome, Klinefelter's syndrome, Noonan's syndrome, yellow nail syndrome, intestinal lymphangiectasia syndrome, and lymphangiomyomatosis.*

**2500. Lymphedema is found in which of the following?**
*Harrison's 20th Ed. Chapter 276 Page 1934*

A. Noonan's syndrome
B. Yellow nail syndrome
C. Klippel-Trenaunay syndrome
D. All of the above

*Patients with a chromosomal aneuploidy (Turner's syndrome, Klinefelter's syndrome) or trisomy 18, 13 or 21 may develop lymphedema. Other disorders include Klippel-Trenaunay syndrome, Parkes-Weber syndrome, Hennekam's syndrome, Noonan's syndrome, yellow nail syndrome, intestinal lymphangiectasia syndrome, lymphangiomyomatosis and neurofibromatosis type 1.*

**2501. Most common cause of secondary lymphedema worldwide is?**
*Harrison's 20th Ed. Chapter 276 Page 1934*

A. Bacterial lymphangitis
B. Filariasis
C. Radiation therapy for breast carcinoma
D. Pregnancy

*Most common cause of secondary lymphedema worldwide is filariasis.*

**2502. Filariasis is caused by?**
*Harrison's 20th Ed. Chapter 276 Page 1934 Table 276-2*

A. Wucheria bancrofti
B. Brugia malayi
C. B. timori
D. Any of the above

**2503. Infectious causes of secondary lymphedema include?**
*Harrison's 20th Ed. Chapter 276 Page 1934*

A. Streptococcal infection
B. Lymphogranuloma venereum
C. Tuberculosis
D. All of the above

**2504. Podoconiosis best relates to?**
*Harrison's 20th Ed. Chapter 276 Page 1934*

A. Surgical excision of axillary and inguinal lymph nodes
B. Irradiation of axillary and inguinal lymph nodes
C. Silicate particles in soil
D. Self-induced or factitious lymphedema

*Podoconiosis refers to absorption of silicate particles in soil derived from volcanic rock following barefoot exposure.*

**2505. Inability to tent the skin at the base of the toes is called?**
*Harrison's 20th Ed. Chapter 276 Page 1934*

A. Stemmer's sign
B. Signet-ring sign
C. Hoover's sign
D. Atoll sign

**2506. Which of the following is related to lymphedema?**
*Harrison's 20th Ed. Chapter 276 Page 1934*

A. Squaring of the toes
B. Peau d'orange
C. Acanthosis and verrucous overgrowths
D. All of the above

**2507. Which of the following disorders cause unilateral leg swelling?**
*Harrison's 20th Ed. Chapter 276 Page 1934*

A. Deep-vein thrombosis
B. Chronic venous insufficiency
C. Lymphedema
D. All of the above

**2508. Sparing of the feet is observed in which of the following?**
*Harrison's 20th Ed. Chapter 276 Page 1934*

A. Myxedema
B. Lipedema
C. Lymphedema
D. All of the above

*Lipedema is usually seen in women and is caused by accumulation of adipose tissue in leg from thigh to the ankle, with sparing of the feet.*

**2509. Which of the following is characteristic of lymphedema on magnetic resonance imaging (MRI)?**
*Harrison's 20th Ed. Chapter 276 Page 1935*

A. Honeycomb pattern in the epifascial compartment
B. Mosaic pattern in the epifascial compartment
C. Crazy paving in the epifascial compartment
D. Eggshell pattern in the epifascial compartment

**2510. In primary lymphedema, lymphatic channels are?**
*Harrison's 20th Ed. Chapter 276 Page 1934*

A. Absent
B. Hypoplastic
C. Ectatic
D. Any of the above

# Pulmonary Hypertension

**2511. In Pulmonary hypertension (PH), mean pulmonary artery pressure is?**
*Harrison's 20th Ed. Chapter 277 Page 1935*

A. > 16 mm Hg
B. > 18 mm Hg
C. > 20 mm Hg
D. > 22 mm Hg

*Pulmonary hypertension (PH) is a spectrum of diseases involving the pulmonary vasculature and is defined as an elevation in pulmonary arterial pressures (mean pulmonary artery pressure >22 mm Hg).*

**2512. In Pulmonary hypertension (PH), the estimated systolic PAP is?**
*Harrison's 20th Ed. Chapter 277 Page 1935*

A. > 28 mm Hg
B. > 32 mm Hg
C. > 36 mm Hg
D. > 40 mm Hg

*In pulmonary hypertension (PH), the estimated systolic PAP is >36 mm Hg.*

**2513. Pulmonary arterial hypertension (PAH) is characterized by symptoms of?**
*Harrison's 20th Ed. Chapter 277 Page 1935*

A. Dyspnea
B. Chest pain
C. Syncope
D. All of the above

*Pulmonary arterial hypertension (PAH) is characterized by dyspnea, chest pain and syncope.*

**2514. Which of the following is the most common symptom attributable to pulmonary hypertension?**
*Harrison's 20th Ed. Chapter 277 Page 1936*

A. Edema
B. Exertional dyspnea
C. Syncope
D. Peripheral edema

*Most common symptom attributable to pulmonary hypertension is exertional dyspnea. Other symptoms are fatigue, angina pectoris (RV ischemia), syncope, near syncope & peripheral edema.*

**2515. Which of the following underlie the development of PAH?**
*Harrison's 20th Ed. Chapter 277 Page 1936*

A. Vascular proliferation
B. Thrombosis
C. Inflammation
D. All of the above

*Vasoconstriction, vascular proliferation, thrombosis, and inflammation underlie the development of PAH.*

**2516. In PH, which of the following characterize the pathological findings in the pulmonary vasculature?**
*Harrison's 20th Ed. Chapter 277 Page 1936*

A. Intimal proliferation & fibrosis
B. Medial hypertrophy
C. In situ thrombosis
D. All of the above

*Intimal proliferation & fibrosis, medial hypertrophy, and in situ thrombosis characterize the pathological findings in the pulmonary vasculature.*

**2517. In PH, with decreased compliance of pulmonary vasculature, the compensatory response is?**
*Harrison's 20th Ed. Chapter 277 Page 1936*

A. Tachypnea
B. Tachycardia
C. Hypertension
D. All of the above

**2518. Which of the following occurs in plexogenic pulmonary arteriopathy?**
*Harrison's 20th Ed. Chapter 277 Page 1936 Figure 277-1*

A. Medial hypertrophy of muscular pulmonary arteries
B. Obstructive lesions of small muscular pulmonary arteries
C. Proliferative lesions of small muscular pulmonary arteries
D. All of the above

**2519. Pathobiologic process that result in pulmonary arterial hypertension is?**
*Harrison's 20th Ed. Chapter 277 Page 1936*

A. Inhibition of voltage-regulated potassium channel
B. Increased serotonin uptake in smooth-muscle cells
C. Hypoxia-induced activation of hypoxia-inducible factor-1α
D. All of the above

*In PAH, abnormalities in molecular pathways regulating the pulmonary vascular endothelial and smooth-muscle cells include inhibition of voltage-regulated potassium channel, mutations in the bone morphogenetic protein-2 receptor, increased serotonin uptake in smooth-muscle cells due to overactivation of the serotonin transporter, hypoxia-induced activation of hypoxia-inducible factor-1α, activation of nuclear factor of activated T cells and excessive thrombin deposition related to a procoagulant state. There is a loss of apoptosis of smooth-muscle cells allowing their proliferation, and emergence of apoptosis-resistant endothelial cells which can obliterate the vascular lumen.*

**2520. Which of the following is the most important initial screening test for the diagnosis of PH?**
*Harrison's 20th Ed. Chapter 277 Page 1937*

A. Doppler echocardiography
B. Echocardiogram with bubble study
C. Cardiopulmonary exercise test (CPET)
D. High-resolution computed tomography (HRCT)

*An echocardiogram with bubble study is the most important initial screening test for the diagnosis of PH.*

**2521. Which of the following can cause PH?**
*Harrison's 20th Ed. Chapter 277 Page 1937*

A. Valvular heart disease
B. Left ventricular systolic & diastolic function
C. Intra-cardiac shunts
D. All of the above

*All forms of PH demonstrate a hypertrophied & dilated right ventricle with elevated estimated pulmonary artery systolic pressure.*

**2522. Which of the following is the gold standard for diagnosis & assessment of disease severity?**
*Harrison's 20th Ed. Chapter 277 Page 1937*

A. Doppler echocardiography
B. CT angiograms
C. Ventilation-perfusion (V/Q) scanning
D. Right heart catheterization (RHC) with pulmonary vasodilator testing

*Invasive hemodynamic monitoring (right heart catheterization) is the gold standard for diagnosis & assessment of disease severity.*

**2523. Classic findings of PH on high-resolution computed tomography include?**
*Harrison's 20th Ed. Chapter 277 Page 1937*

A. Enlarged pulmonary arteries
B. Peripheral pruning of small vessels
C. Enlarged right ventricle & right atrium
D. All of the above

**2524. Centrilobular ground glass infiltrate & thickened septal lines seen in the absence of left heart disease on high-resolution CT suggest?**
*Harrison's 20th Ed. Chapter 277 Page 1937*

A. Emphysema
B. Asthma
C. Pulmonary venous disease
D. Interstitial lung disease

**2525. Which of the following is the classic finding in PAH?**
*Harrison's 20th Ed. Chapter 277 Page 1938*

A. Abnormal Ventilation-perfusion (V/Q) scanning
B. Abnormal CT angiogram
C. Isolated reduction in DLCO
D. All of the above

*An isolated reduction in diffusing capacity of lungs for carbon monoxide (DLCO) is a classic finding in PAH.*

**2526. Which of the finding in right heart catheterization study define precapillary PH or PAH?**
*Harrison's 20th Ed. Chapter 277 Page 1938*

A. Increased mean PAP (mPAP >25 mm Hg)
B. Pulmonary capillary wedge pressure (PCWP) ≤15 mm Hg
C. PVR >3 Wood units
D. All of the above

*An increased mean PAP (mPAP >25 mm Hg), pulmonary capillary wedge pressure (PCWP), left atrial pressure, or left ventricular enddiastolic pressure (LVEDP) ≤15 mm Hg and PVR >3 Wood units define precapillary PH or PAH in right heart catheterization (RHC) study. Post capillary PH is differentiated from precapillary PH by the PCWP being ≥15 mm Hg.*

**2527. In vasodilator testing, decrease in mPAP by how much is considered as a positive pulmonary vasodilator response?**
*Harrison's 20th Ed. Chapter 277 Page 1938*

A. ≥ 3 mm Hg
B. ≥ 5 mm Hg
C. ≥ 10 mm Hg
D. ≥ 15 mm Hg

**2528. Positive responders to vasodilator testing are considered for long-term treatment with?**
*Harrison's 20th Ed. Chapter 277 Page 1938*

A. Angiotensin converting enzyme inhibitors
B. Calcium channel blockers
C. Tadalafil
D. All of the above

*Short acting vasodilators like inhaled nitric oxide (NO) or inhaled epoprostenol are used for vasodilator testing. A decrease in mPAP by ≥10 mm Hg to an absolute level ≤40 mm Hg without a decrease in CO is considered as a positive pulmonary vasodilator response. Positive responders are considered for long-term treatment with calcium channel blockers (CCB).*

**2529. PH due to left heart disease is classified by WHO as?**
*Harrison's 20th Ed. Chapter 277 Page 1939*

A. WHO Group I PH
B. WHO Group II PH
C. WHO Group III PH
D. WHO Group IV PH

*WHO recognizes five categories of PH (I to V), including PAH, PH due to left heart disease, PH due to chronic lung disease, PH associated with chronic thromboemboli, and a group of miscellaneous diseases that only rarely cause PH.*

**2530. Based on RHC, PAH is defined as?**
*Harrison's 20th Ed. Chapter 277 Page 1939*

A. Pulmonary arterial pressure (mPAP) ≥25 mm Hg
B. PVR > 240 dyne-s/cm$^5$
C. PCWP or LVEDP of ≤15 mm Hg
D. All of the above

*Based on RHC, PAH is defined as a sustained elevation in resting mean pulmonary arterial pressure (mPAP) ≥25 mm Hg, PVR > 240 dyne-s/cm$^5$, and PCWP or LVEDP of ≤15 mm Hg.*

**2531. PAH may be associated with?**
*Harrison's 20th Ed. Chapter 277 Page 1939*

A. HIV
B. Connective tissue disease
C. Portal hypertension
D. All of the above

*PAH may be associated with HIV, connective tissue disease, and portal hypertension.*

**2532. Prevalence of PAH is increased in which of the following connective tissue diseases?**
*Harrison's 20th Ed. Chapter 277 Page 1939*

A. Polymyositis
B. Systemic sclerosis
C. Sjögren's syndrome
D. All of the above

**2533. Of the following collagen vascular diseases, PAH is commonest in?**
*Harrison's 20th Ed. Chapter 277 Page 1939*

A. Systemic lupus erythematosus
B. Scleroderma
C. Rheumatoid arthritis
D. Dermatomyositis

*All collagen vascular diseases may be associated with PAH. It is common with CREST syndrome & scleroderma. It is less frequent in SLE, Sjögren's syndrome, dermatomyositis, polymyositis & RA.*

**2534. Prevalence of PAH is increased in?**
*Harrison's 20th Ed. Chapter 277 Page 1939*

A. Scleroderma renal crisis
B. Limited cutaneous scleroderma
C. Diffuse cutaneous scleroderma
D. Scleromyxedema

**2535. CREST syndrome includes all except?**
*Harrison's 20th Ed. Chapter 363 Page 2621*

A. Calcinosis
B. Raynaud's phenomenon
C. Sclerodactyly
D. Thrombosis

CREST syndrome includes Calcinosis, Raynaud's phenomenon, Esophageal involvement, Sclerodactyly, and Telangiectasia.

**2536. Portopulmonary hypertension is observed in?**
*Harrison's 20th Ed. Chapter 277 Page 1939*

A. Primary biliary cholangitis
B. Autoimmune hepatitis
C. Hepatocellular carcinoma
D. None of the above

Portopulmonary hypertension occurs in 2 - 10% of patients with established portal hypertension. Its occurrence is independent of the cause of liver disease & is seen in patients with non-hepatic causes of portal hypertension.

**2537. Which of the following is the characteristic event in portopulmonary hypertension?**
*Harrison's 20th Ed. Chapter 277 Page 1939*

A. Medial hyperplasia
B. Intrapulmonary shunting
C. Intimal fibrosis
D. Pulmonary venous obliteration

In portopulmonary hypertension, there occurs an abnormal vasodilation of pulmonary vasculature leading to intrapulmonary shunting.

**2538. WHO Group II PH includes patients with?**
*Harrison's 20th Ed. Chapter 277 Page 1939*

A. Left heart systolic dysfunction
B. Aortic and mitral valve disease
C. Heart failure with preserved ejection fraction (HFpEF)
D. All of the above

**2539. The hallmark of Group II PH is?**
*Harrison's 20th Ed. Chapter 277 Page 1939*

A. Intrinsic pulmonary arterial disease
B. Pulmonary venous hypertension
C. Obstruction of the pulmonary vasculature
D. All of the above

The hallmark of Group II PH is elevated left atrial pressure with resulting pulmonary venous hypertension, although transpulmonary gradient and PVR remain normal.

**2540. Which of the following carry a higher overall risk of PH?**
*Harrison's 20th Ed. Chapter 277 Page 1939*

A. Left heart systolic dysfunction
B. Aortic and mitral valve disease
C. Heart failure with preserved ejection fraction (HFpEF)
D. All of the above

Studies suggest that HFpEF may carry a higher overall risk of PH.

**2541. Which of the following can produce pulmonary hypertension?**
*Harrison's 20th Ed. Chapter 277 Page 1939*

A. Portal Hypertension
B. Obstructive sleep apnea (OSA)
C. Sickle cell disease
D. All of the above

**2542. Sleep-disordered breathing is classified by WHO as?**
*Harrison's 20th Ed. Chapter 277 Page 1939*

A. WHO Group I PH
B. WHO Group II PH
C. WHO Group III PH
D. WHO Group IV PH

Sleep-disordered breathing is included in Group III PH.

**2543. Globally, which of the following is one of the most common causes of PH?**
*Harrison's 20th Ed. Chapter 277 Page 1939*

A. Schistosomiasis
B. Chronic thromboembolic disease
C. Left heart systolic dysfunction
D. Pulmonary arterial hypertension

Globally, schistosomiasis is one of the most common causes of PH.

**2544. Which of the following is the action of Prostacyclin (PGI$_2$)?**
*Harrison's 20th Ed. Chapter 277 Page 1940*

A. Vasodilation
B. Antiproliferative effects on vascular smooth muscle
C. Inhibits platelet aggregation
D. All of the above

**2545. Which of the following reduces pulmonary artery pressure acutely with little effect on systemic vascular bed?**
*Harrison's 19th Ed. 1660*

A. Inhaled nitric oxide
B. Intravenous adenosine
C. Intravenous epoprostenol
D. All of the above

Inhaled nitric oxide, IV adenosine & IV epoprostenol reduce pulmonary artery pressure acutely which is a fall in mean pulmonary artery pressure (MPAP) >=10 mm Hg & a final MPAP <40 mm Hg.

**2546. Conventional therapy for pulmonary arterial hypertension includes?**
*Harrison's 19th Ed. Page 1660*

A. Anticoagulation
B. Diuretics

C. Calcium channel blockers
D. All of the above

*Anticoagulant therapy is advocated for all patients with PAH as warfarin increases survival of patients with PAH. Diuretic therapy relieves peripheral edema & reduces RV volume overload in presence of tricuspid regurgitation. Patients who have substantial reductions in pulmonary arterial pressure in response to short-acting vasodilators at the time of cardiac catheterization should be treated initially with calcium channel blockers.*

**2547. Phosphodiesterase-5 is responsible for the hydrolysis of which of the following in pulmonary vascular smooth muscle?**
*Harrison's 20th Ed. Chapter 277 Page 1940*

A. Cyclic GMP
B. Cyclic AMP
C. Endothelin-1
D. Inositol 1,4,5-trisphosphate ($IP_3$)

*Phosphodiesterase-5 (PDE-5) is responsible for the hydrolysis of cyclic 3',5'-guanosine monophosphate (cyclic GMP) in pulmonary vascular smooth muscle which induces relaxation of smooth muscle. Inhibitors of PDE-5 such as sildenafil, vardenafil, and tadalafil reduce the breakdown of cyclic GMP. Nitric oxide increases the production of cyclic GMP.*

**2548. Which of the following prostacyclins is used for treatment of PAH?**
*Harrison's 20th Ed. Chapter 277 Page 1940*

A. Iloprost
B. Epoprostenol
C. Treprostinil
D. All of the above

**2549. Which of the following is an 'Endothelin Receptor Antagonist' used in the treatment of pulmonary arterial hypertension?**
*Harrison's 20th Ed. Chapter 277 Page 1940*

A. Epoprostenol
B. Treprostinil
C. Bosentan
D. Sildenafil

*Endothelin receptor antagonists bosentan and ambrisentan are approved for treatment of PAH. Liver functions must be monitored monthly throughout the duration of use. Bosentan is contraindicated in patients who are on cyclosporine or glyburide concurrently. Sildenafil is a phosphodiesterase-5 inhibitor. Treprostinil is an analogue of epoprostenol.*

**2550. Which of the following is an ET receptor antagonist?**
*Harrison's 20th Ed. Chapter 277 Page 1940*

A. Ambrisentan
B. Bosentan
C. Macitentan
D. All of the above

*Ambrisentan is a selective ET-A receptor antagonist while Bosentan and Macitentan are non-selective ET receptor antagonists.*

**2551. Selexipag best relates to?**
*Harrison's 20th Ed. Chapter 277 Page 1940*

A. Prostaglandin $I_2$ (IP) receptor
B. Endothelin-1 (ET-1) receptor
C. β2-receptor
D. Adenosine $A_1$-receptor

*Selexipag is an oral nonprostanoid diphenylpyrazine derived selective IP prostacyclin receptor agonist that binds the prostaglandin I2 (IP) receptor.*

**2552. Which of the following about Nitric oxide (NO) is false?**
*Harrison's 20th Ed. Chapter 277 Page 1940*

A. Derives from endothelial cells
B. Activate guanylyl cyclase to generates cGMP
C. Induces vasodilation, inhibits platelet activation
D. None of the above

**2553. Phosphodiesterase type 5 enzymes metabolize?**
*Harrison's 20th Ed. Chapter 277 Page 1940*

A. cGMP
B. cAMP
C. CREB
D. All of the above

*Nitric oxide (NO) derived from endothelial cells activate guanylyl cyclase that generates cGMP in vascular smooth muscle cells & platelets. cGMP induces vasodilation through relaxation of arterial smooth muscle cells & inhibits platelet activation. Phosphodiesterase-5 (PDE5) inhibitors increase cyclic guanosine monophosphate (cGMP) levels.*

**2554. Riociguate increases the production of?**
*Harrison's 20th Ed. Chapter 277 Page 1940*

A. Prostacyclin ($PGI_2$)
B. Nitric oxide
C. Endothelin
D. All of the above

*Riociguat is a soluble guanylyl cyclase stimulator acting synergistically with endogenous NO, and also directly stimulating soluble guanylyl cyclase independent of NO availability. Riociugat acts by increasing the production of nitric oxide.*

**2555. Which of the following best relates to familial pulmonary arterial hypertension?**
*Harrison's 20th Ed. Chapter 476 Page 3517*

A. Tumor necrosis factor (TNF) receptor superfamily
B. Serine protease inhibitor (serpin) superfamily
C. Transforming growth factor β (TGF-β) superfamily
D. GPCR superfamily

**2556. Which of the following is a member of transforming growth factor β (TGF-β) superfamily?**
*Harrison's 20th Ed. Chapter 476 Page 3517-8*

A. Bone morphogenetic protein receptor-2 (BMPR-2)
B. Activin receptor-like kinase-1 (Alk-1)
C. Endoglin
D. All of the above

## ANSWERS

| | | | | | |
|---|---|---|---|---|---|
| 1. D | 46. D | 91. A | 136. D | 181. B | 226. B |
| 2. D | 47. A | 92. C | 137. D | 182. D | 227. A |
| 3. D | 48. D | 93. C | 138. A | 183. A | 228. A |
| 4. D | 49. D | 94. D | 139. D | 184. B | 229. B |
| 5. B | 50. B | 95. D | 140. C | 185. C | 230. C |
| 6. A | 51. B | 96. D | 141. D | 186. C | 231. B |
| 7. D | 52. C | 97. A | 142. B | 187. B | 232. B |
| 8. D | 53. A | 98. C | 143. B | 188. D | 233. A |
| 9. C | 54. A | 99. B | 144. D | 189. B | 234. D |
| 10. D | 55. A | 100. D | 145. D | 190. D | 235. A |
| 11. C | 56. B | 101. B | 146. D | 191. A | 236. C |
| 12. B | 57. C | 102. A | 147. C | 192. C | 237. C |
| 13. C | 58. D | 103. A | 148. B | 193. D | 238. D |
| 14. D | 59. A | 104. D | 149. D | 194. D | 239. D |
| 15. D | 60. D | 105. D | 150. D | 195. B | 240. D |
| 16. C | 61. C | 106. D | 151. D | 196. B | 241. D |
| 17. C | 62. B | 107. C | 152. C | 197. A | 242. C |
| 18. A | 63. D | 108. A | 153. C | 198. D | 243. A |
| 19. C | 64. D | 109. B | 154. D | 199. B | 244. D |
| 20. C | 65. D | 110. B | 155. A | 200. D | 245. B |
| 21. D | 66. D | 111. C | 156. B | 201. B | 246. C |
| 22. D | 67. C | 112. D | 157. A | 202. A | 247. A |
| 23. A | 68. D | 113. D | 158. C | 203. D | 248. A |
| 24. A | 69. C | 114. C | 159. A | 204. D | 249. B |
| 25. D | 70. B | 115. B | 160. A | 205. A | 250. B |
| 26. D | 71. A | 116. D | 161. B | 206. C | 251. B |
| 27. A | 72. B | 117. D | 162. B | 207. B | 252. C |
| 28. A | 73. C | 118. D | 163. B | 208. D | 253. B |
| 29. B | 74. D | 119. B | 164. C | 209. D | 254. C |
| 30. C | 75. C | 120. A | 165. B | 210. A | 255. B |
| 31. A | 76. D | 121. C | 166. C | 211. D | 256. B |
| 32. D | 77. A | 122. D | 167. B | 212. D | 257. D |
| 33. D | 78. D | 123. A | 168. D | 213. B | 258. A |
| 34. B | 79. C | 124. D | 169. B | 214. A | 259. D |
| 35. C | 80. D | 125. D | 170. A | 215. B | 260. A |
| 36. D | 81. D | 126. D | 171. C | 216. D | 261. D |
| 37. B | 82. C | 127. B | 172. B | 217. C | 262. D |
| 38. A | 83. D | 128. C | 173. B | 218. A | 263. B |
| 39. D | 84. C | 129. D | 174. B | 219. C | 264. D |
| 40. D | 85. A | 130. D | 175. C | 220. D | 265. D |
| 41. D | 86. D | 131. D | 176. A | 221. A | 266. D |
| 42. D | 87. A | 132. B | 177. C | 222. B | 267. D |
| 43. B | 88. B | 133. A | 178. A | 223. C | 268. B |
| 44. C | 89. D | 134. A | 179. D | 224. B | 269. A |
| 45. D | 90. B | 135. D | 180. D | 225. C | 270. D |

## ANSWERS

| | | | | | |
|---|---|---|---|---|---|
| 271. D | 316. D | 361. D | 406. D | 451. D | 496. C |
| 272. A | 317. D | 362. D | 407. D | 452. B | 497. D |
| 273. B | 318. D | 363. D | 408. C | 453. C | 498. A |
| 274. D | 319. C | 364. D | 409. A | 454. D | 499. A |
| 275. D | 320. C | 365. D | 410. B | 455. D | 500. D |
| 276. D | 321. C | 366. D | 411. C | 456. C | 501. D |
| 277. D | 322. A | 367. D | 412. D | 457. C | 502. A |
| 278. B | 323. D | 368. C | 413. C | 458. D | 503. B |
| 279. D | 324. D | 369. C | 414. A | 459. A | 504. B |
| 280. D | 325. B | 370. A | 415. D | 460. D | 505. B |
| 281. D | 326. D | 371. A | 416. B | 461. B | 506. D |
| 282. B | 327. C | 372. B | 417. C | 462. A | 507. D |
| 283. D | 328. D | 373. D | 418. B | 463. C | 508. D |
| 284. A | 329. A | 374. D | 419. D | 464. D | 509. D |
| 285. B | 330. D | 375. C | 420. D | 465. D | 510. D |
| 286. B | 331. B | 376. D | 421. A | 466. B | 511. C |
| 287. D | 332. D | 377. D | 422. D | 467. C | 512. C |
| 288. B | 333. D | 378. D | 423. D | 468. D | 513. C |
| 289. A | 334. D | 379. B | 424. C | 469. D | 514. D |
| 290. D | 335. B | 380. D | 425. D | 470. B | 515. D |
| 291. C | 336. B | 381. B | 426. D | 471. B | 516. D |
| 292. C | 337. A | 382. B | 427. A | 472. A | 517. D |
| 293. D | 338. B | 383. A | 428. B | 473. C | 518. D |
| 294. C | 339. C | 384. D | 429. A | 474. C | 519. C |
| 295. B | 340. D | 385. B | 430. C | 475. C | 520. D |
| 296. D | 341. C | 386. A | 431. D | 476. D | 521. D |
| 297. A | 342. B | 387. D | 432. D | 477. A | 522. A |
| 298. C | 343. D | 388. C | 433. C | 478. B | 523. A |
| 299. C | 344. D | 389. D | 434. D | 479. C | 524. B |
| 300. C | 345. D | 390. A | 435. D | 480. A | 525. D |
| 301. A | 346. D | 391. B | 436. D | 481. D | 526. D |
| 302. C | 347. C | 392. D | 437. D | 482. C | 527. D |
| 303. B | 348. A | 393. D | 438. D | 483. D | 528. D |
| 304. C | 349. A | 394. A | 439. D | 484. D | 529. D |
| 305. D | 350. C | 395. A | 440. D | 485. D | 530. A |
| 306. B | 351. D | 396. B | 441. C | 486. A | 531. D |
| 307. D | 352. C | 397. C | 442. D | 487. C | 532. B |
| 308. C | 353. C | 398. D | 443. A | 488. B | 533. C |
| 309. D | 354. D | 399. D | 444. B | 489. D | 534. D |
| 310. D | 355. C | 400. C | 445. A | 490. A | 535. B |
| 311. A | 356. C | 401. D | 446. D | 491. C | 536. B |
| 312. A | 357. D | 402. D | 447. D | 492. C | 537. A |
| 313. A | 358. D | 403. B | 448. A | 493. D | 538. D |
| 314. D | 359. D | 404. D | 449. A | 494. A | 539. D |
| 315. C | 360. D | 405. D | 450. B | 495. A | 540. D |

## ANSWERS

| | | | | | |
|---|---|---|---|---|---|
| 541. D | 586. C | 631. A | 676. A | 721. D | 766. A |
| 542. B | 587. B | 632. B | 677. D | 722. B | 767. B |
| 543. B | 588. D | 633. D | 678. B | 723. D | 768. A |
| 544. B | 589. A | 634. D | 679. A | 724. C | 769. C |
| 545. D | 590. C | 635. D | 680. B | 725. D | 770. D |
| 546. A | 591. B | 636. D | 681. C | 726. D | 771. D |
| 547. B | 592. D | 637. C | 682. D | 727. B | 772. B |
| 548. C | 593. A | 638. D | 683. D | 728. D | 773. D |
| 549. D | 594. D | 639. C | 684. A | 729. D | 774. A |
| 550. D | 595. D | 640. B | 685. C | 730. D | 775. A |
| 551. A | 596. C | 641. D | 686. D | 731. A | 776. D |
| 552. D | 597. C | 642. D | 687. D | 732. D | 777. C |
| 553. B | 598. D | 643. C | 688. D | 733. D | 778. D |
| 554. A | 599. D | 644. D | 689. C | 734. D | 779. B |
| 555. C | 600. B | 645. D | 690. D | 735. D | 780. B |
| 556. A | 601. B | 646. D | 691. A | 736. D | 781. D |
| 557. D | 602. D | 647. D | 692. D | 737. B | 782. D |
| 558. B | 603. D | 648. C | 693. D | 738. C | 783. D |
| 559. D | 604. D | 649. A | 694. D | 739. D | 784. C |
| 560. D | 605. D | 650. D | 695. D | 740. A | 785. D |
| 561. D | 606. A | 651. A | 696. D | 741. D | 786. D |
| 562. C | 607. D | 652. D | 697. A | 742. D | 787. D |
| 563. B | 608. D | 653. C | 698. A | 743. D | 788. D |
| 564. D | 609. D | 654. D | 699. D | 744. D | 789. B |
| 565. D | 610. D | 655. B | 700. D | 745. D | 790. C |
| 566. D | 611. D | 656. D | 701. D | 746. D | 791. B |
| 567. D | 612. D | 657. B | 702. D | 747. D | 792. D |
| 568. A | 613. A | 658. C | 703. D | 748. A | 793. C |
| 569. A | 614. D | 659. B | 704. D | 749. D | 794. D |
| 570. D | 615. A | 660. B | 705. D | 750. D | 795. D |
| 571. C | 616. A | 661. B | 706. A | 751. D | 796. D |
| 572. D | 617. B | 662. D | 707. D | 752. D | 797. C |
| 573. D | 618. A | 663. B | 708. A | 753. D | 798. C |
| 574. C | 619. B | 664. D | 709. B | 754. D | 799. D |
| 575. C | 620. D | 665. D | 710. B | 755. D | 800. A |
| 576. D | 621. D | 666. D | 711. B | 756. D | 801. D |
| 577. D | 622. B | 667. D | 712. D | 757. D | 802. A |
| 578. D | 623. A | 668. D | 713. D | 758. D | 803. D |
| 579. D | 624. D | 669. D | 714. B | 759. D | 804. D |
| 580. D | 625. D | 670. B | 715. D | 760. D | 805. D |
| 581. C | 626. C | 671. D | 716. D | 761. D | 806. D |
| 582. D | 627. D | 672. A | 717. D | 762. D | 807. D |
| 583. D | 628. C | 673. D | 718. B | 763. B | 808. D |
| 584. D | 629. D | 674. D | 719. D | 764. D | 809. D |
| 585. B | 630. D | 675. D | 720. D | 765. C | 810. A |

## ANSWERS

| | | | | | |
|---|---|---|---|---|---|
| 811. D | 856. A | 901. D | 946. D | 991. B | 1036. D |
| 812. C | 857. A | 902. D | 947. D | 992. A | 1037. D |
| 813. D | 858. D | 903. D | 948. C | 993. C | 1038. C |
| 814. D | 859. D | 904. D | 949. B | 994. D | 1039. D |
| 815. D | 860. B | 905. B | 950. D | 995. D | 1040. C |
| 816. D | 861. B | 906. C | 951. D | 996. D | 1041. D |
| 817. A | 862. B | 907. B | 952. C | 997. D | 1042. B |
| 818. D | 863. A | 908. D | 953. B | 998. D | 1043. D |
| 819. B | 864. A | 909. D | 954. D | 999. C | 1044. C |
| 820. D | 865. D | 910. D | 955. D | 1000. D | 1045. C |
| 821. A | 866. A | 911. C | 956. B | 1001. C | 1046. D |
| 822. D | 867. C | 912. A | 957. C | 1002. C | 1047. B |
| 823. D | 868. B | 913. D | 958. C | 1003. D | 1048. D |
| 824. D | 869. C | 914. D | 959. C | 1004. D | 1049. C |
| 825. B | 870. D | 915. A | 960. C | 1005. D | 1050. D |
| 826. B | 871. A | 916. B | 961. C | 1006. B | 1051. B |
| 827. C | 872. C | 917. A | 962. D | 1007. D | 1052. B |
| 828. D | 873. D | 918. B | 963. D | 1008. C | 1053. D |
| 829. C | 874. D | 919. D | 964. A | 1009. A | 1054. C |
| 830. D | 875. D | 920. D | 965. D | 1010. D | 1055. C |
| 831. B | 876. A | 921. D | 966. A | 1011. A | 1056. B |
| 832. A | 877. D | 922. D | 967. D | 1012. D | 1057. A |
| 833. B | 878. D | 923. D | 968. C | 1013. D | 1058. D |
| 834. C | 879. D | 924. D | 969. D | 1014. B | 1059. B |
| 835. D | 880. D | 925. B | 970. B | 1015. C | 1060. D |
| 836. D | 881. D | 926. D | 971. D | 1016. A | 1061. D |
| 837. B | 882. D | 927. D | 972. D | 1017. C | 1062. D |
| 838. D | 883. C | 928. D | 973. D | 1018. D | 1063. C |
| 839. B | 884. A | 929. D | 974. D | 1019. C | 1064. D |
| 840. C | 885. C | 930. D | 975. D | 1020. C | 1065. C |
| 841. D | 886. C | 931. A | 976. A | 1021. D | 1066. B |
| 842. D | 887. D | 932. D | 977. D | 1022. A | 1067. D |
| 843. A | 888. D | 933. B | 978. D | 1023. D | 1068. A |
| 844. A | 889. B | 934. D | 979. C | 1024. B | 1069. D |
| 845. A | 890. B | 935. C | 980. B | 1025. C | 1070. A |
| 846. D | 891. B | 936. D | 981. B | 1026. A | 1071. B |
| 847. D | 892. D | 937. D | 982. D | 1027. A | 1072. B |
| 848. D | 893. B | 938. B | 983. D | 1028. D | 1073. C |
| 849. A | 894. C | 939. D | 984. C | 1029. D | 1074. D |
| 850. D | 895. D | 940. D | 985. B | 1030. B | 1075. D |
| 851. D | 896. D | 941. D | 986. C | 1031. B | 1076. C |
| 852. B | 897. C | 942. A | 987. B | 1032. C | 1077. B |
| 853. A | 898. D | 943. B | 988. D | 1033. D | 1078. B |
| 854. B | 899. D | 944. D | 989. D | 1034. D | 1079. B |
| 855. A | 900. C | 945. A | 990. A | 1035. D | 1080. D |

## ANSWERS

| | | | | | |
|---|---|---|---|---|---|
| 1081. C | 1126. D | 1171. B | 1216. B | 1261. B | 1306. C |
| 1082. B | 1127. C | 1172. B | 1217. C | 1262. B | 1307. C |
| 1083. A | 1128. D | 1173. C | 1218. D | 1263. D | 1308. B |
| 1084. D | 1129. D | 1174. C | 1219. B | 1264. D | 1309. A |
| 1085. C | 1130. B | 1175. B | 1220. A | 1265. D | 1310. D |
| 1086. D | 1131. D | 1176. D | 1221. D | 1266. D | 1311. D |
| 1087. D | 1132. C | 1177. A | 1222. B | 1267. B | 1312. D |
| 1088. D | 1133. B | 1178. D | 1223. C | 1268. C | 1313. B |
| 1089. A | 1134. A | 1179. D | 1224. C | 1269. B | 1314. D |
| 1090. D | 1135. C | 1180. A | 1225. C | 1270. D | 1315. D |
| 1091. B | 1136. D | 1181. D | 1226. C | 1271. D | 1316. C |
| 1092. D | 1137. D | 1182. D | 1227. D | 1272. B | 1317. C |
| 1093. A | 1138. D | 1183. D | 1228. A | 1273. C | 1318. D |
| 1094. D | 1139. D | 1184. C | 1229. A | 1274. C | 1319. D |
| 1095. A | 1140. C | 1185. D | 1230. A | 1275. A | 1320. D |
| 1096. D | 1141. C | 1186. B | 1231. D | 1276. D | 1321. D |
| 1097. D | 1142. D | 1187. D | 1232. D | 1277. B | 1322. D |
| 1098. C | 1143. D | 1188. C | 1233. D | 1278. D | 1323. D |
| 1099. D | 1144. D | 1189. D | 1234. A | 1279. D | 1324. D |
| 1100. D | 1145. A | 1190. B | 1235. A | 1280. B | 1325. D |
| 1101. C | 1146. B | 1191. A | 1236. C | 1281. D | 1326. C |
| 1102. C | 1147. D | 1192. A | 1237. B | 1282. D | 1327. C |
| 1103. D | 1148. D | 1193. D | 1238. B | 1283. D | 1328. B |
| 1104. D | 1149. A | 1194. C | 1239. A | 1284. D | 1329. A |
| 1105. B | 1150. D | 1195. C | 1240. B | 1285. C | 1330. D |
| 1106. C | 1151. D | 1196. C | 1241. A | 1286. D | 1331. D |
| 1107. D | 1152. B | 1197. D | 1242. C | 1287. D | 1332. D |
| 1108. D | 1153. A | 1198. C | 1243. C | 1288. A | 1333. C |
| 1109. A | 1154. D | 1199. D | 1244. C | 1289. D | 1334. B |
| 1110. D | 1155. A | 1200. A | 1245. D | 1290. C | 1335. D |
| 1111. A | 1156. D | 1201. A | 1246. D | 1291. D | 1336. C |
| 1112. A | 1157. D | 1202. B | 1247. C | 1292. D | 1337. D |
| 1113. D | 1158. D | 1203. D | 1248. C | 1293. C | 1338. D |
| 1114. B | 1159. D | 1204. C | 1249. B | 1294. D | 1339. D |
| 1115. D | 1160. B | 1205. D | 1250. D | 1295. D | 1340. D |
| 1116. C | 1161. C | 1206. D | 1251. C | 1296. D | 1341. D |
| 1117. C | 1162. D | 1207. D | 1252. B | 1297. D | 1342. C |
| 1118. D | 1163. D | 1208. A | 1253. C | 1298. D | 1343. C |
| 1119. A | 1164. D | 1209. A | 1254. D | 1299. D | 1344. D |
| 1120. D | 1165. D | 1210. B | 1255. C | 1300. D | 1345. C |
| 1121. D | 1166. D | 1211. B | 1256. B | 1301. A | 1346. D |
| 1122. A | 1167. D | 1212. A | 1257. A | 1302. C | 1347. C |
| 1123. C | 1168. D | 1213. C | 1258. D | 1303. B | 1348. D |
| 1124. B | 1169. C | 1214. D | 1259. D | 1304. B | 1349. A |
| 1125. B | 1170. C | 1215. A | 1260. B | 1305. D | 1350. C |

## ANSWERS

| | | | | | |
|---|---|---|---|---|---|
| 1351. D | 1396. D | 1441. D | 1486. D | 1531. D | 1576. D |
| 1352. B | 1397. D | 1442. C | 1487. D | 1532. D | 1577. D |
| 1353. C | 1398. D | 1443. A | 1488. D | 1533. A | 1578. D |
| 1354. D | 1399. C | 1444. C | 1489. B | 1534. D | 1579. D |
| 1355. C | 1400. D | 1445. C | 1490. B | 1535. D | 1580. C |
| 1356. C | 1401. D | 1446. D | 1491. B | 1536. D | 1581. D |
| 1357. D | 1402. A | 1447. D | 1492. D | 1537. D | 1582. D |
| 1358. C | 1403. D | 1448. D | 1493. D | 1538. B | 1583. D |
| 1359. C | 1404. D | 1449. C | 1494. B | 1539. D | 1584. D |
| 1360. D | 1405. D | 1450. D | 1495. D | 1540. C | 1585. D |
| 1361. A | 1406. A | 1451. D | 1496. D | 1541. C | 1586. A |
| 1362. D | 1407. C | 1452. D | 1497. D | 1542. B | 1587. D |
| 1363. A | 1408. D | 1453. B | 1498. D | 1543. B | 1588. B |
| 1364. D | 1409. C | 1454. D | 1499. D | 1544. D | 1589. C |
| 1365. D | 1410. B | 1455. A | 1500. D | 1545. D | 1590. C |
| 1366. B | 1411. D | 1456. C | 1501. D | 1546. B | 1591. D |
| 1367. D | 1412. D | 1457. D | 1502. D | 1547. D | 1592. B |
| 1368. D | 1413. B | 1458. A | 1503. C | 1548. C | 1593. B |
| 1369. D | 1414. D | 1459. D | 1504. D | 1549. C | 1594. D |
| 1370. B | 1415. D | 1460. A | 1505. B | 1550. D | 1595. C |
| 1371. D | 1416. B | 1461. B | 1506. A | 1551. C | 1596. A |
| 1372. B | 1417. C | 1462. C | 1507. A | 1552. D | 1597. A |
| 1373. B | 1418. B | 1463. B | 1508. D | 1553. D | 1598. C |
| 1374. A | 1419. B | 1464. C | 1509. D | 1554. D | 1599. B |
| 1375. B | 1420. B | 1465. C | 1510. C | 1555. D | 1600. B |
| 1376. B | 1421. D | 1466. C | 1511. D | 1556. D | 1601. D |
| 1377. C | 1422. C | 1467. D | 1512. D | 1557. D | 1602. D |
| 1378. A | 1423. C | 1468. C | 1513. D | 1558. A | 1603. C |
| 1379. D | 1424. A | 1469. D | 1514. C | 1559. A | 1604. B |
| 1380. B | 1425. D | 1470. C | 1515. B | 1560. D | 1605. C |
| 1381. D | 1426. D | 1471. D | 1516. B | 1561. D | 1606. D |
| 1382. B | 1427. D | 1472. A | 1517. D | 1562. D | 1607. A |
| 1383. D | 1428. B | 1473. B | 1518. D | 1563. D | 1608. A |
| 1384. D | 1429. B | 1474. A | 1519. D | 1564. D | 1609. C |
| 1385. D | 1430. D | 1475. A | 1520. D | 1565. D | 1610. A |
| 1386. A | 1431. A | 1476. B | 1521. D | 1566. D | 1611. C |
| 1387. B | 1432. D | 1477. B | 1522. D | 1567. D | 1612. D |
| 1388. B | 1433. D | 1478. D | 1523. D | 1568. C | 1613. B |
| 1389. D | 1434. D | 1479. D | 1524. D | 1569. D | 1614. B |
| 1390. D | 1435. D | 1480. B | 1525. A | 1570. D | 1615. D |
| 1391. D | 1436. D | 1481. A | 1526. D | 1571. D | 1616. B |
| 1392. B | 1437. D | 1482. D | 1527. D | 1572. D | 1617. C |
| 1393. C | 1438. C | 1483. D | 1528. D | 1573. B | 1618. A |
| 1394. A | 1439. B | 1484. C | 1529. C | 1574. D | 1619. A |
| 1395. D | 1440. B | 1485. D | 1530. C | 1575. D | 1620. A |

## ANSWERS

| | | | | | |
|---|---|---|---|---|---|
| 1621. D | 1666. B | 1711. D | 1756. A | 1801. D | 1846. D |
| 1622. B | 1667. B | 1712. D | 1757. C | 1802. B | 1847. D |
| 1623. C | 1668. D | 1713. D | 1758. B | 1803. B | 1848. D |
| 1624. D | 1669. B | 1714. D | 1759. D | 1804. D | 1849. D |
| 1625. A | 1670. D | 1715. D | 1760. D | 1805. C | 1850. D |
| 1626. A | 1671. D | 1716. D | 1761. B | 1806. D | 1851. D |
| 1627. A | 1672. D | 1717. A | 1762. C | 1807. D | 1852. A |
| 1628. A | 1673. B | 1718. A | 1763. C | 1808. D | 1853. D |
| 1629. B | 1674. C | 1719. C | 1764. D | 1809. C | 1854. D |
| 1630. D | 1675. D | 1720. B | 1765. C | 1810. D | 1855. C |
| 1631. B | 1676. A | 1721. B | 1766. A | 1811. D | 1856. D |
| 1632. A | 1677. C | 1722. B | 1767. D | 1812. D | 1857. A |
| 1633. A | 1678. D | 1723. A | 1768. A | 1813. D | 1858. A |
| 1634. D | 1679. D | 1724. D | 1769. D | 1814. D | 1859. D |
| 1635. C | 1680. A | 1725. A | 1770. C | 1815. D | 1860. C |
| 1636. D | 1681. C | 1726. D | 1771. D | 1816. D | 1861. D |
| 1637. D | 1682. D | 1727. D | 1772. D | 1817. B | 1862. B |
| 1638. A | 1683. C | 1728. C | 1773. B | 1818. B | 1863. D |
| 1639. D | 1684. C | 1729. D | 1774. D | 1819. D | 1864. D |
| 1640. D | 1685. C | 1730. D | 1775. D | 1820. B | 1865. C |
| 1641. B | 1686. D | 1731. D | 1776. D | 1821. A | 1866. D |
| 1642. B | 1687. C | 1732. D | 1777. D | 1822. D | 1867. C |
| 1643. C | 1688. D | 1733. D | 1778. C | 1823. C | 1868. D |
| 1644. D | 1689. D | 1734. D | 1779. B | 1824. A | 1869. A |
| 1645. D | 1690. A | 1735. C | 1780. D | 1825. D | 1870. C |
| 1646. A | 1691. D | 1736. D | 1781. A | 1826. D | 1871. B |
| 1647. D | 1692. B | 1737. C | 1782. D | 1827. C | 1872. D |
| 1648. D | 1693. C | 1738. B | 1783. A | 1828. C | 1873. D |
| 1649. B | 1694. B | 1739. D | 1784. D | 1829. D | 1874. B |
| 1650. D | 1695. D | 1740. B | 1785. D | 1830. C | 1875. D |
| 1651. B | 1696. A | 1741. B | 1786. D | 1831. B | 1876. D |
| 1652. B | 1697. D | 1742. C | 1787. B | 1832. B | 1877. B |
| 1653. D | 1698. D | 1743. A | 1788. D | 1833. D | 1878. A |
| 1654. A | 1699. D | 1744. D | 1789. B | 1834. D | 1879. B |
| 1655. D | 1700. B | 1745. B | 1790. D | 1835. B | 1880. B |
| 1656. D | 1701. C | 1746. D | 1791. D | 1836. C | 1881. B |
| 1657. D | 1702. A | 1747. B | 1792. D | 1837. B | 1882. A |
| 1658. D | 1703. C | 1748. D | 1793. D | 1838. D | 1883. D |
| 1659. D | 1704. C | 1749. B | 1794. A | 1839. C | 1884. C |
| 1660. B | 1705. B | 1750. D | 1795. D | 1840. D | 1885. B |
| 1661. D | 1706. A | 1751. C | 1796. D | 1841. C | 1886. C |
| 1662. D | 1707. D | 1752. B | 1797. A | 1842. C | 1887. B |
| 1663. D | 1708. A | 1753. D | 1798. A | 1843. C | 1888. C |
| 1664. C | 1709. D | 1754. C | 1799. B | 1844. A | 1889. A |
| 1665. C | 1710. B | 1755. C | 1800. A | 1845. A | 1890. B |

## ANSWERS

| | | | | | |
|---|---|---|---|---|---|
| 1891. C | 1936. B | 1981. B | 2026. D | 2071. D | 2116. D |
| 1892. B | 1937. A | 1982. A | 2027. D | 2072. D | 2117. D |
| 1893. D | 1938. D | 1983. B | 2028. D | 2073. A | 2118. A |
| 1894. D | 1939. C | 1984. B | 2029. A | 2074. D | 2119. A |
| 1895. B | 1940. B | 1985. C | 2030. D | 2075. C | 2120. A |
| 1896. A | 1941. D | 1986. B | 2031. D | 2076. D | 2121. B |
| 1897. B | 1942. B | 1987. C | 2032. B | 2077. B | 2122. B |
| 1898. D | 1943. A | 1988. B | 2033. B | 2078. A | 2123. A |
| 1899. D | 1944. A | 1989. D | 2034. B | 2079. D | 2124. B |
| 1900. C | 1945. D | 1990. D | 2035. D | 2080. D | 2125. C |
| 1901. C | 1946. D | 1991. D | 2036. D | 2081. B | 2126. D |
| 1902. B | 1947. B | 1992. D | 2037. C | 2082. D | 2127. D |
| 1903. D | 1948. B | 1993. D | 2038. D | 2083. D | 2128. D |
| 1904. A | 1949. D | 1994. C | 2039. A | 2084. B | 2129. D |
| 1905. B | 1950. A | 1995. B | 2040. D | 2085. B | 2130. C |
| 1906. D | 1951. D | 1996. B | 2041. A | 2086. A | 2131. A |
| 1907. D | 1952. B | 1997. B | 2042. D | 2087. B | 2132. B |
| 1908. D | 1953. C | 1998. D | 2043. D | 2088. D | 2133. B |
| 1909. B | 1954. D | 1999. C | 2044. D | 2089. D | 2134. A |
| 1910. D | 1955. B | 2000. C | 2045. D | 2090. D | 2135. C |
| 1911. D | 1956. B | 2001. D | 2046. B | 2091. B | 2136. D |
| 1912. D | 1957. D | 2002. D | 2047. B | 2092. D | 2137. C |
| 1913. D | 1958. D | 2003. A | 2048. D | 2093. D | 2138. C |
| 1914. D | 1959. D | 2004. D | 2049. A | 2094. D | 2139. B |
| 1915. D | 1960. C | 2005. C | 2050. A | 2095. C | 2140. C |
| 1916. C | 1961. C | 2006. A | 2051. A | 2096. D | 2141. D |
| 1917. D | 1962. D | 2007. D | 2052. B | 2097. B | 2142. C |
| 1918. D | 1963. D | 2008. A | 2053. B | 2098. D | 2143. D |
| 1919. D | 1964. D | 2009. D | 2054. A | 2099. A | 2144. D |
| 1920. A | 1965. B | 2010. D | 2055. C | 2100. C | 2145. D |
| 1921. D | 1966. D | 2011. D | 2056. A | 2101. D | 2146. D |
| 1922. B | 1967. D | 2012. A | 2057. D | 2102. D | 2147. A |
| 1923. B | 1968. D | 2013. C | 2058. B | 2103. C | 2148. C |
| 1924. D | 1969. B | 2014. D | 2059. A | 2104. A | 2149. D |
| 1925. D | 1970. B | 2015. C | 2060. D | 2105. C | 2150. B |
| 1926. D | 1971. A | 2016. A | 2061. C | 2106. C | 2151. D |
| 1927. B | 1972. D | 2017. C | 2062. C | 2107. D | 2152. C |
| 1928. D | 1973. C | 2018. C | 2063. B | 2108. C | 2153. A |
| 1929. B | 1974. C | 2019. D | 2064. D | 2109. A | 2154. C |
| 1930. C | 1975. C | 2020. B | 2065. D | 2110. D | 2155. D |
| 1931. A | 1976. B | 2021. D | 2066. C | 2111. D | 2156. D |
| 1932. B | 1977. C | 2022. D | 2067. C | 2112. C | 2157. A |
| 1933. B | 1978. B | 2023. D | 2068. A | 2113. D | 2158. D |
| 1934. C | 1979. D | 2024. C | 2069. C | 2114. B | 2159. B |
| 1935. D | 1980. B | 2025. A | 2070. D | 2115. B | 2160. C |

## ANSWERS

| | | | | | |
|---|---|---|---|---|---|
| 2161. D | 2206. A | 2251. A | 2296. B | 2341. A | 2386. B |
| 2162. D | 2207. C | 2252. D | 2297. C | 2342. D | 2387. D |
| 2163. C | 2208. D | 2253. B | 2298. C | 2343. D | 2388. A |
| 2164. D | 2209. B | 2254. C | 2299. B | 2344. D | 2389. B |
| 2165. D | 2210. A | 2255. D | 2300. B | 2345. D | 2390. D |
| 2166. A | 2211. D | 2256. B | 2301. B | 2346. D | 2391. B |
| 2167. A | 2212. D | 2257. A | 2302. B | 2347. D | 2392. B |
| 2168. A | 2213. C | 2258. A | 2303. C | 2348. D | 2393. D |
| 2169. D | 2214. B | 2259. C | 2304. D | 2349. B | 2394. D |
| 2170. D | 2215. B | 2260. B | 2305. C | 2350. B | 2395. C |
| 2171. D | 2216. B | 2261. D | 2306. D | 2351. B | 2396. B |
| 2172. D | 2217. C | 2262. B | 2307. D | 2352. A | 2397. D |
| 2173. B | 2218. D | 2263. B | 2308. D | 2353. B | 2398. B |
| 2174. C | 2219. D | 2264. A | 2309. D | 2354. B | 2399. C |
| 2175. D | 2220. D | 2265. C | 2310. D | 2355. D | 2400. C |
| 2176. B | 2221. B | 2266. B | 2311. D | 2356. D | 2401. D |
| 2177. D | 2222. D | 2267. D | 2312. C | 2357. B | 2402. A |
| 2178. D | 2223. D | 2268. D | 2313. A | 2358. D | 2403. D |
| 2179. D | 2224. C | 2269. D | 2314. D | 2359. C | 2404. C |
| 2180. A | 2225. D | 2270. A | 2315. C | 2360. D | 2405. A |
| 2181. A | 2226. B | 2271. B | 2316. D | 2361. D | 2406. B |
| 2182. A | 2227. D | 2272. A | 2317. C | 2362. A | 2407. C |
| 2183. A | 2228. C | 2273. C | 2318. A | 2363. D | 2408. B |
| 2184. D | 2229. A | 2274. C | 2319. B | 2364. D | 2409. D |
| 2185. C | 2230. D | 2275. C | 2320. C | 2365. B | 2410. D |
| 2186. C | 2231. C | 2276. B | 2321. D | 2366. A | 2411. B |
| 2187. A | 2232. C | 2277. D | 2322. B | 2367. D | 2412. D |
| 2188. D | 2233. D | 2278. A | 2323. D | 2368. A | 2413. C |
| 2189. D | 2234. D | 2279. D | 2324. B | 2369. D | 2414. C |
| 2190. B | 2235. D | 2280. D | 2325. C | 2370. D | 2415. A |
| 2191. D | 2236. C | 2281. D | 2326. D | 2371. B | 2416. D |
| 2192. D | 2237. D | 2282. B | 2327. B | 2372. D | 2417. D |
| 2193. A | 2238. D | 2283. D | 2328. B | 2373. C | 2418. C |
| 2194. D | 2239. D | 2284. D | 2329. D | 2374. B | 2419. A |
| 2195. D | 2240. D | 2285. D | 2330. D | 2375. D | 2420. D |
| 2196. A | 2241. C | 2286. A | 2331. D | 2376. B | 2421. B |
| 2197. D | 2242. D | 2287. D | 2332. D | 2377. C | 2422. D |
| 2198. D | 2243. A | 2288. D | 2333. C | 2378. D | 2423. D |
| 2199. B | 2244. D | 2289. D | 2334. C | 2379. B | 2424. C |
| 2200. B | 2245. D | 2290. D | 2335. D | 2380. A | 2425. D |
| 2201. B | 2246. D | 2291. D | 2336. C | 2381. B | 2426. D |
| 2202. C | 2247. C | 2292. D | 2337. A | 2382. C | 2427. C |
| 2203. D | 2248. D | 2293. B | 2338. D | 2383. D | 2428. D |
| 2204. D | 2249. A | 2294. D | 2339. B | 2384. A | 2429. D |
| 2205. A | 2250. C | 2295. A | 2340. C | 2385. C | 2430. D |

## ANSWERS

| | | | | | |
|---|---|---|---|---|---|
| 2431. B | 2452. B | 2473. D | 2494. D | 2515. D | 2536. D |
| 2432. D | 2453. D | 2474. D | 2495. C | 2516. D | 2537. B |
| 2433. D | 2454. D | 2475. A | 2496. D | 2517. B | 2538. D |
| 2434. D | 2455. D | 2476. D | 2497. A | 2518. D | 2539. B |
| 2435. A | 2456. D | 2477. D | 2498. D | 2519. D | 2540. C |
| 2436. A | 2457. D | 2478. D | 2499. D | 2520. B | 2541. D |
| 2437. D | 2458. D | 2479. C | 2500. D | 2521. D | 2542. C |
| 2438. D | 2459. C | 2480. D | 2501. B | 2522. D | 2543. A |
| 2439. D | 2460. D | 2481. B | 2502. D | 2523. D | 2544. D |
| 2440. D | 2461. C | 2482. D | 2503. D | 2524. C | 2545. D |
| 2441. A | 2462. C | 2483. D | 2504. C | 2525. C | 2546. D |
| 2442. C | 2463. D | 2484. B | 2505. A | 2526. D | 2547. A |
| 2443. B | 2464. D | 2485. B | 2506. D | 2527. C | 2548. D |
| 2444. D | 2465. D | 2486. A | 2507. D | 2528. B | 2549. C. |
| 2445. B | 2466. D | 2487. B | 2508. B | 2529. B | 2550. D |
| 2446. B | 2467. C | 2488. D | 2509. A | 2530. D | 2551. A |
| 2447. A | 2468. D | 2489. D | 2510. D | 2531. D | 2552. D |
| 2448. C | 2469. C | 2490. B | 2511. D | 2532. B | 2553. A |
| 2449. D | 2470. A | 2491. A | 2512. C | 2533. B | 2554. D |
| 2450. D | 2471. D | 2492. B | 2513. D | 2534. B | 2555. C |
| 2451. C | 2472. D | 2493. A | 2514. B | 2535. D | 2556. D |